Methods in Enzymology

Volume 420
STEM CELL TOOLS AND OTHER
EXPERIMENTAL PROTOCOLS

METHODS IN ENZYMOLOGY

EDITORS-IN-CHIEF

John N. Abelson Melvin I. Simon

DIVISION OF BIOLOGY
CALIFORNIA INSTITUTE OF TECHNOLOGY
PASADENA, CALIFORNIA

FOUNDING EDITORS

Sidney P. Colowick and Nathan O. Kaplan

Methods in Enzymology

Volume 420

Stem Cell Tools and Other Experimental Protocols

EDITED BY

Irina Klimanskaya

Robert Lanza

ADVANCED CELL TECHNOLOGY
WORCESTER, MASSACHUSETTS

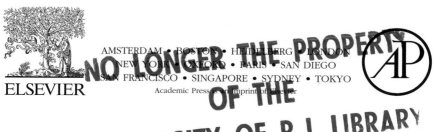

AMSTERDAM • BOSTON • HEIDELBERG • LONDON
NEW YORK • OXFORD • PARIS • SAN DIEGO
SAN FRANCISCO • SINGAPORE • SYDNEY • TOKYO
Academic Press is an imprint of Elsevier

ELSEVIER

Working together to grow
libraries in developing countries

www.elsevier.com | www.bookaid.org | www.sabre.org

ELSEVIER   BOOK AID
              International   Sabre Foundation

To Richard Latsis, the Teacher
　　　　　　　　　　–Irina

Table of Contents

Section I. *In Vitro* Experimentation and Research Tools

Section II. Tissue Engineering and Regenerative Medicine

Contributors to Volume 420

Article numbers are in parentheses following the names of contributors. Affiliations listed are current.

SADHANA AGARWAL (12), *Molecular and Cell Biology, Advanced Cell Technology, Inc., Worcester, Massachusetts*

MICHAL AMIT (3), *Department of Obstetrics and Gynecology, Rambam Medical Center, Sohnis and Forman Families Stem Cell Center, Technion–Israel Institute of Technology, Haifa, Israel*

KONSTANTINOS ANASTASSIADIS (7), *Genomics, Technische Universitaet Dresden, Am Tatzberg 47, Dresden, Germany*

ANTHONY ATALA (9, 13), *Wake Forest Institute for Regenerative Medicine, Winston Salem, North Carolina*

YILIN CAO (17), *Department of Plastic Surgery, Shanghai 9th People's Hospital, Shanghai, People's Republic of China*

HOWARD Y. CHANG (10), *Program in Epithelial Biology, Stanford University School of Medicine, Stanford, California*

XIN CHEN (10), *Department of Biopharaceutical Sciences, University of California, San Francisco, San Francisco, California*

SHAHAR COHEN (14), *Stem Cell Center, Bruce Rappaport Faculty of Medicine, Technion – Israel, Haifa, Israel*

LEI CUI (17), *Department of Plastic Surgery, Shanghai 9th People's Hospital, Shanghai, People's Republic of China*

GEORGE Q. DALEY (4), *Children's Hospital Boston, Harvard Medical School, Boston, Massachusetts*

MICHA DRUKKER (19), *Department of Pathology, Stanford University School of Medicine, Stanford, California*

DANIEL EBERLI (13), *Wake Forest Institute for Regenerative Medicine, Winston Salem, North Carolina*

TREVOR EPP (8), *Institute of Biomaterials and Biomedical Engineering, University of Toronto, Toronto, Ontario, Canada*

MARGARET A. GOODELL (11), *Center for Cell and Gene Therapy, Baylor College of Medicine, Houston, Texas*

MICHAL GROPP (5), *Fodyn Savad Institute of Gene Therapy and Department of Bostetrics and Gynecology, Hadassah University Hospital, EinKerem, Jerusalem, Israel*

XI-MIN GUO (15), *Institute of Basic Medical Sciences and Tissue Engineering Research Center, Academy of Military Medical Sciences, Bejing, People's Republic of China*

JASON HIPP (9), *Department of Urology, Wake Forest Institute for Regenerative Medicine, Winston-Salem, North Carolina*

JEFF HOLST (6), *Gene and Stem Cell Therapy Program, Centenary Institute of Cancer Medicine and Cell Biology, Newtown, Australia*

JOSEPH ITSKOVITZ-ELDOR (3, 14), *Department of Obstetrics and Gynecology, Rambam Medical Center, Sohnis and Forman Families Stem Cell Center, Bruce Rappaport Faculty of Medicine, Technion–Israel Institute of Technology, Haifa, Israel*

LUCY LESHANSKI (14), *Stem Cell Center, Bruce Rappaport Faculty of Medicine, Technion – Israel, Haifa, Israel*

SHULAMIT LEVENBERG (18), *Biomedical Engineering Department, Technion, Haifa, Israel*

K. K. LIN (11), *Stem Cells and Regenerative Medicine Center, Baylor College of Medicine, Houston, Texas*

WEI LIU (17), *Department of Plastic Surgery, Shanghai 9th People's Hospital, Shanghai, People's Republic of China*

JEREMY J. MAO (16), *College of Dental Medicine – Fu Foundation School of Engineering and Applied Sciences, Columbia University, New York, New York*

NICHOLAS W. MARION (16), *College of Dental Medicine – Fu Foundation School of Engineering and Applied Sciences, Columbia University, New York, New York*

AMPARO MERCADER (1), *Instituo Valenciano de Infertilidad, Instituto Universitario, Valencia, Spain*

JOHN E. J. RASKO (6), *Gene and Stem Cell Therapy Program, Centenary Institute of Cancer Medicine and Cell Biology, Newtown, Australia*

TAMMY REID (8), *Institute of Biomaterials and Biomedical Engineering, University of Toronto, Toronto, Ontario, Canada*

BENJAMIN REUBINOFF (5), *Fodyn Savad Institute of Gene Therapy and Department of Bostetrics and Gynecology, Hadassah University Hospital, EinKerem, Jerusalem, Israel*

JANET ROSSANT (8), *Samuel Lunenfeld Research Institute, University of Toronto, Mount Sinai Hospital, Toronto, Ontario, Canada*

FRANK SCHNÜTGEN (7), *Department for Molecular Hematology, University of Frankfurt Medical School, Frankfurt am Main, Germany*

CARLOS SIMÓN (1), *Instituo Valenciano de Infertilidad, Fundacion IVI Instituto Universitario, Valencia, Spain*

WILLIAM L. STANFORD (8), *Institute of Biomaterials and Biomedical Engineering, University of Toronto, Toronto, Ontario, Canada*

A. FRANCIS STEWART (7), *Genomics, Am Tatzberg 47, Technische Universitaet Dresden, Dresden, Germany*

JAMES A. THOMSON (10), *Genome Center of Wisconsin and Department of Anatomy, Wisconsin National Primate Research Center, Madison, Wisconsin*

X. CINDY TIAN (15), *Center for Regenerative Biology, University of Connecticut, Storrs, Connecticut*

DIANA VALBUENA (1), *Instituo Valenciano de Infertilidad, Fundacion IVI Instituto Universitario, Valencia, Spain*

HARALD VON MELCHNER (7), *Department for Molecular Hematology, University of Frankfurt Medical School, Frankfurt am Main, Germany*

CHANG-YONG WANG (15), *Academy of Military Medical Sciences, Institute of Basic Medical Sciences and Tissue Engineering Research Center, Bejing, People's Republic of China*

DARIN J. WEBER (20), *The Biologics Consulting Group, Inc., Seattle, Washington*

CHUNHUI XU (2), *Geron Corporation, Menlo Park, California*

XIANGZHONG YANG (15), *Center for Regenerative Biology, University of Connecticut, Storrs, Connecticut*

HOLM ZAEHRES (4), *Children's Hospital Boston, Harvard Medical School, Boston, Massachusetts*

JANET ZOLDAN (18), *Biomedical Engineering Department, Technion, Haifa, Israel*

Preface

Stem cells are of great interest to scientists and clinicians due to their unique ability to differentiate into various tissues of the body. In addition to being a promising source of cells for transplantation and regenerative medicine, they also serve as an excellent model of vertebrate development. In the recent years, the interest in stem cell research has spread beyond the scientific community to the public at large as a result of heated political and ethical debate.

There are two broad categories of stem cells – "embryonic" and "adult." Embryonic stem cells – also known as *pluripotent* stem cells – are derived from preimplantation-stage embryos and retain the capacity to grow in culture indefinitely, as well as to differentiate into virtually all the tissues of the body. Adult stem cells are found in most tissues of the adult organism; scientists are beginning to learn how to isolate, culture, and differentiate them into a range of tissue-specific types (and are thus considered *multipotent*).

Growing stem cells in culture and differentiating them on demand requires specific skills and knowledge beyond basic cell culture techniques. We have tried to assemble the most robust and current techniques (including both conventional and novel methods) in the stem cell field and invited the world's leading scientists with hands-on expertise to write the chapters on methods they are experts in or even established themselves. Volume 418, "Embryonic Stem Cells," offers a variety of know-how from derivation to differentiation of embryonic stem cells, including such sought-after methods as human embryonic stem cell derivation and maintenance, morula- and single blastomere-derived ES cells, ES cells created via parthenogenesis and nuclear transfer, as well as techniques for derivation of ES cells from other species, including mouse, bovine, zebrafish, and avian. The second section of this volume covers the recent advances in differentiation and maintenance of ES cell derivatives from all three germ layers: cells of neural lineage, retinal pigment epithelium, cardiomyocytes, haematopoietic and vascular cells, oocytes and male germ cells, pulmonary and insulin-producing cells, among others.

Volume 419, "Adult Stem Cells," covers stem cells of all three germ layers and organ systems. The methods include isolation, maintenance, analysis, and differentiation of a wide range of adult stem cell types, including neural, retinal, epithelial cells, dental, skeletal, and haematopoietic cells, as well as ovarian, spermatogonial, lung, pancreatic, intestinal, throphoblast, germ, cord blood, amniotic fluid, and placental stem cells.

Volume 420, "Tools for Stem Cell Research and Tissue Engineering," has collected specific stem cells applications as well as a variety of techniques, including gene trapping, gene expression profiling, RNAi and gene delivery, embryo culture for human ES cell derivation, characterization and purification of stem cells, and cellular reprogramming. The second section of this volume addresses tissue engineering using derivatives of adult and embryonic stem cells, including important issues such as immunogenicity and clinical applications of stem cell derivatives.

Each chapter is written as a short review of the field followed by an easy-to-follow set of protocols that enables even the least experienced researchers to successfully establish the techniques in their laboratories.

We wish to thank the contributors to all three volumes for sharing their invaluable expertise in comprehensive and easy to follow step-by-step protocols. We also would like to acknowledge Cindy Minor at Elsevier for her invaluable assistance assembling this three-volume series.

IRINA KLIMANSKAYA
ROBERT LANZA

Foreword

As stem cell researchers, we are frequently asked by politicians, patients, reporters, and other non-scientists about the relative merits of studying embryonic stem cells *versus* adult stem cells, and when stem cells will provide novel therapies for human diseases. The persistence of these two questions and the passion with which they are asked reveals the extent to which stem cells have penetrated the vernacular, captured public attention, and become an icon for the scientific, social, and political circumstances of our times.

Focusing first on the biological context of stem cells, it is clear that the emergence of stem cells as a distinct research field is one of the most important scientific initiatives of the 'post-genomic' era. Stem cell research is the confluence between cell and developmental biology. It is shaped at every turn by the maturing knowledge base of genetics and biochemistry and is accelerated by the platform technologies of recombinant DNA, monoclonal antibodies, and other biotechnologies. Stem cells are interesting and useful because of their dual capacity to differentiate and to proliferate in an undifferentiated state. Thus, they are expected to yield insights not only into pluripotency and differentiation, but also into cell cycle regulation and other areas, thereby having an impact on fields ranging from cancer to aging.

This directs us to why it is necessary to study different types of stem cells, including those whose origins from early stages of development confers ethical complexity (embryonic stem cells) and those that are difficult to find, grow, or maintain as undifferentiated populations (most types of adult stem cells). The question itself veils a deeper purpose for studying the biology of stem cells, which is to gain a fundamental understanding of the nature of cell fate decisions during development. We still have a relatively shallow understanding of how stem cells maintain their undifferentiated state for prolonged periods and then 'choose' to specialize along the pathways they are competent to pursue. Achieving a precise understanding of such 'stemness' and of differentiation will require information from as wide a variety of sources as possible. This process of triangulation could be compared to how global positioning satellites enable us to locate ourselves: signal from a single satellite tells us relatively little, and precision is achieved only when we acquire signals from three or more. Similarly, it is necessary to study multiple types of stem cells and their progeny if we are to evaluate the outcome of cellular development *in vitro* in comparison with normal development.

An answer to the question of when stem cells will yield novel clinical outcomes requires us to define the likely therapeutic achievements. Of course, adult and neonatal blood stem cells have been used in transplantation for many years, and it is likely that new sources and applications for them will emerge from current studies. It is less likely, however, that transplantation will be the first application of research on other adult stem cell types or of research on the differentiated progeny of embryonic stem cells. This reflects in part the degree of characterization of such progeny that will be needed to ensure their long-term safety and efficacy when transplanted to humans. It is their use as *in vitro* cellular models that is more likely to pioneer novel clinical applications of the specialized human cell types that can be derived from stem cells. These cells, including cultured neurons, cardiomyocytes, kidney cells, lung cells, and numerous others, will imminently provide a novel platform technology for drug discovery and testing. The applications of such cellular models are likely to be extensive, leading to development of new medicines for a myriad of human health problems. The wide availability of these specialized human cells will also provide an opportunity to evaluate the stability and function of stem cell progeny in the Petri dish well before they are used in transplantation. Finally, we should not overlook the importance of stem cells and their progeny as models for understanding human developmental processes. While we cannot foresee the impact of a profound understanding of human cellular differentiation, it has the potential of transcending even the most remarkable applications that we can imagine involving transplantation.

Despite the links of stem cell research to other fields of biology and to established technologies, growing and differentiating stem cells systematically in culture requires specific skills and knowledge beyond basic cell and developmental biology techniques. These *Methods in Enzymology* volumes include the most current techniques in the stem cell field, written by leading scientists with hands-on expertise in methods they have developed or in which they are recognized as experts. Each chapter is written as a short review of outcomes from the particular method, with an easy-to-follow set of protocols that should enable less experienced researchers to successfully establish the method in their laboratories. Together, the three volumes cover the spectrum of both embryonic and adult stem cells and provide tools for extending the uses of stem cells to tissue engineering. It is hoped that the availability and wide dissemination of these methods will provide wider access to the stem cell field, thereby accelerating acquisition of the knowledge needed to apply stem cell research in novel ways to improve our understanding of human biology and health.

ROGER A. PEDERSEN, PH.D.
PROFESSOR OF REGENERATIVE MEDICINE
UNIVERSITY OF CAMBRIDGE

METHODS IN ENZYMOLOGY

VOLUME 262. DNA Replication
Edited by JUDITH L. CAMPBELL

VOLUME 263. Plasma Lipoproteins (Part C: Quantitation)
Edited by WILLIAM A. BRADLEY, SANDRA H. GIANTURCO, AND JERE P. SEGREST

VOLUME 264. Mitochondrial Biogenesis and Genetics (Part B)
Edited by GIUSEPPE M. ATTARDI AND ANNE CHOMYN

VOLUME 265. Cumulative Subject Index Volumes 228, 230–262

VOLUME 266. Computer Methods for Macromolecular Sequence Analysis
Edited by RUSSELL F. DOOLITTLE

VOLUME 267. Combinatorial Chemistry
Edited by JOHN N. ABELSON

VOLUME 268. Nitric Oxide (Part A: Sources and Detection of NO; NO Synthase)
Edited by LESTER PACKER

VOLUME 269. Nitric Oxide (Part B: Physiological and Pathological Processes)
Edited by LESTER PACKER

VOLUME 270. High Resolution Separation and Analysis of Biological Macromolecules (Part A: Fundamentals)
Edited by BARRY L. KARGER AND WILLIAM S. HANCOCK

VOLUME 271. High Resolution Separation and Analysis of Biological Macromolecules (Part B: Applications)
Edited by BARRY L. KARGER AND WILLIAM S. HANCOCK

VOLUME 272. Cytochrome P450 (Part B)
Edited by ERIC F. JOHNSON AND MICHAEL R. WATERMAN

VOLUME 273. RNA Polymerase and Associated Factors (Part A)
Edited by SANKAR ADHYA

VOLUME 274. RNA Polymerase and Associated Factors (Part B)
Edited by SANKAR ADHYA

VOLUME 275. Viral Polymerases and Related Proteins
Edited by LAWRENCE C. KUO, DAVID B. OLSEN, AND STEVEN S. CARROLL

VOLUME 276. Macromolecular Crystallography (Part A)
Edited by CHARLES W. CARTER, JR., AND ROBERT M. SWEET

VOLUME 277. Macromolecular Crystallography (Part B)
Edited by CHARLES W. CARTER, JR., AND ROBERT M. SWEET

VOLUME 278. Fluorescence Spectroscopy
Edited by LUDWIG BRAND AND MICHAEL L. JOHNSON

VOLUME 279. Vitamins and Coenzymes (Part I)
Edited by DONALD B. MCCORMICK, JOHN W. SUTTIE, AND CONRAD WAGNER

Section I

In Vitro Experimentation and Research Tools

[1] Human Embryo Culture

By Amparo Mercader,
Diana Valbuena, and Carlos Simón

Abstract

Human embryonic stem cells (hESCs) are derived from preimplantation embryos. Approximately 60% of human embryos are blocked during *in vitro* development. Although statistics are inconclusive, experience demonstrates that hESCs are more effectively derived from high-quality embryos. In this way, optimal human embryo culture conditions are a crucial aspect in any derivation laboratory. Embryos can be cultured solely with sequential media or cocultured on a monolayer of a given cell type.

This chapter explores general aspects of human embryonic development, the concept of sequential culture and coculture, and specific protocols and procedures in which the authors are experienced, including the results obtained.

Introduction

Human embryonic stem cells (hESCs) are derived from preimplantation-stage embryos, a process that involves culturing embryos to the blastocyst stage (Thomson *et al.*, 1998). HESCs have also been isolated from morula-stage embryos (Strelchenko *et al.*, 2004) and even from later-stage blastocysts (7–8 days) (Stojkovic *et al.*, 2004). Although hESC lines have been derived from embryos of poor quality (Mitalipova *et al.*, 2003), it is clear that hESCs are more efficiently derived from high-quality embryos (Oh *et al.*, 2005; Simon *et al.*, 2005).

To optimize embryo development *in vitro*, it is essential to adopt a global approach to the embryo culture system that takes into account the media, gas phase, type of medium overlay, culture vessel, incubation chamber, ambient air quality, and the embryologists themselves. The concept of an embryo culture system highlights the interactions that exist not only between the embryo and its physical surroundings but also with all the parameters present in the laboratory. Only by taking such a holistic approach we can optimize embryo development *in vitro* as the previous step for optimal hESC derivation.

Initially, the zygote cleaves into two daughter cells, which subsequently divide to form the morula 4 days later. The transcription of the embryonic genome first occurs between the four-and eight-cell stages (Braude *et al.*,

METHODS IN ENZYMOLOGY, VOL. 420
0076-6879/06 $35.00
DOI: 10.1016/S0076-6879(06)20001-6

1988), which constitutes a critical moment. Compaction of the individual blastomeres follows, and finally develop to the blastocyst stage. Approximately 40–50% of embryos arrest during *in vitro* development.

Today, human embryology laboratories are faced not only with a multitude of embryo culture media from which to choose but also with various possibilities of how to use defined media or coculture systems.

Human Embryo Development

In the laboratory, embryo development from oocyte retrieval to the blastocyst stage occurs as follows:

Day 0: The human oocyte is retrieved from the follicle.

Day 1: Fertilization day. Polar bodies and pronuclei are visualized. Only fertilized eggs with two polar bodies and two pronuclei are considered to be correctly fertilized.

Day 2: First cleavage. The embryos generally have two to four cells. Embryos are evaluated for number of blastomeres (n), rate (%) and type (n) of fragmentation, symmetry (n), compaction (n), and multinucleation and are classified accordingly (Fig. 1A). Example: an embryo with four cells, 10% of fragmentation equally distributed throughout, with blastomeres of a similar size, without compaction and with one cell with two nuclei is classified as 4, 10, III, 2, 0, 1 × 2.

Day 3: The embryos have six to eight cells and are evaluated as indicated previously (Fig. 1B).

Day 4: Subsequent divisions form a 16–32-cell embryo: the morula stage. Individual blastomeres become indistinguishable as they come into close contact with each other. This phenomenon is named compaction. On day 4, the type of morula is classified as either morula or compacted morula (Fig. 1C).

Day 5: Spaces appear between the compacting cells, resulting in the formation of an external layer of cells, known as the trophoblast, and a group of centrally located cells, known as the inner cell mass (ICM). At this stage of development, the embryo is called a blastocyst (Fig. 1D).

Day 6: The blastocoelic cavity enlarges and causes the embryo to grow and begin to hatch out from the zona pellucida (ZP). Blastocyst expansion thins the ZP because of a series of expansions and contractions.

Blastocysts are classified morphologically as follows:

• Early blastocyst: when spaces appear between the compaction (Fig. 2A).

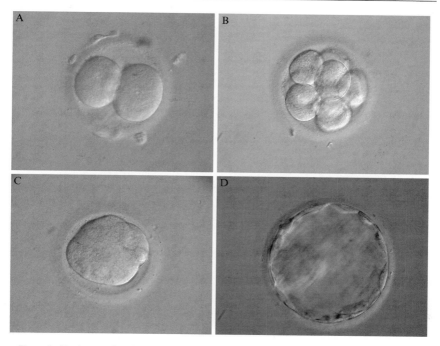

Fɪɢ. 1. Embryo development. (A) Two-cell embryo. (B) Eight-cell embryo. (C) Compacted morula. (D) Expanded blastocyst.

- Cavitated blastocyst: when the blastocoelic cavity is more than 50% of the total volume (Fig. 2B).
- Expanded blastocyst: when the blastocoelic cavity enlarges in size, the embryo and a monolayer, also known as the trophectoderm (TE), and an ICM can be differentiated (Fig. 2C).
- Hatching blastocyst: the embryo begins to hatch out of the ZP.
- Hatched blastocyst: the embryo is outside the zona pellucida (Fig. 2D).

The different parts of the blastocysts—ICM and TE—can also be classified morphologically.

Inner Cell Mass

There are four types of ICM:

A. Dense and compact with many cells (Fig. 3A).
B. Several cells and not compact (Fig. 3B).

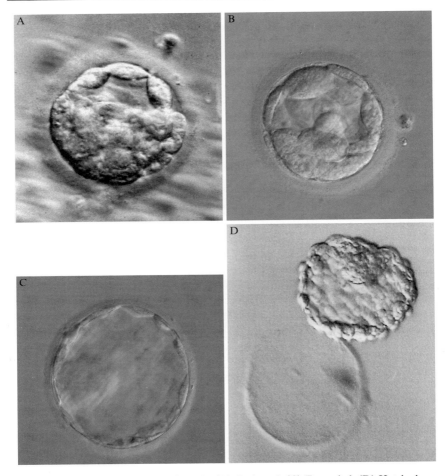

FIG. 2. Types of blastocyst. (A) Early. (B) Cavitated. (C) Expanded. (D) Hatched.

C. Very few cells (Fig. 3C).
D. Absence of a true ICM (pseudoblastocyst) (Fig. 3D).

Trophectoderm

There are four types:

A. Complete, with a monolayer of cells; forming a cohesive epithelium (Fig. 3E).
B. Incomplete, with a lineal zone (Fig. 3F).

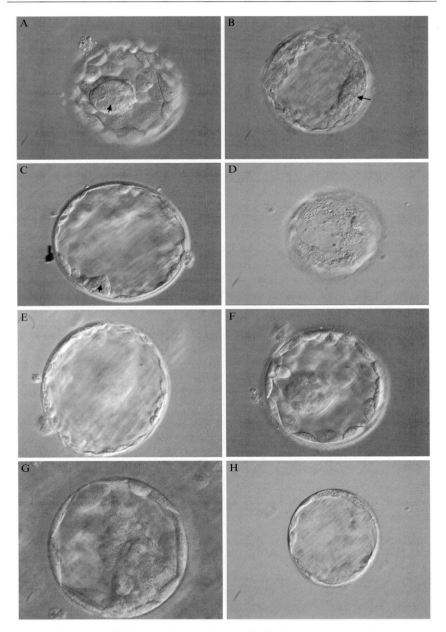

FIG. 3. (A–D) Types of inner cell mass. (E–H) Types of trophectoderm.

C. With few large cells (Fig. 3G).

D. With degenerated cells (Fig. 3H).

Example: An expanded blastocyst with an ICM of very few cells and a trophectoderm with a lineal zone is classified as BE (C, B).

Embryo development does not always follow an "ideal" pattern, sometimes becoming delayed or blocked because of low quality or accelerating inappropriately because of chromosomal abnormalities. Furthermore, morphology can vary considerably and is difficult to interpret at the expected developmental stage.

Human Embryo Culture: General Considerations

The dramatic changes in embryo physiology, nutrient requirements, and nutrient gradients in the female reproductive tract have led to the formulation of two culture media that are applied at different stages of human embryo development. This is the practice of sequential culture media. On the other hand, the concept of "cells helping cells," extended throughout many areas of cell biology, has prompted embryologists to coculture human embryos in the presence of other types of cells (feeder cells), resulting in the development of the coculture system (Simon *et al.*, 1999; Mercader *et al.*, 2003).

Sequential Culture

Several detailed treatises have been written on the composition of embryo culture media, focusing particularly on four components: glucose, amino acids, ethylenediaminetetraacetic acid (EDTA), and macromolecules. Studies in mammals, including humans (Conaghan *et al.*, 1993; Quinn, 1995), have demonstrated the importance of relatively high concentrations of pyruvate and lactate and a relatively low level of glucose in the early stages, whereas the opposite metabolic conditions have been shown to be required at the blastocyst stage. Amino acids contained in culture media enhance human embryo development up until the blastocyst stage (Devreker *et al.*, 1998). In particular, a switch occurs in amino acid requirements during embryo development (Lane and Gardner, 1997). The beneficial effects of divalent cation EDTA in embryo culture media have been extensively reported (Mehta *et al.*, 1990), although said benefits are confined to the cleavage stage (Gardner and Lane, 1996; Gardner *et al.*, 2000a). A commonly used protein source in human IVF and embryo culture has been patient serum, which is added to the culture medium at a concentration of 5–20%. However, recombinant human serum albumin (HSA) is now available, eliminating the problems associated with transfusion and permitting the standardization of media formulation (Gardner *et al.*, 2000b).

In general, the sequential culture is composed of two different media designed to meet metabolic requirements throughout embryo development. The first of these media is designed to support the development of the zygote to the eight-cell stage, whereas the second aids development from the eight-cell stage to the blastocyst stage.

Coculture System

Even though the formulations of embryo culture media have improved significantly over the years and have, for the most part, a more physiological composition, embryo development *in vitro* still lags behind that *in vivo*. For this reason, the sequential system has been opened up to include the coculture strategy.

The suggested beneficial effects of coculture include the secretion of embryotrophic factors such as nutrients and substrates, growth factors and cytokines (for a review, see Bavister [1995]), and the elimination of potentially harmful substances such as heavy metals and ammonium and free radical formation, thereby detoxifying the culture medium.

Multiple cell types have been used for this purpose, including human reproductive tissues such as oviducts (Bongso *et al.*, 1992, 1989; Ouhibi *et al.*, 1989; Walker *et al.*, 1997; Weichselbaum *et al.*, 2002; Yeung *et al.*, 1996), human endometrium (Barmat *et al.*, 1998; De los Santos *et al.*, 2003; Desai *et al.*, 1994; Jayot *et al.*, 1995; Liu *et al.*, 1999; Simón *et al.*, 1999; Spandorfer *et al.*, 2002), oviduct–endometrial sequential coculture (Bongso *et al.*, 1994), cumulus cells (Carrell *et al.*, 1999; Quinn and Margalit, 1996; Saito *et al.*, 1994), granulosa cells (Fabbri *et al.*, 2000; Plachot *et al.*, 1993), non–human cells (Wiemer *et al.*, 1993), non–human cell lines (D'Estaing *et al.*, 2001; Hu *et al.*, 1997, 1998; Magli *et al.*, 1995; Menezo *et al.*, 1990, 1992; Sakkas *et al.*, 1994; Schillaci *et al.*, 1994; Turner and Lenton, 1996; Van Blerkom, 1993; Veiga *et al.*, 1999), and even cells from ovarian carcinoma (Ben-Chetrit *et al.*, 1996). As a consequence, the reported effects of this technology on embryonic development are cell, tissue, and species nonspecific. We have developed a coculture system using autologous human endometrial epithelial cells (Simon *et al.*, 1999), and we routinely use this system as a clinical program in our center (Mercader *et al.*, 2003).

Protocols

Protocol of Sequential Culture

1. On day 0 (oocyte retrieval day), culture dishes with human tubal fluid (HTF) (IVI, Barcelona, Spain) culture drops of 50 μl, overlaid with oil, are incubated overnight in a 5% CO_2 incubator.

2. On day 1, embryo fertilization is assessed. All correctly fertilized oocytes are rinsed with the HTF in the culture dish before being transferred to the culture drops.
3. On day 2, embryos are assessed to identify whether they have reached the cleavage stage. Culture drops containing 50 μl of CCM medium (Vitrolife AB, Kungsbacka, Sweden) are placed in a culture dish and overlaid with oil. The culture dish is placed in the incubator overnight.
4. On day 3, embryo cleavage is assessed. Embryos are transferred from the HTF medium into the CCM medium, where they remain until derivation (day 5 or 6).
5. On day 4, the embryos are maintained in CCM. Culture drops containing 50 μl of CCM medium are placed in a culture dish and overlaid with oil. The culture dish is placed in the incubator overnight.
6. On days 5 and 6, embryos are assessed according to the morphological classification previously indicated. Derivation is performed when good quality blastocysts are achieved at day 5 or 6.

Protocols for the Embryo Coculture System with Human Endometrial Epithelial Cells (Simon et al., 1999; Mercader et al., 2003)

Reagents for Endometrial Culture

COLLAGENASE TYPE IA. The digestion is performed with 0.1% collagenase in DMEM.

1. Add 10 ml of water for embryo transfer to 100 mg of collagenase.
2. Stock concentration is 10 mg/ml.
3. Digestion volume is 10 ml; therefore, add 0.1 ml collagenase stock (10×) to 0.9 ml DMEM (10×) to obtain 0.1 % collagenase in DMEM.
4. Store in 1-ml aliquots at $-20°$.

DULBECCO'S MODIFIED EAGLE'S MEDIUM (DMEM). This is a liquid media, and no supplements are added.

MCDB-105. This is a powdered medium. Prepare with water for embryo transfer as described in the following. Store in the dark at 2–8°.

1. Measure 90% of the final required volume of embryo transfer water.
2. Add the powdered medium. Stir until dissolved, but do not heat. The medium is yellow in color.
3. Rinse original package with a small amount of water to remove all traces of powder. Add to solution.

4. Adjust the pH of the medium. The pH at room temperature must be 5.1 ± 0.3. Although the final pH should be 7.4, we adjust it to 7.2 because at 37°, pH increases 0.1–0.3 units. Add 4–5 ml of 1 M NaOH and check pH. Add 1 M NaOH until pH = 7.2.
5. Add additional water to bring the solution to final volume.
6. Sterilize immediately by filtration using a membrane with a porosity of 0.22 μm.

FUNGIZONE. The vial contains 250 μg/ml of Amphotericin B.

1. Rehydrate with 20 ml of embryo transfer water.
   The recommended final concentration is between 0.25 and 2.5 μg/ml. Our working dilution is 0.5 μg/ml; therefore, add 2 μl/ml to the medium.

GENTAMICIN. The vial contains 50 mg/ml. Our working concentration is 100 μg/ml; therefore, add 2 μl/ml to the medium.

INSULIN. Insulin promotes the uptake of glucose and amino acids and has a mitogenic effect. It is stable at 2–8° for 1 year. Soluble insulin is available in acidified water. Our working dilution is 5 μg/ml.

1. For a vial of 100 mg, to prepare a 10-mg/ml stock solution, add 10 ml of acidified water (pH ≤ 2.0) (add 100 μl of glacial acetic acid).
2. Add 0.5 μl/ml to the medium to obtain the correct working concentration.

HUMAN SERUM ALBUMIN. This serum is used to promote cell attachment. Appropriate aliquots (volume recommended is 40 ml) should be prepared using sterile containers. The serum should be stored at −20°.

Preparation of Endometrial Epithelial Cell Medium

We use two basic media (DMEM and MCDB-105), supplemented with 10% HSA and insulin. In addition, antibiotics and antimycotics are added to control possible contamination.

The medium is composed of: 3 DMEM:1 MCDB-105 supplemented with 10% HSA, gentamicin (100 μg/ml), Fungizone (0.5 μg/ml), and insulin (5 μg/ml).

It is sterilized by passing it through a 0.22-μm filter and is then stored in aliquots at 4°.

ENDOMETRIAL CULTURE. Endometrial biopsy specimens are obtained in the luteal phase with a catheter (Gynetics, Amsterdam, The Netherlands).

Epithelial and stromal endometrial cells are isolated as described in the following:

1. Mince the biopsy specimens into small pieces of less than 1 mm in length.
2. The minced biopsy pieces are placed in a conical tube with 10 ml of 0.1% collagenase type IA.
3. The biopsy is exposed to mild collagenase digestion through agitation for 1 h in a 37° water bath.
4. Stand the tube in a vertical position for 10 min in a horizontal laminar flow.
5. Remove the supernatant (with stromal cells) and wash by resuspending the pellet (glandular and epithelial cells) three times, for 5 min each time, in 3–5 ml of DMEM.
6. Finally, resuspend the pellet in 4–5 ml of 1% HSA in DMEM. Recover the mixture into a culture flask (Falcon, Becton Dickinson, NJ). Incubate the flask for 15 min.
7. Recover the supernatant into a fresh flask and add 3 ml of 1% HSA in DMEM. Incubate this second flask for 15 min.
8. Recover all the supernatant and place it in a tube. Check the volume.
9. Prepare 800–700 μl of endometrial epithelial cell medium and add 200–300 μl of recovered supernatant with cells into culture wells.
10. Glandular–epithelial cells are cultured for approximately 4–6 days until confluent (monolayer) (Fig. 4). The monolayer of endometrial epithelial cells is used for embryo coculture.

Protocol for Embryo Coculture on Human Endometrial Epithelial Cells

On day 0 (oocyte retrieval day), culture dishes with IVF medium (Vitrolife AB, Kungsbacka, Sweden) are placed in the incubator. Culture drops of 50 μl are placed in a culture dish and overlaid with oil. The medium is incubated overnight in 5% CO_2.

On day 1, embryo fertilization is assessed. All correctly fertilized oocytes are rinsed in the drops in the culture dish before being transferred to the IVF culture drops. IVF and CCM media are left in the incubator (0.5 ml of each one/zygote) overnight.

On day 2, embryos are assessed to detect whether they have reached the cleavage stage. A single embryo is cocultured with 1 ml of IVF:CCM (1:1) on an endometrial epithelial monolayer in individual wells on a 24-multiwell tissue culture plate (Falcon, Becton Dickinson).

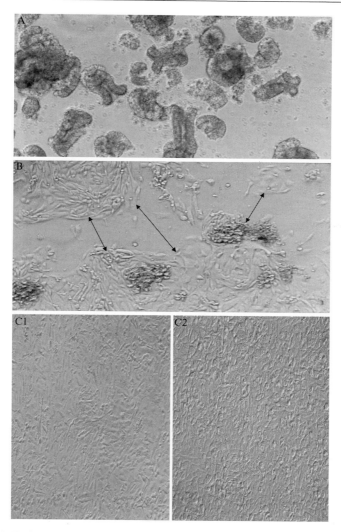

FIG. 4. Endometrial epithelial cells culture. (A) On day 0. (B) Proliferation. (C) Monolayer. On days 4–6.

On day 3, embryo development is assessed. Embryos are transferred to CCM drops, and the culture dish is placed for 10–15 min in the incubator. The embryos are then assessed. The IVF:CCM medium is removed, and 1 ml of CCM medium is placed in each well with one embryo.

On day 4, embryo development is assessed.
On days 5 and 6, embryos are morphologically classified.

Results

Human embryonic development using the two previously described culture systems was compared in a total of 3508 embryos from 474 patients attending the Instituto Valenciano de Infertilidad between January and December 2004. Patients were treated for infertility and divided into two groups according to whether they use their own oocytes (IVF) or receive ova from donors (ovum donation program). In addition, each group was divided into two subgroups in accordance with the culture system used: coculture versus sequential culture. We have analyzed, at different stages of development, the blastocyst rates achieved with sequential culture versus our coculture system with endometrial epithelial cells. A chi-square probability test was used to analyze the blastocyst rates of each group. P values < 0.05 were considered to be statistically significant.

In patients with IVF, statistical differences were observed in the rates of expanded blastocysts ($p < 0.05$) obtained and in the total blastocyst rates in coculture versus sequential media (56.2 vs. 47.3% [$p < 0.01$], respectively) (Table I). In patients with ovum donation (Table II), a statistical increase in cavitated and hatching blastocysts ($p < 0.05$) was obtained with the coculture system, whereas the total blastocyst rate augmented differently, depending on the culture system used: 65.2% (coculture) vs. 51.9% (sequential) ($p < 0.0001$).

In conclusion, the experience acquired in the IVF laboratory over the past decades allows us to optimize the culture system for human embryos and therefore improve both implantation and derivation success rates. Many embryos used for hESC derivation have been frozen and must

TABLE I
COMPARATIVE EMBRYO DEVELOPMENT IN PATIENTS UNDERGOING *IN VITRO* FERTILIZATION

Type of blastocyst	Coculture system (%)	Sequential (%)	p
Early	31 (9.4)	70 (8.1)	ns
Cavitated	36 (10.9)	96 (11.1)	ns
Expanded	83 (25.1)	161 (18.5)	< 0.05
Hatching	35 (10.5)	76 (8.7)	ns
Hatched	1 (0.3)	8 (0.9)	ns
Total	186 (56.2)	411 (47.3)	< 0.01

TABLE II
COMPARATIVE EMBRYO DEVELOPMENT IN PATIENTS UNDERGOING OOCYTE DONATION

Type of blastocyst	Coculture system (%)	Sequential (%)	p
Early	57 (7.3)	104 (6.8)	ns
Cavitated	128 (16.5)	160 (10.4)	< 0.0001
Expanded	207 (26.6)	355 (23.2)	ns
Hatching	104 (13.4)	159 (10.4)	< 0.05
Hatched	11 (1.4)	18 (1.1)	ns
Total	507 (65.2)	796 (51.9)	< 0.0001

therefore be thawed following a specific protocol, after which the indicated culture systems can be applied.

Acknowledgments

We express our gratitude to Miodrag Stojkovic for critical proofreading of this manuscript.

References

Barmat, L. I., Liu, H. C., Spandorfer, S. D., Xu, K., Veeck, L., Damario, M. A., and Rosenwaks, Z. (1998). Human preembryo development on autologous endometrial coculture versus conventional medium. *Fertil. Steril.* **70,** 1109–1113.

Bavister, B. D. (1995). Culture of preimplantation embryos: facts and artifacts. *Hum. Reprod. Update* **1,** 91–148.

Ben-Chetrit, A., Jurisicova, A., and Casper, R. F. (1996). Coculture with ovarian cancer cell enhances human blastocyst formation *in vitro. Fertil. Steril.* **65,** 664–666.

Bongso, A., Fong, C. Y., Ng, S. C., and Ratnam, S. (1994). Human embryonic behaviour in a sequential human oviduct–endometrial coculture system. *Fertil. Steril.* **61,** 976–978.

Bongso, A., Ng, S. C., Fong, C. Y., Anandakumar, C., Marshall, B., Edirisinghe, R., and Ratnam, S. (1992). Improved pregnancy rate after transfer of embryos grown in human fallopian tubal cell coculture. *Fertil. Steril.* **58,** 569–574.

Bongso, A., Soon-Chye, N., Sathananthan, H., Lian, N. P., Rauff, M., and Ratnam, S. (1989). Improved quality of human embryos when co-cultured with human ampullary cells. *Hum. Reprod.* **4,** 706–713.

Braude, P., Bolton, V., and Moore, S. (1988). Human gene expression first occurs between the four- and eight-cell stages of preimplantation development. *Nature* **332,** 459–461.

Carrell, D. T., Peterson, C. M., Jones, K. P., Hatasaka, H. H., Udoff, L. C., Cornwell, C. E., Thorp, C., Kuneck, P., Erickson, L., and Campbell, B. (1999). A simplified coculture system using homologous, attached cumulus tissue results in improved human embryo morphology and pregnancy rates during *in vitro* fertilization. *J. Assist. Reprod. Genet.* **16,** 344–349.

Conaghan, J., Handyside, A. H., Winston, R. M., and Leese, H. J. (1993). Effects of pyruvate and glucose on the development of human preimplantation embryos *in vitro. J. Reprod. Fertil.* **99,** 87–95.

D'Estaing, S. G., Lornage, J., Hadj, S., Boulieu, D., Salle, B., and Guerin, J. F. (2001). Comparison of two blastocyst culture systems: Coculture on Vero cells and sequential media. *Fertil. Steril.* **76,** 1032–1035.

Desai, N. N., Kennard, E. A., Kniss, D. A., and Friedman, C. I. (1994). Novel human endometrial cell line promotes blastocyst development. *Fertil. Steril.* **61,** 760–766.

Devreker, F., Winston, R. M., and Hardy, K. (1998). Glutamine improves human preimplantation development *in vitro. Fertil. Steril.* **69,** 293–299.

Fabbri, R., Porcu, E., Marsella, T., Primavera, M. R., Cecconi, S., Nottola, S. A., Motta, P. M., Venturoli, S., and Flamigni, C. (2000). Human embryo development and pregnancies in a homologous granulosa cell coculture system. *J. Assist. Reprod. Genet.* **17,** 1–12.

Gardner, D. K., and Lane, M. (1996). Alleviation of the "2-cell block" and development to the blastocyst of CF1mouse embryos: Role of amino acids, EDTA and physical parameters. *Hum. Reprod.* **11,** 2703–2712.

Gardner, D. K., Lane, M. W., and Lane, M. (2000a). EDTA stimulates cleavage stage bovine embryo development in culture but inhibits blastocyst development and differentiation. *Mol. Reprod. Dev.* **57,** 256–261.

Gardner, D. K., and Lane, M. (2000b). Recombinant human serum albumin and hyaluronan can replace blood-derived albumin in embryo culture media. *Fertil. Steril.* **74**(Suppl. 3), O86.

Hu, Y., Maxson, W., Hoffman, D. J., Ory, S., Eager, S., Dupre, J., and Worrilow, K. (1998). Co-culture with assisted hatching of human embryos using buffalo rat liver cells. *Hum. Reprod.* **13,** 165–168.

Hu, Y., Maxson, W., Hoffman, D. J., Eager, S., and Dupre, J. (1997). Coculture of human embryos with buffalo rat liver cells for women with decreased prognosis in *in vitro* fertilization. *Am. J. Obstet. Gynecol.* **177,** 358–362.

Jayot, S., Parneix, I., Verdaguer, S., Discamps, G., Audebert, A., and Emperaire, J. C. (1995). Coculture of embryos on homologous endometrial cells in patients with repeated failures of implantation. *Fertil. Steril.* **63,** 109–114.

Lane, M., and Gardner, D. K. (1997). Differential regulation of mouse embryo development and viability by amino acids. *J. Reprod. Fertil.* **109,** 153–164.

Liu, H. C., He, Z. Y., Mele, C. A., Veeck, L., Davis, O., and Rosenwaks, Z. (1999). Human endometrial stromal cells improve embryo quality by enhancing the expression of insulin-like growth factors and their receptors in cocultured human preimplantation embryos. *Fertil. Steril.* **71,** 361–367.

Magli, M. C., Gianaroli, L., Ferraretti, A. P., Fortini, D., Fiorentino, A., and D'Errico, A. (1995). Human embryo co-culture: Results of a randomised prospective study. *Int. J. Fertil. Menopausal Stud.* **40,** 254–259.

Mehta, T. S., and Kiessling, A. A. (1990). Development potential of mouse embryos conceived *in vitro* and cultured in ethylenediaminetetraacetic acid with or without amino acids or serum. *Biol. Reprod* **43,** 600–606.

Menezo, Y., Hazout, A., Dumont, M., Herbaut, N., and Nicollet, B. (1992). Coculture of embryos on Vero cells and transfer of blastocysts in humans. *Hum. Reprod.* **7,** 101–106.

Menezo, Y. J. R., Guerin, J. F., and Czyba, J. C. (1990). Improvement of human early embryo development *in vitro* by coculture on monolayers of Vero cells. *Biol. Reprod.* **42,** 301–306.

Mercader, A., Garcia-Velasco, J. A., Escudero, E., Remohi, J., Pellicer, A., and Simon, C. (2003). Clinical experience and perinatal outcome of blastocyst transfer after coculture of human embryos with human endometrial epithelial cells: A 5-year follow-up study. *Fertil. Steril.* **80,** 1162–1168.

Mitalipova, M., Calhoun, J., Shin, S., Wininger, D., Schulz, T., Noggle, S., Venable, A., Lyons, I., Robins, A., and Stice, S. (2003). Human embryonic stem cell lines derived from discarded embryos. *Stem Cells* **21,** 521–526.

Oh, S. K., Kim, H. S., Ahn, H. J., Seol, H. W., Kim, Y. Y., Park, Y. B., Yoon, C. J., Kim, D. W., Kim, S. H., and Moon, S. Y. (2005). Derivation and characterization of new human embryonic stem cell lines: SNUhES1, SNUhES2, and SNUhES3. *Stem Cells* **23,** 211–219.

Ouhibi, N., Menezo, Y., Benet, G., and Nicollet, B. (1989). Culture of epithelial cells derived from the oviduct of different species. *Hum. Reprod.* **4,** 229–235.

Plachot, M., Antoine, J. M., Alvarez, S., Firmin, C., Pfister, A, Mandelbaum, J., Junca, A. M., and Salat-Baroux, J. (1993). Granulosa cells improve human embryo development *in vitro. Hum. Reprod.* **8,** 2133–2140.

Quinn, P., and Margalit, R. (1996). Beneficial effects of coculture with cumulus cells on blastocyst formation in a prospective trial with supernumerary human embryos. *J. Assist. Reprod. Genet.* **13,** 9–14.

Quinn, P. (1995). Enhanced results in mouse and human embryo culture using a modified human tubal fluid medium lacking glucose and phosphate. *J. Assist. Reprod. Genet.* **12,** 97–105.

Saito, H., Hirayama, T., Koike, K., Saito, T., Nohara, M., and Hiroi, M. (1994). Cumulus mass maintains embryo quality. *Fertil. Steril.* **62,** 555–558.

Sakkas, D., Jaquenoud, N., Leppens, G., and Campana, A. (1994). Comparison of results after *in vitro* fertilized human embryos are cultured in routine medium and in coculture on Vero cells: A randomized study. *Fertil. Steril.* **61,** 521–525.

Schillaci, R., Ciriminna, R., and Cefalù, E. (1994). Vero cell effect on *in vitro* human blastocyst development: Preliminary results. *Hum. Reprod.* **9,** 1131–1135.

Simon, C., Escobedo, C., Valbuena, D., Genbacev, O., Galan, A., Krtolica, A., Asensi, A., Sanchez, E., Esplugues, J., Fisher, S., and Pellicer, A. (2005). First derivation in Spain of human embryonic stem cell lines: Use of long-term cryopreserved embryos and animal-free conditions. *Fertil. Steril.* **83,** 246–249.

Simon, C., Mercader, A., Garcia-Velasco, J., Nikas, G., Moreno, C., Remohi, J., and Pellicer, A. (1999). Coculture of human embryos with autologous human endometrial epithelial cells in patients with implantation failure. *J. Clin. Endocrinol. Metab.* **84,** 2638–2646.

Spandorfer, S. D., Barmat, L., Navarro, J., Burmeister, L., Veeck, L., Clarke, R., Liu, H. C., and Rosenwaks, Z. (2002). Autologous endometrial coculture in patients with a previous history of poor quality embryos. *J. Assist. Reprod. Genet.* **19,** 309–312.

Stojkovic, M., Lako, M., Stojkovic, P., Stewart, R., Przyborski, S., Armstrong, L., Evans, J., Herbert, M., Hyslop, L., Ahmad, S., Murdoch, A., and Strachan, T. (2004). Derivation of human embryonic stem cells from day-8 blastocysts recovered after three-step *in vitro* culture. *Stem Cells* **22,** 790–797.

Strelchenko, N., Verlinsky, O., Kukharenko, V., and Verlinsky, Y. (2004). Morula-derived human embryonic stem cells. *Reprod. Biomed. Online.* **9,** 623–629.

Thomson, J. A., Itskovitz-Eldor, J., Shapiro, S. S., Waknitz, M. A., Swiergiel, J. J., Marshall, V. S., and Jones, J. M. (1998). Embryonic stem cell lines derived from human blastocysts. *Science* **282,** 1145–1147.

Turner, K., and Lenton, E. A. (1996). The influence of Vero cell culture on human embryo development and chorionic gonadotrophin production *in vitro. Hum. Reprod.* **11,** 1966–1974.

Van Blerkom, J. (1993). Development of human embryos to the hatched blastocyst stage in the presence or absence of a monolayer of Vero cells. *Hum. Reprod.* **8,** 1525–1539.

Veiga, A., Torrello, M. J., Menezo, Y., Busquets, A., Sarrias, O., Coroleu, B., and Barri, P. N. (1999). Use of co-culture of human embryos on Vero cells to improve clinical implantation rate. *Hum. Reprod.* **14,** 112–120.

Walker, D. J., Vlad, M. T., and Kennedy, C. R. (1997). Establishment of human tubal epithelial cells for coculture in an IVF program. *J. Assist. Reprod. Genet.* **14,** 83–87.

Weichselbaum, A., Paltieli, Y., Philosoph, R., Rivnay, B., Coleman, R., Seibel, M. M., and Bar-Ami, S. (2002). Improved development of very-poor-quality human preembryos by coculture with human fallopian ampullary cells. *J. Assist. Reprod. Genet.* **19,** 7–13.

Wiemer, K. E., Hoffman, D. I., Maxson, W. S., Eager, S, Muhlberger, B., Fiore, I., and Cuervo, M. (1993). Embryonic morphology and rate of implantation of human embryos following co-culture on bovine oviductal epithelial cells. *Hum. Reprod.* **8,** 97–101.

Yeung, W. S., Lau, E. Y., Chan, S. T., and Ho, P. C. (1996). Coculture with homologous oviductal cells improved the implantation of human embryos—a prospective randomized control trial. *J. Assist. Reprod.Genet.* **13,** 762–767.

[2] Characterization and Evaluation of Human Embryonic Stem Cells

By CHUNHUI XU

Abstract

Human embryonic stem cells (hESCs) provide great opportunities for regenerative medicine, pharmacological and toxicological investigation, and the study of human embryonic development. These applications require proper derivation, maintenance, and extensive characterization of undifferentiated cells before being used for differentiation into cells of interest. Undifferentiated hESCs possess several unique features, including their extensive proliferation capacity in the undifferentiated state, ability to maintain a normal karyotype after long-term culture, expression of markers characteristic of stem cells, high constitutive telomerase activity, and capacity to differentiate into essentially all somatic cell types. This chapter will summarize the current development in culture conditions and provide technical details for the evaluation and characterization of hESCs.

Introduction

hESCs were first successfully isolated from inner cell masses (ICMs) of preimplantation embryos or blastocysts (Thomson *et al.*, 1998). ICMs were obtained by removal of trophoblast, the outer layer of blastocysts, through immunosurgery, and the cells were plated onto a layer of mitotically inactivated mouse embryonic fibroblast (MEF) feeders to prevent cells

METHODS IN ENZYMOLOGY, VOL. 420   0076-6879/06 $35.00
Copyright 2006, Elsevier Inc. All rights reserved.   DOI: 10.1016/S0076-6879(06)20002-8

from spontaneously differentiating. The cells were further passaged by enzymatic dissociation and replated onto new feeders for expansion. Additional hESC lines have since been isolated by several laboratories using various methods, such as culturing cells in other feeders or feeder-free conditions and extracting cells from frozen embryos instead of fresh ones (Hoffman and Carpenter, 2005; Klimanskaya et al., 2005).

Since the original derivation of hESCs, culture conditions for the growth of undifferentiated cells have been significantly improved. An earlier modification of the culture method is the development of a feeder-free culture system, where cells are maintained on Matrigel or laminin in medium conditioned by MEF (MEF-CM) (Carpenter et al., 2004; Lebkowski et al., 2001; Rosler et al., 2004; Xu et al., 2001). To minimize the risk of pathogen contamination, additional efforts have been devoted to screening human feeder cells, matrices, and medium supplements for the maintenance of undifferentiated cells. This led to the identification of human cells derived from a variety of tissues (Amit et al., 2003; Cheng et al., 2003; Genbacev et al., 2005; Hovatta et al., 2003; Inzunza et al., 2005; Miyamoto et al., 2004; Richards et al., 2002) or hESC derivatives (Stojkovic et al., 2005b; Wang et al., 2005c; Xu et al., 2004) for their capability to serve as feeders directly or as a source of conditioned medium. Human serum, extracellular matrices extracted from MEFs, and fibronectin have been identified as alternative matrices to Matrigel or laminin (Amit et al., 2004; Klimanskaya et al., 2005; Stojkovic et al., 2005a). In addition, several growth factors such as basic fibroblast growth factor (bFGF) (Wang et al., 2005a,b; Xu et al., 2005a,b) and transforming growth factor beta (TGFβ)/activin/nodal signaling pathway (Amit et al., 2004; Beattie et al., 2005; James et al., 2005; Vallier et al., 2004) have been identified for their involvement in self-renewal of undifferentiated hESCs. Another development in refining culture condition is the use of a defined serum-free medium XVIVO 10 (Cambrex, Walkerville, MD) containing only human and recombinant proteins, supplemented with high concentration of bFGF (Li et al., 2005). More recently, culture and derivation of hESCs were achieved in defined conditions in which medium and matrixes contain proteins solely derived from recombinant sources or purified from human materials (Ludwig et al., 2006). These improvements have provided solid groundwork for the generation of undifferentiated hESCs in a reproducible fashion with well-defined, qualified materials.

Characterization of Undifferentiated hESCs

Cardinal features of undifferentiated hESCs are the extensive proliferation capacity of the cells in the undifferentiated state (self-renewal) and the ability of the cells to differentiate into multiple cell types (pluripotency)

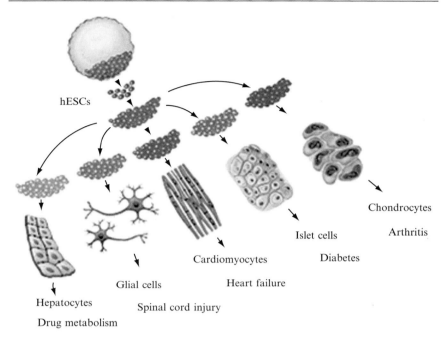

hESCs

Chondrocytes

Islet cells   Arthritis

Cardiomyocytes   Diabetes

Glial cells   Heart failure

Hepatocytes   Spinal cord injury

Drug metabolism

Fig. 1. Fundamental features of undifferentiated hESCs. hESCs derived from the inner cell mass have the ability to proliferate in the undifferentiated state (self-renewal) and to differentiate into multiple cell types (pluripotency). These derivatives include glial cells, cardiomyocytes, islet cells, chondrocytes, and hepatocytes that are valuable for treatment of diseases and drug discovery.

that are useful for regenerative medicine and drug discovery (Fig. 1). Characterization of hESCs is an essential process when deriving a new hESC line or developing a new culture procedure for undifferentiated hESCs. This process had been carried out in the experiments described previously that aimed to optimize culture conditions. For example, it was demonstrated that even after long-term culture, cells maintained on Matrigel or laminin in MEF-CM retained a normal karyotype and a stable proliferation rate, had high telomerase activity, and expressed markers associated with undifferentiated hESCs (Xu *et al.*, 2001). In addition, they had been induced to differentiate into cell types representing the three germ layers both *in vitro* and *in vivo,* including neural progenitors (Carpenter *et al.*, 2001), cardiomyocytes (Xu *et al.*, 2002a), trophoblast (Xu *et al.*, 2002b), hepatocyte-like cells (Rambhatla *et al.*, 2003), oligodendrocytes (Nistor *et al.*, 2003) and hematopoietic progenitors (Chadwick *et al.*, 2003). Characterization of the cells cultured under other feeder-free conditions is summarized in Table I.

Following is a detailed description of the methods for the characterization of hESCs, using cells maintained in the feeder-free system as examples, if not specified otherwise.

Cell Morphology

Growth of undifferentiated hESCs requires specific and optimal culture conditions to prevent them from undergoing spontaneous differentiation. Nevertheless, current culture protocols with feeders or feeder-free conditions usually give rise to a mixed population of cells with various morphologies because of spontaneous differentiation. Typically, undifferentiated hESCs form compact colonies with cells tightly associated with each other through functional gap junctions (Carpenter *et al.*, 2004; Wong *et al.*, 2004; Xu *et al.*, 2004) and show a high nuclear cytoplasmic ratio with prominent nucleoli. In early passage cultures (usually <50 passages in our laboratory), some of the colonies are compact and contain cells with typical undifferentiated morphology, whereas others are a mixture of undifferentiated cells and differentiated cell types (Fig. 2A–C). These differentiated cells show 3-D embryonic body (EB)–like structures or are flat and large, which can be observed within or at the edge of the colonies. Most of the colonies are surrounded by a monolayer of differentiated stromal-like or fibroblast-like cells. After a longer period of maintenance (>50 passages), very few stromal-like cells remain in cultures. When reaching confluence, undifferentiated colonies fuse with each other and form a relatively uniform-looking sheet-llike monolayer that is observable under a microscope at a low magnification. Compared with earlier passage cells, these cultures usually show a higher percentage of cells expressing markers associated with undifferentiated hESCs, suggesting selective survival of undifferentiated hESCs over long-term cultures (Fig. 2D). Because the morphology of the hESC colonies may be correlated with the degree of differentiation within the culture, it is good practice to monitor cell morphology at each passage in conjunction with marker analysis as discussed in the following.

Markers for Undifferentiated hESCs

Undifferentiated hESCs express several surface markers that were initially identified on human embryonic carcinoma cells using monoclonal antibodies, such as stage-specific embryonic antigen-3 (SSEA-3) and SSEA-4 for glycolipids, TRA-1–60 and TRA-1–81 for keratan sulfate–related proteoglycan antigens, and GCTM-2 for the protein core of a

TABLE I

EXAMPLES OF LONG-TERM FEEDER-FREE CULTURES OF hESCs

Cells	Matrix	Media	Characterization	References
H1, H7, H9, H14	Matrigel or human laminin	MEF-CM using medium containing 20% SR and 4–8 ng/ml bFGF	>1 year; morphology; expression of SSEA-4, TRA-1-60, TRA-1-81, OCT3/4, hTERT, CRIPTO and alkaline phosphatase; gene profiling analysis; telomerase activity; proliferation; karyotype analysis; EB formation; teratoma formation; cryopreservation; cardiomyocyte differentiation; neuron differentiation; hepatocyte-like cell differentiation; trophoblast differentiation; osteoblast differentiation; oligodendrocyte differentiation; hematopoietic cell differentiation; genetic modification	Carpenter *et al.*, 2001; Chadwick *et al.*, 2003; Lebkowski *et al.*, 2001; Ma *et al.*, 2003; Nistor *et al.*, 2003; Rambhatla *et al.*, 2003; Sottile *et al.*, 2003; Xu *et al.*, 2001, 2002a,b; Zwaka and Thomson, 2003
H7, H9	Matrigel	CM from immortalized hESC-derived fibroblast-like cells using medium containing 20% SR and 4–8 ng/ml bFGF	10 passages; morphology; expression of SSEA-4, TRA-1-60, TRA-1-81, OCT3/4, hTERT, CRIPTO and alkaline phosphatase; telomerase activity; karyotype analysis; EB formation; teratoma formation	Xu *et al.*, 2004
I-6, I-3, H9	Human or bovine fibronectin	Medium containing 15% SR, 4 ng/ml bFGF and 0.12 ng/ml TGFb1	50 passages; morphology; expression of SSEA-4, SSEA3, TRA-1-60, TRA-1-81 and OCT3/4-cloning efficiency; EB formation; teratoma formation	Amit *et al.*, 2004
H7, H9	Matrigel	Medium containing 20% SR and 40 ng/ml bFGF	15 passages; morphology; expression of SSEA-4, TRA-1-60, OCT3/4, hTERT and CRIPTO; telomerase activity; proliferation; karyotype analysis; EB formation; teratoma formation	Xu *et al.*, 2005a

Cell lines	Substrate	Medium	Characterization	Reference
H1, H9, H14	Human laminin	Medium containing 20% SR, 40 ng/ml bFGF and 500 ng/ml noggin	27 passages; morphology; expression of SSEA-4, TRA-1-60, OCT3/4, NANOG, and ZFP42; proliferation; karyotype analysis; EB formation; teratoma formation; trophoblast differentiation; cryopreservation	Xu et al., 2005b
H1, H9	Matrigel	Medium containing 20% SR and 24–36 ng/ml bFGF	>30 passages; morphology; expression of TRA-1-60, TRA-1-81, OCT3/4, and alkaline phosphatase; proliferation; karyotype analysis; EB formation; hematopoietic cell differentiation	Wang et al., 2005b
H1	Matrigel or human laminin	Medium containing XVIVO10, and 80 ng/ml bFGF	>20 passages; morphology; expression of SSEA-4, TRA-1-60, OCT3/4, hTERT, and CRIPTO; telomerase activity; proliferation; karyotype analysis; EB formation; teratoma formation; cryopreservation	Li et al., 2005
HSF6	Laminin	Medium containing 20% SR, 50 ng/ml activin A, 50 ng/ml KGF and 10 mM nicotinamide	>20 passages; morphology; expression of SSEA4, TRA-1-60, OCT3/4, hTERT, and NANOG; proliferation; karyotype analysis; EB formation; teratoma formation	Beattie et al., 2005
H9, HSF6	FBS	CDM (Johansson and Wiles, 1995) supplemented with 12 ng/ml bFGF and 10 ng/ml activin A or 12 ng/ml bFGF and 100 ng/ml Nodal	10 passages; morphology; expression of TRA-1-60, SSEA-3, SSEA-4, OCT3/4, and CRIPTO	Vallier et al., 2005
H1, H7, H9, H14, WA15, WA16	Matrigel or a combination of collagen IV, fibronectin, laminin, and vitronectin	Defined TeSR1 medium containing bFGF, LiCl, γ-aminobutyric acid, pipecolic acid and TGFβ1	>7 months; morphology; expression of SSEA4, TRA-1-60, TRA-1-81, OCT3/4, Rex1, hTERT and NANOG; proliferation; cloning efficiency; karyotype analysis; teratoma formation; derivation of new cell lines; sialic acid contamination	Ludwig et al., 2006

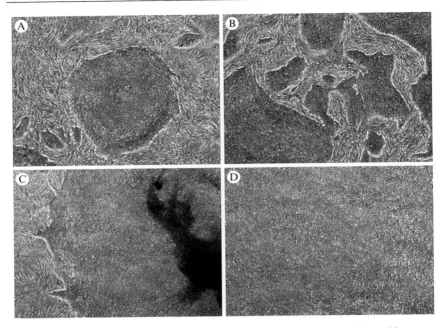

Fɪɢ. 2. Morphology of hESCs maintained on Matrigel in medium conditioned by mouse embryonic fibroblasts (MEF-CM). (A–C) H7 passage 39 culture showed that undifferentiated colonies with different shapes were surrounded by fibroblast or stromal-like cells. Differentiated cells were also found in the center of a colony in C. (D) H7 passage 52 culture showed relative uniform undifferentiated cell morphology.

keratan sulfate/chondroitin sulfate pericellular matrix proteoglycan (Andrews *et al.*, 1996; Badcock *et al.*, 1999; Pera *et al.*, 1988; Reubinoff *et al.*, 2000; Thomson *et al.*, 1998; Xu *et al.*, 2001). hESCs also express a number of generic molecular markers of pluripotent stem cells that are shared with other cells, some of which seem to be critical for their self-renewal. These include OCT3/4, a POU transcription factor; hTERT, the catalytic component of telomerase; CRIPTO (TDGF1), a growth factor; NANOG, homeobox transcription factor; SOX2, a HMG-box transcription factor; UTF-1, undifferentiated embryonic cell transcription factor; and REX1, zinc finger protein 42 (Abeyta *et al.*, 2004; Bhattacharya *et al.*, 2004; Boyer *et al.*, 2005; Brandenberger *et al.*, 2004a,b; Miura *et al.*, 2004; Richards *et al.*, 2004; Sperger *et al.*, 2003). A subset of hESCs also express CD133 (AC133) (Miraglia *et al.*, 1997; Uchida *et al.*, 2000; Yin *et al.*, 1997), a transmembrane glycoprotein expressed by hematopoietic stem cells, neural stem cells, and endothelial cells; CD9 (Oka *et al.*, 2002), a transmembrane protein expressed by undifferentiated mouse ESCs; and CD90 (Thy-1), a surface marker for hematopoietic stem cells and neural cells (Carpenter *et al.*, 2004; Draper *et al.*, 2002; Kaufman *et al.*, 2001; Rosler *et al.*, 2004). In addition, undifferentiated hESC colonies display strong alkaline phosphatase activity that is also present in other pluripotent cells (Reubinoff *et al.*, 2000; Thomson *et al.*, 1998; Xu *et al.*, 2001). Together, they represent a panel of markers that are associated with pluripotent hESCs.

During differentiation, expression of undifferentiated cell markers is down-regulated and, concomitantly, that of differentiated cell markers is up-regulated. For example, SSEA-1 is undetectable in undifferentiated hESCs, but its expression is elevated on differentiation (Henderson *et al.*, 2002; Reubinoff *et al.*, 2000; Thomson *et al.*, 1998). In practice, these markers are useful for monitoring the status of undifferentiated cells in culture and for comparing culture conditions. Flow cytometry analysis, immunocytochemical analysis, and/or real-time reverse transcriptase-polymerase chain reaction (RT-PCR) analysis may be used to assess expression of these markers, and alkaline phosphatase activity can be measured with a specific substrate for the enzyme. Examples of these analyses are described in the following.

Immunocytochemistry for Markers of Undifferentiated hESCs

Immunocytochemical analysis allows one to monitor expression of undifferentiated hESC markers in conjunction with cell morphology and provides detailed information about the location of an antigen. It is recommended to determine optimal concentrations for each specific lot of antibodies using a positive control cell line, which can be a human embryonic carcinoma cell line or an established hESC line.

For surface marker staining, a live cell–staining procedure is preferred. First, cells are seeded onto chamber slides (Nunc, Rochester, NY) that have been pretreated as follows. For feeder-free cultures, chamber slides are precoated with matrix such as Matrigel, laminin, or fibonectin. For cultures with feeders, irradiated- or mitomycin C–treated feeders are seeded onto the chamber slides. The cells can be maintained for 2–7 days before immunocytochemical analysis. After the culture, remove the medium and incubate the cells with primary antibodies (SSEA-1, SSEA-4, TRA-1–60, or TRA-1–81), diluted in warm knockout Dulbecco modified Eagle medium (DMEM) (Invitrogen, Carlsbad, CA) at 37° for 30 min. Antibodies against SSEA-1 and SSEA-4 can be obtained from the Developmental Studies Hybridoma Bank (University of Iowa, Iowa City, IA) or Chemicon (Temecule, CA), where antibodies against TRA-1–60 and TRA-1–81 are also available. For double staining, choose primary antibodies with different isotypes (e.g., IgG3-type SSEA-4 antibody together with IgM-type TRA-1–60 antibody). After the incubation, wash the slides twice (for 5 min each) with knockout DMEM and then fix the cells with 2% paraformaldehyde in phosphate-buffered saline (PBS) for 15 min. The slide is then washed with PBS and incubated in 5% normal goat serum (NGS) in PBS at room temperature for 30 min to prevent the nonspecific binding of antibodies, followed by incubation with the fluorescein isothiocyanate (FITC)-conjugated goat anti-mouse IgG (Sigma, St. Louis, MO), diluted in PBS containing 1% NGS, at room temperature for 30–60 min. For double staining, secondary antibodies against specific isotypes of the primary antibodies conjugated with different fluorescence dyes can be used. For example, goat anti-mouse IgG3 conjugated with Alexa 488 and goat anti-mouse IgM conjugated with Alexa 594 (Invitrogen) can be used to double stain SSEA-4 and TRA-1-60. After the incubation, wash the cells with PBS three times (for 5 min each), and then mount the slide with Vectashield mounting media for fluorescence (Vector Laboratories, Inc., Burlingame, CA) that contains DAPI to counterstain nuclei and antibleaching compounds to prevent quenching fluorescence. Other DNA binding dyes, such as Hoechst, can also be used to stain nuclei. The slide is then examined under an ultraviolet microscope.

To detect intracellular antigens such as OCT3/4 and NANOG, cells need to be fixed and permeabilized before antibody detection. First fix cells on a slide in 2–4% paraformaldehyde at room temperature for 20 min. After washing, the cells are permeabilized for 2 min in 100% ethanol. After another washing, the slide is incubated in 5% donkey serum in PBS at room temperature for 2 h or at 4° overnight.

Incubate the slide at room temperature for 2 h with a goat antibody against OCT3/4 (Santa Cruz Biotechnology, Inc., Santa Cruz, CA) diluted with 1% donkey serum in PBS. Cells are then washed three times with PBS (5–10 min for each washing). The slide is then incubated with FITC-conjugated donkey anti-goat IgG (Jackson ImmunoResearch Laboratories, Inc., West Grove, PA) and diluted in PBS containing 1% donkey serum at room temperature for 1 h. After the incubation, wash the cells three times with PBS (5–10 min for each wash), then mount the slide with Vectashield mounting media for microscope examination.

Flow Cytometry Analysis of Surface Markers

Flow cytometry analysis provides quantitative information regarding the percentage of cells expressing stem cell markers in culture and the staining intensity. A profile of multiple markers can be simultaneously obtained by this method.

After growing cells in a tissue culture plate, remove culture medium, and incubate the cells with collagenase IV (200 units/ml) (Invitrogen) in knockout DMEM at 37° for 5 min. Collagenase IV is then removed, and the cells are incubated with 0.5 m*M* ethylenediamine tetraacetic acid (EDTA) in PBS at 37° for 5–10 min. Alternately, cells can be washed with PBS and dissociated with 0.5% trypsin/EDTA (Invitrogen). Gently pipet the cells several times, spin to collect the cells, and resuspend them in PBS containing 0.1% BSA (diluent) to ∼1×10^7 cells/ml. For each test, add 50 μl primary antibodies against SSEA-1, SSEA-4, TRA-1–60 or TRA-1–81, as well as isotype controls, diluted appropriately, to 50 μl of the resuspended cells, and incubate them at room temperature for 30 min. Wash the cells with the diluent, and resuspend them in the diluent containing rat anti-mouse kappa chain antibodies conjugated with polyethylene glycol (PE) (Becton Dickinson, San Jose, CA). After incubation at 4° for 30 min, cells are washed with 1 ml of the diluent and analyzed on FACScalibur Flow Cytometer (Becton Dickinson) using the CellQuest software. Follow this procedure when performing multicolor flow cytometry analysis, except that different primary antibodies with different isotypes (e.g., IgG3 SSEA-4 and IgM TRA-1–60) are added together and that secondary antibodies against each of the isotypes conjugated with different fluorescence dyes are used. In addition, as compensation controls, single marker staining for each of the antigens needs to be carried out separately. For both the single and multiple marker analyses, the secondary antibody incubation may be skipped if a primary antibody directly conjugated with a specific dye or different antibodies directly conjugated with different dyes are available. The latter method is recommended when developing more throughput assays.

Detection of Alkaline Phosphatase

Culture cells on Matrigel or laminin-coated chamber slides overnight or longer. To detect alkaline phosphatase activity, first remove the culture medium, wash the slide with PBS, and then fix the cells with 4% paraformaldehyde for 15 min. After another wash with PBS, incubate the cells with alkaline phosphatase substrate (Vector Laboratories, Inc.) at room temperature in the dark for 1 h or until colonies show a pink color. Rinse the slide gently once for 2–5 min in 100% ethanol before mounting and observing under a light or ultraviolet microscopy.

Quantitative RT-PCR analysis of OCT3/4, hTERT, NANOG, and CRIPTO

Quantitative RT-PCR analysis is an alternative method to determine relative gene expression, particularly when specific antibodies are lacking.

Cells may be cultured in a 6-well plate (Qiagen, Valencia, CA). After removal of the culture medium, harvest the cells by adding 350–700 μl lysis buffer to each well, and isolate RNA using Qiagen RNeasy kit (Qiagen) following the tissue isolation procedure recommended for the QiaShredder

(Qiagen). Before RT-PCR analysis, treat RNA samples with DNase I (Ambion, Austin, TX) to remove contaminating genomic DNA. Set up TaqMan one-step RT-PCR using the master mix (Applied Biosystems, Foster City, CA) and specific primers and probes for OCT3/4, hTERT, NANOG, or CRIPTO listed in Table II. Each reaction mixture contains

TABLE II

PRIMERS AND PROBES FOR REAL-TIME RT-PCR TAQMAN ASSAYS

Genes	Sequences
Undifferentiated cells:	
OCT3/4 forward	GAAACCCACACTGCAGCAGA
probe	FAM-CAGCCACATCGCCCAGCAGC-TAM
reverse	CACATCCTTCTCGAGCCCA
hTERT primers	Purchased from Applied Biosystems
and probe	(Assay Number 4319447F)
CRIPTO forward	TGAGCACGATGTGCGC
probe	FAM-AGAGAACTGTGGGTCTGTGCCCCATG-TAM
reverse	TTCTTGGGCAGCCAGGTG
NANOG forward	GCAGAAGGCCTCAGCACCTA
probe	FAM-CTACCCCAGCCTTTACTCTTCCTACCACCA-TAM
reverse	AGTCGGGTTCACCAGGCAT
Mesoderm:	
Nkx2.5 forward	ACCCAGCCAAGGACCCTAGA
probe	FAM-CGAAAAGAAAGAGCTGTGC-MGB
reverse	CTCCACCGCCTTCTGCAG
Tbx5 primers	Purchased from Applied Biosystems
and probe	(Assay Number Hs00361155 m1)
MEF2C forward	CACATCGACCTCCAAGTGCA
probe	FAM-AACACAGGTGGTCTGAT-MGB
reverse	CCAGACGTGAGGTCTCCACC
Endoderm:	
HNF3β forward	CCGACTGGAGCAGCTACTATG
probe	FAM-CAGAGCCCGAGGGCTACTCCTCC-TAM
reverse	TACGTGTTCATGCCGTTCAT
Sox17 forward	CAGCAGAATCCAGACCTGCA
probe	FAM-ACGCCGAGTTGAGCAAGATGCTGG-TAM
reverse	GTCAGCGCCTTCCACGACT
Ectoderm:	
NeuroD1forward	TCACTGCTCAGGACCTACTAACA
probe	FAM-TACAGCGAGAGTGGGCTGATGGG-TAM
reverse	GAGGACCTTGGGGCTGAG
Pax 6 primers	Purchased from Applied Biosystem
and probe	(Assay Number Hs00242217_m1)
Control:	
18S primers	Purchased from Applied Biosystems
and probe	(Assay Number 4319413E)

$1\times$ RT-master mix, 300 nM of each primer, and 80 nM of probe, and approximately 50 ng of total RNA in a final volume of 50 μl. Perform real-time RT-PCR on the ABI Prism 7700 Sequence Detection System (Applied Biosystems) using the following conditions: RT at 48° for 30 min; denaturation and AmpliTaq gold activation at 95° for 10 min; and amplification for 40 cycles at 95° for 15 sec and 60° for 1 min. As a control, the samples are also subjected to the analysis of 18S ribosomal RNA by real-time RT-PCR using a kit from Applied Biosystems. Analyze the reactions by the software from ABI Prism 7700 Sequence Detection System. The relative quantitation of gene expression can be done by normalization against endogenous 18S ribosomal RNA using the $\Delta\Delta C_T$ method described in the ABI User Bulletin #2, Relative Quantitation of Gene Expression, 1997. Triplicate cultures are recommended to derive the relative level of OCT3/4, hTERT, NANOG, or CRIPTO in mean ± standard deviation.

Proliferation

Unlike somatic cells, hESCs display extensive proliferative properties without undergoing senescence. Theoretically, these cells are functionally immortal and have an unrestricted life span. Information regarding proliferation capacity of the cells is useful for many applications. For example, in the case of cell transplantation, it allows one to estimate the length of culture time required to expand undifferentiated cells to the desired amount for differentiation into certain cell types. Several methods can be used to monitor proliferation capacity of hESCs. Analysis of DNA content by flow cytometry can provide cell cycle profile, and measurement of BrdU or 3H thymidine incorporation can give specific information regarding cells in the S phase (Beattie *et al.*, 2005). These assays are, however, not useful to determine the exact cell expansion. A straightforward measurement of cell expansion can be performed by direct cell counting. Cells are generally passaged by collagenase IV dissociation, which usually only gives rise to cell clumps. For cell counting purpose, cells in a duplicate well are dissociated into single cells using trypsin/ EDTA (Li *et al.*, 2005). Cell expansion can then be calculated on the basis of the number of cells harvested compared with the number of cells initially inoculated. Cell proliferation rate can also be assessed by counting cells in triplicate cultures every 1–2 days for 1 week to obtain the growth curve, which is then used to derive population doubling time (Xu *et al.*, 2001).

An important feature of hESCs is their capacity to expand from a single cell. Two clonal cell lines, H9.1 and H9.2, have been successfully subcloned from H9 cells (Amit *et al.*, 2000). Single cell cloning has also been achieved using H1, H13, I3, and I6 cell lines (Amit and Itskovitz-Eldor, 2002).

Undifferentiated hESCs have high telomerase activity, which is consistent with their prolonged proliferation capacity and expression of hTERT. Telomerase activity can be detected by telomeric repeat amplification protocol (TRAP), as described (Kim *et al.*, 1994; Weinrich *et al.*, 1997).

Karyotype Analysis

Karyotype analysis of hESC cultures should be routinely performed, because abnormal karyotypes have been reported in certain cultures maintained both on feeders and in feeder-free conditions (Draper *et al.*, 2004). In our laboratory, cultures are examined for karyotype by the standard G-banding method performed by a qualified cytogenetic laboratory (Oakland Children's Hospital, Oakland, CA).

Differentiation Capacity

Undifferentiated hESCs can be induced to differentiate into a broad range of cell types that may be of potential use for treatment of degenerative diseases such as heart disease, spinal cord injury, Parkinson's disease, and diabetes. So far, cardiomyocytes, neural progenitors, oligodendrocytes, trophoblasts, endothelial cells, hematopoietic lineages, hepatocytes, osteoblasts, insulin-expressing cells, and other cell types have been derived from hESCs using specific procedures (for examples, see Assady *et al.*, 2001; Carpenter *et al.*, 2001; Chadwick *et al.*, 2003b; He *et al.*, 2003; Kehat *et al.*, 2001; Lebkowski *et al.*, 2001; Levenberg *et al.*, 2002; Mummery *et al.*, 2002; Odorico *et al.*, 2001; Rambhatla *et al.*, 2003; Schuldiner *et al.*, 2000; Sottile *et al.*, 2003; Xu *et al.*, 2002a,b; Zhang *et al.*, 2001). When injected into immunodeficient mice, undifferentiated hESCs cells undergo differentiation, leading to the generation of tumors called teratomas consisting of multiple cell types with highly organized structures. These tissues represent those derived from all three germ layers (ectoderm, mesoderm, and endoderm), such as cartilage, bone, toothlike structure, secretary epithelium, primitive neuroepithelial tubule, skin, gastrointestinal epithelium, and respiratory epithelium.

In Vivo *Differentiation through Teratoma Formation*

When cells reach confluence, harvest them by incubating in collagenase IV (200 units/ml) at 37° for 5 min. Collect the cells as clumps by gentle scraping and transfer to a tube. The cells are then washed in PBS and resuspended in PBS to 5×10^7 cells/ml. Inject the cells intramuscularly into the anterior tibialis (hind limbs) of SCID/beige mice ($\sim 5 \times 10^6$ cells in 100 μl per site) or other immunodeficient mice. Tumor formation is then monitored, at least once a week, for a period up to 1 year. When a tumor is formed or reaches 50–100 mm^3 (usually after $\sim$70–90 days in our laboratory), the animal is then euthanized, and the tumor is excised and processed for histological analysis.

In Vitro *Differentiation through Embryoid Bodies*

In vitro spontaneous differentiation can be induced by culturing hESCs in suspension to form EBs. Multiple cell types, including neurons, cardiomyocytes, endoderm cells, and epithelial cells, can be detected in the EB outgrowths generated using the following procedure. After cells reach confluence, add collagenase IV (200 U/ml) dissolved in knockout DMEM into 6-well plates (1 ml/well) or T225 flasks (15 ml/flask), and incubate at 37° for 5 min. After the incubation, aspirate the collagenase IV, and add differentiation medium consisting of 80% knockout DMEM, 20% non–heat-inactivated FBS (Sigma), 1% nonessential amino acids (Invitrogen), 1 mM L-glutamine (Invitrogen), and 0.1 mM ß-mercaptoethanol (Sigma) into the culture (2 ml/well in 6-well plates, 30 ml/T225 flask). The cells are then harvested with a cell scraper or pipet and transferred as clumps to 6-well low–attachment plates (Corning, cat# 29443-030) (1:1 split, one well of 6-well plates into one well of the low-attachment plates, 1 T225 into three low–attachment plates; the split ratio for this procedure should be adjusted so that each well receives ~3 × 10^6 cells). Add differentiation medium to each well to give a total volume of 4 ml per well. After overnight culture in suspension, cells form floating aggregates known as EBs. The differentiation medium should be changed every 2–3 days. To change the medium, transfer EBs into 15-ml or 50-ml tubes and let the aggregates settle for ~5 min, aspirate the supernatant, replace with fresh differentiation medium (4 ml/well), and then transfer to low–attachment, 6-well plates for further culture. During the first few days, the EBs are small with irregular outlines and increase in size by day 4 in suspension. The EBs can be maintained in suspension for more than 10 days. Alternately, EBs at different stages can be transferred to adherent tissue culture plates for further induction of differentiation. Note that the EB formation becomes less efficient when cells maintained in the feeder-free condition reach high passages (>50 passages). These cultures usually lack stromal cells and become a sheetlike monolayer containing high percentages of cells expressing undifferentiated cell markers. To improve EB formation from high–passage cells, first seed cells onto matrix in MEF-CM and then switch to the differentiation medium. The cells are then grown to confluence in differentiation medium for 5–6 days before initiation of the suspension culture.

To examine the differentiated culture, immunocytochemical or RT-PCR analyses can be used to detect cell type-specific markers. Useful diagnostic markers are β-tubulin III for neurons, α-fetoprotein (AFP) for endoderm cells, cardiac troponin I (cTnI) for cardiomyocytes, and pan-cytokeratins for epithelial cells. For immunocytochemistry, EBs are plated onto gelatin-coated chamber slides for differentiation and subsequent analysis. Fix and permeablize the differentiated cultures as described in the preceding section for detecting intracellular antigens. After blocking with 5% NGS in PBS, the cells are incubated at room temperature for 2 h with a monoclonal antibody against β-tubulin III (Sigma), AFP (Sigma), cTnI (Spectral Diagnostic Inc., Toronto, Ontario, Canada), or pan-cytokeratins (Dako Corporation, Carpinteria, CA) diluted appropriately in 1% NGS in PBS. After washing, incubate the cells with FITC-conjugated goat anti-mouse IgG (Sigma), diluted in PBS containing 1% NGS, at room temperature for 30 min–1 h. Alternately, goat anti-mouse IgG1 conjugated with Alexa 488 or goat anti-mouse IgG1 conjugated with Alexa 594 (Invitrogen) can be used. Cells are then washed three times with PBS (5–10 min/washing) and mounted with Vectashield mounting media for examination with ultraviolet microscopy. Alternately, real-time RT-PCR analysis is performed instead of immunocytochemistry to detect markers associated with cell types derived from mesoderm, endoderm, and ectoderm. Table II lists primers and probes for suggested markers. It should be noted that more in-depth analyses of functional phenotypes are required to confirm the differentiation of specific cell types, details of which can be found elsewhere.

Although the EB formation procedure has been commonly used to assess *in vitro* spontaneous differentiation, other protocols without the requirement of EB formation may also be used to induce hESCs into specific cell types, particularly when EB formation is inefficient or unable to give rise to particular cells of interest. For example, two hESC lines, HES-1 and HES-2, fail to form EBs with the hanging drop method or simple suspension but have been induced to generate contracting cardiomyocytes after prolonged culture on MEF feeders (Reubinoff *et al.*, 2000) or after coculture with the endoderm-like cell line END-2 derived from mouse embryonic carcinoma cells (mECs) (Mummery *et al.*, 2002, 2003).

Conclusion

Research on hESCs continues to advance rapidly on various fronts, including derivation of additional hESC lines and development of novel methods to culture undifferentiated cells. Potential application of these cells demands assurance of the highest quality as expected, which can be monitored by the methods described previously and should be carried out in a comprehensive manner. As our understanding of human stem cell biology expands, it is of no doubt that additional methods, such as those at a genomic level, will be developed. These and the existing methods should be helpful to providing confidence for hESCs to be used in a clinical setting.

Acknowledgments

I thank Drs. Jane Lebkowski, Calvin Harley, and Joseph Gold for their critical review of this manuscript and my colleagues for their invaluable contribution to our studies.

References

Abeyta, M. J., Clark, A. T., Rodriguez, R. T., Bodnar, M. S., Pera, R. A., and Firpo, M. T. (2004). Unique gene expression signatures of independently-derived human embryonic stem cell lines. *Hum. Mol. Genet.* **13,** 601–608.

Amit, M., Carpenter, M. K., Inokuma, M. S., Chiu, C. P., Harris, C. P., Waknitz, M. A., Itskovitz-Eldor, J., and Thomson, J. A. (2000). Clonally derived human embryonic stem cell lines maintain pluripotency and proliferative potential for prolonged periods of culture. *Dev. Biol.* **227,** 271–278.

Amit, M., and Itskovitz-Eldor, J. (2002). Derivation and spontaneous differentiation of human embryonic stem cells. *J. Anat.* **200,** 225–232.

Amit, M., Margulets, V., Segev, H., Shariki, K., Laevsky, I., Coleman, R., and Itskovitz-Eldor, J. (2003). Human feeder layers for human embryonic stem cells. *Biol. Reprod.* **68,** 2150–2156.

Amit, M., Shariki, C., Margulets, V., and Itskovitz-Eldor, J. (2004). Feeder layer- and serum-free culture of human embryonic stem cells. *Biol. Reprod.* **70,** 837–845.

Andrews, P. W., Casper, J., Damjanov, I., Duggan-Keen, M., Giwercman, A., Hata, J., von Keitz, A., Looijenga, L. H., Millan, J. L., Oosterhuis, J. W., Pera, M., Sawada, M., Schmoll, H. J., Skakkebaek, N. E., van Putten, W., and Stern, P. (1996). Comparative analysis of cell surface antigens expressed by cell lines derived from human germ cell tumours. *Int. J. Cancer* **66,** 806–816.

Assady, S., Maor, G., Amit, M., Itskovitz-Eldor, J., Skorecki, K. L., and Tzukerman, M. (2001). Insulin production by human embryonic stem cells. *Diabetes* **50,** 1691–1697.

Badcock, G., Pigott, C., Goepel, J., and Andrews, P. W. (1999). The human embryonal carcinoma marker antigen TRA-1–60 is a sialylated keratan sulfate proteoglycan. *Cancer Res.* **59,** 4715–4719.

Beattie, G. M., Lopez, A. D., Bucay, N., Hinton, A., Firpo, M. T., King, C. C., and Hayek, A. (2005). Activin A maintains pluripotency of human embryonic stem cells in the absence of feeder layers. *Stem Cells* **23,** 489–495.

Bhattacharya, B., Miura, T., Brandenberger, R., Mejido, J., Luo, Y., Yang, A. X., Joshi, B. H., Ginis, I., Thies, R. S., Amit, M., Lyons, I., Condie, B. G., Itskovitz-Eldor, J., Rao, M. S., and Puri, R. K. (2004). Gene expression in human embryonic stem cell lines: Unique molecular signature. *Blood* **103,** 2956–2964.

Boyer, L. A., Lee, T. I., Cole, M. F., Johnstone, S. E., Levine, S. S., Zucker, J. P., Guenther, M. G., Kumar, R. M., Murray, H. L., Jenner, R. G., Gifford, D. K., Melton, D. A., Joenisch, R., and Young, R. A. (2005). Core transcriptional regulatory circuitry in human embryonic stem cells. *Cell* **122,** 947–956.

Brandenberger, R., Khrebtukova, I., Thies, R. S., Miura, T., Jingli, C., Puri, R., Vasicek, T., Lebkowski, J., and Rao, M. (2004a). MPSS profiling of human embryonic stem cells. *BMC Dev. Biol.* **4,** 10.

Brandenberger, R., Wei, H., Zhang, S., Lei, S., Murage, J., Fisk, G. J., Li, Y., Xu, C., Fang, R., Guegler, K., Rao, M. S., Mandalam, R., Lebkowski, J., and Stanton, L. W. (2004b). Transcriptome characterization elucidates signaling networks that control human ES cell growth and differentiation. *Nat. Biotechnol.* **22,** 707–716.

Carpenter, M. K., Inokuma, M. S., Denham, J., Mujtaba, T., Chiu, C. P., and Rao, M. S. (2001). Enrichment of neurons and neural precursors from human embryonic stem cells. *Exp. Neurol.* **172,** 383–397.

Carpenter, M. K., Rosler, E. S., Fisk, G. J., Brandenberger, R., Ares, X., Miura, T., Lucero, M., and Rao, M. S. (2004). Properties of four human embryonic stem cell lines maintained in a feeder-free culture system. *Dev. Dyn.* **229,** 243–258.

Chadwick, K., Wang, L., Li, L., Menendez, P., Murdoch, B., Rouleau, A., and Bhatia, M. (2003). Cytokines and BMP-4 promote hematopoietic differentiation of human embryonic stem cells. *Blood* **102,** 906–915.

Cheng, L., Hammond, H., Ye, Z., Zhan, X., and Dravid, G. (2003). Human adult marrow cells support prolonged expansion of human embryonic stem cells in culture. *Stem Cells* **21,** 131–142.

Draper, J. S., Pigott, C., Thomson, J. A., and Andrews, P. W. (2002). Surface antigens of human embryonic stem cells: Changes upon differentiation in culture. *J. Anat.* **200,** 249–258.

Draper, J. S., Smith, K., Gokhale, P., Moore, H. D., Maltby, E., Johnson, J., Meisner, L., Zwaka, T. P., Thomson, J. A., and Andrews, P. W. (2004). Recurrent gain of chromosomes 17q and 12 in cultured human embryonic stem cells. *Nat. Biotechnol.* **22,** 53–54.

Genbacev, O., Krtolica, A., Zdravkovic, T., Brunette, E., Powell, S., Nath, A., Caceres, E., McMaster, M., McDonagh, S., Li, Y., Mandalam, R., Lebkowski, J., and Fisher, S. J. (2005). Serum-free derivation of human embryonic stem cell lines on human placental fibroblast feeders. *Fertil. Steril.* **83,** 1517–1529.

He, J. Q., Ma, Y., Lee, Y., Thomson, J. A., and Kamp, T. J. (2003). Human embryonic stem cells develop into multiple types of cardiac myocytes: Action potential characterization. *Circ. Res.* **93,** 32–39.

Henderson, J. K., Draper, J. S., Baillie, H. S., Fishel, S., Thomson, J. A., Moore, H., and Andrews, P. W. (2002). Preimplantation human embryos and embryonic stem cells show comparable expression of stage-specific embryonic antigens. *Stem Cells* **20,** 329–337.

Hoffman, L. M., and Carpenter, M. K. (2005). Characterization and culture of human embryonic stem cells. *Nat. Biotechnol.* **23,** 699–708.

Hovatta, O., Mikkola, M., Gertow, K., Stromberg, A. M., Inzunza, J., Hreinsson, J., Rozell, B., Blennow, E., Andang, M., and Ahrlund-Richter, L. (2003). A culture system using human foreskin fibroblasts as feeder cells allows production of human embryonic stem cells. *Hum. Reprod.* **18,** 1404–1409.

Inzunza, J., Gertow, K., Stromberg, M. A., Matilainen, E., Blennow, E., Skottman, H., Wolbank, S., Ahrlund-Richter, L., and Hovatta, O. (2005). Derivation of human embryonic stem cell lines in serum replacement medium using postnatal human fibroblasts as feeder cells. *Stem Cells* **23,** 544–549.

James, D., Levine, A. J., Besser, D., and Hemmati-Brivanlou, A. (2005). TGF{beta}/activin/nodal signaling is necessary for the maintenance of pluripotency in human embryonic stem cells. *Development* **132,** 1273–1282.

Johansson, B. M., and Wiles, M. V. (1995). Evidence for involvement of activin A and bone morphogenetic protein 4 in mammalian mesoderm and hematopoietic development. *Mol. Cell Biol.* **15,** 141–151.

Kaufman, D. S., Hanson, E. T., Lewis, R. L., Auerbach, R., and Thomson, J. A. (2001). Hematopoietic colony-forming cells derived from human embryonic stem cells. *Proc. Natl. Acad. Sci. USA* **98,** 10716–10721.

Kehat, I., Kenyagin-Karsenti, D., Snir, M., Segev, H., Amit, M., Gepstein, A., Livne, E., Binah, O., Itskovitz-Eldor, J., and Gepstein, L. (2001). Human embryonic stem cells can differentiate into myocytes with structural and functional properties of cardiomyocytes. *J. Clin. Invest.* **108,** 407–414.

Kim, N. Y., Piatyszek, M. A., Prowse, K. R., Harley, C. B., West, M. D., Ho, P. L., Coviello, G. M., Wright, W. E., Weinrich, S. L., and Shay, J. W. (1994). Specific association of human telomerase activity with immortal cell lines and cancer. *Science* **266**, 2011–2015.

Klimanskaya, I., Chung, Y., Meisner, L., Johnson, J., West, M. D., and Lanza, R. (2005). Human embryonic stem cells derived without feeder cells. *Lancet* **365**, 1636–1641.

Lebkowski, J. S., Gold, J., Xu, C., Funk, W., Chiu, C. P., and Carpenter, M. K. (2001). Human embryonic stem cells: Culture, differentiation, and genetic modification for regenerative medicine applications. *Cancer J.* **7**(Suppl. 2), S83–S93.

Levenberg, S., Golub, J. S., Amit, M., Itskovitz-Eldor, J., and Langer, R. (2002). Endothelial cells derived from human embryonic stem cells. *Proc. Natl. Acad. Sci. USA* **99**, 4391–4396.

Li, Y., Powell, S., Brunette, E., Lebkowski, J., and Mandalam, R. (2005). Expansion of human embryonic stem cells in defined serum-free medium devoid of animal-derived products. *Biotechnol. Bioeng.* **91**, 688–698.

Ludwig, T. E., Levenstein, M. E., Jones, J. M., Berggren, W. T., Mitchen, E. R., Frane, J. L., Crandall, L. J., Daigh, C. A., Conard, K. R., Piekarczyk, M. S., Llanas, R. A., and Thomson, J. A. (2006). Derivation of human embryonic stem cells in defined conditions. *Nat. Biotechnol.*

Ma, Y., Ramezani, A., Lewis, R., Hawley, R. G., and Thomson, J. A. (2003). High-level sustained transgene expression in human embryonic stem cells using lentiviral vectors. *Stem Cells* **21**, 111–117.

Miraglia, S., Godfrey, W., Yin, A. H., Atkins, K., Warnke, R., Holden, J. T., Bray, R. A., Waller, E. K., and Buck, D. W. (1997). A novel five-transmembrane hematopoietic stem cell antigen: Isolation, characterization, and molecular cloning. *Blood* **90**, 5013–5021.

Miura, T., Luo, Y., Khrebtukova, I., Brandenberger, R., Zhou, D., Thies, R. S., Vasicek, T., Young, H., Lebkowski, J., Carpenter, M. K., and Rao, M. S. (2004). Monitoring early differentiation events in human embryonic stem cells by massively parallel signature sequencing and expressed sequence tag scan. *Stem Cells Dev.* **13**, 694–715.

Miyamoto, K., Hayashi, K., Suzuki, T., Ichihara, S., Yamada, T., Kano, Y., Yamabe, T., and Ito, Y. (2004). Human placenta feeder layers support undifferentiated growth of primate embryonic stem cells. *Stem Cells* **22**, 433–440.

Mummery, C., Ward, D., van den Brink, C. E., Bird, S. D., Doevendans, P. A., Opthof, T., Brutel de la Riviere, A., Tertoolen, L., van der Heyden, M., and Pera, M. (2002). Cardiomyocyte differentiation of mouse and human embryonic stem cells. *J. Anat.* **200**, 233–242.

Mummery, C., Ward-van Oostwaard, D., Doevendans, P., Spijker, R., van den Brink, S., Hassink, R., van der Heyden, M., Opthof, T., Pera, M., de la Riviere, A. B., Passier, R., and Tertoolen, L. (2003). Differentiation of human embryonic stem cells to cardiomyocytes: Role of coculture with visceral endoderm-like cells. *Circulation* **107**, 2733–2740.

Nistor, I. G., Totoiu, M. O., Haque, N., Carpenter, M. K., and Keirstead, H. S. (2003). Human embryonic stem cells differentiate into oligodendrocytes in high purity and myelinate after spinal cord transplantation. *Glia* **29**, 385–396.

Odorico, J. S., Kaufman, D. S., and Thomson, J. A. (2001). Multilineage differentiation from human embryonic stem cell lines. *Stem Cells* **19**, 193–204.

Oka, M., Tagoku, K., Russell, T. L., Nakano, Y., Hamazaki, T., Meyer, E. M., Yokota, T., and Terada, N. (2002). CD9 is associated with leukemia inhibitory factor-mediated maintenance of embryonic stem cells. *Mol. Biol. Cell* **13**, 1274–1281.

Pera, M. F., Blasco-Lafita, M. J., Cooper, S., Mason, M., Mills, J., and Monaghan, P. (1988). Analysis of cell-differentiation lineage in human teratomas using new monoclonal antibodies to cytostructural antigens of embryonal carcinoma cells. *Differentiation* **39**, 139–149.

Rambhatla, L., Chiu, C. P., Kundu, P., Peng, Y., and Carpenter, M. K. (2003). Generation of hepatocyte-like cells from human embryonic stem cells. *Cell Transplant.* **12**, 1–11.

Reubinoff, B. E., Pera, M. F., Fong, C. Y., Trounson, A., and Bongso, A. (2000). Embryonic stem cell lines from human blastocysts: Somatic differentiation *in vitro. Nat. Biotechnol.* **18**, 399–404.

Richards, M., Fong, C. Y., Chan, W. K., Wong, P. C., and Bongso, A. (2002). Human feeders support prolonged undifferentiated growth of human inner cell masses and embryonic stem cells. *Nat. Biotechnol.* **20**, 933–936.

Richards, M., Tan, S. P., Tan, J. H., Chan, W. K., and Bongso, A. (2004). The transcriptome profile of human embryonic stem cells as defined by SAGE. *Stem Cells* **22**, 51–64.

Rosler, E. S., Fisk, G. J., Ares, X., Irving, J., Miura, T., Rao, M. S., and Carpenter, M. K. (2004). Long-term culture of human embryonic stem cells in feeder-free conditions. *Dev. Dyn.* **229**, 259–274.

Schuldiner, M., Yanuka, O., Itskovitz-Eldor, J., Melton, D. A., and Benvenisty, N. (2000). Effects of eight growth factors on the differentiation of cells derived from human embryonic stem cells. *Proc. Natl. Acad. Sci. USA* **92**, 11307–11312.

Sottile, V., Thomson, A., and McWhir, J. (2003). *In vitro* osteogenic differentiation of human ES cells. *Cloning Stem Cells* **5**, 149–155.

Sperger, J. M., Chen, X., Draper, J. S., Antosiewicz, J. E., Chon, C. H., Jones, S. B., Brooks, J. D., Andrews, P. W., Brown, P. O., and Thomson, J. A. (2003). Gene expression patterns in human embryonic stem cells and human pluripotent germ cell tumors. *Proc. Natl. Acad. Sci. USA* **100**, 13350–13355.

Stojkovic, P., Lako, M., Przyborski, S., Stewart, R., Armstrong, L., Evans, J., Zhang, X., and Stojkovic, M. (2005a). Human-serum matrix supports undifferentiated growth of human embryonic stem cells. *Stem Cells* **23**, 895–902.

Stojkovic, P., Lako, M., Stewart, R., Przyborski, S., Armstrong, L., Evans, J., Murdoch, A., Strachan, T., and Stojkovic, M. (2005b). An autogeneic feeder cell system that efficiently supports growth of undifferentiated human embryonic stem cells. *Stem Cells* **23**, 306–314.

Thomson, J. A., Itskovitz-Eldor, J., Shapiro, S. S., Waknitz, M. A., Swiergiel, J. J., Marshall, V. S., and Jones, J. M. (1998). Embryonic stem cell lines derived from human blastocysts. *Science* **282**, 1145–1147.

Uchida, N., Buck, D. W., He, D., Reitsma, M. J., Masek, M., Phan, T. V., Tsukamoto, A. S., Gage, F. H., and Weissman, I. L. (2000). Direct isolation of human central nervous system stem cells. *Proc. Natl. Acad. Sci. USA* **97**, 14720–14725.

Vallier, L., Alexander, M., and Pedersen, R. A. (2005). Activin/Nodal and FGF pathways cooperate to maintain pluripotency of human embryonic stem cells. *J. Cell Sci.* **118**, 4495–4509.

Vallier, L., Reynolds, D., and Pedersen, R. A. (2004). Nodal inhibits differentiation of human embryonic stem cells along the neuroectodermal default pathway. *Dev. Biol.* **275**, 403–421.

Wang, G., Zhang, H., Zhao, Y., Li, J., Cai, J., Wang, P., Meng, S., Feng, J., Miao, C., Ding, M., Li, D., and Deng, H. (2005a). Noggin and bFGF cooperate to maintain the pluripotency of human embryonic stem cells in the absence of feeder layers. *Biochem. Biophys. Res. Commun.* **330**, 934–942.

Wang, L., Li, L., Menendez, P., Cerdan, C., and Bhatia, M. (2005b). Human embryonic stem cells maintained in the absence of mouse embryonic fibroblasts or conditioned media are capable of hematopoietic development. *Blood* **105**, 4598–4603.

Wang, Q., Fang, Z., Jin, F., Lu, Y., Gai, H., and Sheng, H. Z. (2005c). Derivation and growing human embryonic stem cells on feeders. *Stem Cells* **23**, 1221–1227.

Weinrich, S. L., Pruzan, R., Ma, L., Ouellette, M., Tesmer, V. M., Holt, S. E., Bodnar, A. G., Lichtsteiner, S., Kim, N. W., Trager, J. B., Taylor, R. D., Carlos, R., Andrews, W. H., Wright, W. E., Shay, J. W., Harley, C. B., and Morin, G. B. (1997). Reconstitution of human telomerase with the template RNA component hTR and the catalytic protein subunit hTRT. *Nat. Genet.* **17,** 498–502.

Wong, R. C., Pebay, A., Nguyen, L. T., Koh, K. L., and Pera, M. F. (2004). Presence of functional gap junctions in human embryonic stem cells. *Stem Cells* **22,** 883–889.

Xu, C., Inokuma, M. S., Denham, J., Golds, K., Kundu, P., Gold, J. D., and Carpenter, M. K. (2001). Feeder-free growth of undifferentiated human embryonic stem cells. *Nat. Biotech.* **19,** 971–974.

Xu, C., Jiang, J., Sottile, V., McWhir, J., Lebkowski, J., and Carpenter, M. K. (2004). Immortalized fibroblast-like cells derived from human embryonic stem cells support undifferentiated cell growth. *Stem Cells* **22,** 972–980.

Xu, C., Police, S., Rao, N., and Carpenter, M. K. (2002a). Characterization and enrichment of cardiomyocytes derived from human embryonic stem cells. *Circ. Res.* **91,** 501–508.

Xu, C., Rosler, E., Jiang, J., Lebkowski, J. S., Gold, J. D., O'Sullivan, C., Delavan-Boorsma, K., Mok, M., Bronstein, A., and Carpenter, M. K. (2005a). Basic fibroblast growth factor supports undifferentiated human embryonic stem cell growth without conditioned medium. *Stem Cells* **23,** 315–323.

Xu, R. H., Chen, X., Li, D. S., Li, R., Addicks, G. C., Glennon, C., Zwaka, T. P., and Thomson, J. A. (2002b). BMP4 initiates human embryonic stem cell differentiation to trophoblast. *Nat. Biotechnol.* **20,** 1261–1264.

Xu, R.-H., Peck, R. M., Li, D. S., Feng, X., Ludwig, T., and Thomson, J. A. (2005b). Basic FGF and suppression of BMP signaling sustain undifferentiated proliferation of human ES cells. *Nat. Methods* **3,** 185–190.

Yin, A. H., Miraglia, S., Zanjani, E. D., Almeida-Porada, G., Ogawa, M., Leary, A. G., Olweus, J., Kearney, J., and Buck, D. W. (1997). AC133, a novel marker for human hematopoietic stem and progenitor cells. *Blood* **90,** 5002–5012.

Zhang, S. C., Wernig, M., Duncan, I. D., Brustle, O., and Thomson, J. A. (2001). *In vitro* differentiation of transplantable neural precursors from human embryonic stem cells. *Nat. Biotechnol.* **19,** 1129–1133.

Zwaka, T. P., and Thomson, J. A. (2003). Homologous recombination in human embryonic stem cells. *Nat. Biotechnol.* **21,** 319–321.

[3] Feeder-Free Culture of Human Embryonic Stem Cells

By MICHAL AMIT and JOSEPH ITSKOVITZ-ELDOR

Abstract

In addition to their contribution to research fields such as early human development, self-renewal, and differentiation mechanisms, human embryonic stem cells (hESCs) may serve as a tool for drug testing and for the study of cell-based therapies. Traditionally, these cells have been cultured with mouse embryonic fibroblast (MEF) feeder layers, which allow their continuous growth in an undifferentiated state. However, for future clinical

0076-6879/06 $35.00
DOI: 10.1016/S0076-6879(06)20003-X

applications, hESCs should be cultured under defined conditions, preferably in a xeno-free culture system, where exposure to animal pathogens is prevented. To this end, different culture methods for hESCs, based on serum replacement and free of supportive cell layers, were developed. This chapter discusses a simple, feeder-free culture system on the basis of medium supplemented with transforming growth factor $\beta1$ (TGF$\beta1$), basic fibroblast growth factor (bFGF) and fibronectin as matrix.

Introduction

Embryonic stem cells (ESCs) are pluripotent cells derived from the inner cell mass (ICM) of embryos at the blastocyst stage. The first ESC lines were derived from mouse embryos in 1981 by two separate groups (Evans and Kaufman, 1981; Martin, 1981). In their 25 years of existence, mouse ESCs were extensively used for the study of directed differentiation into specific cell types, self-maintenance processes, early developmental events, and more. Since these pioneering studies, ESC lines have been derived from three nonhuman primates (Suemori *et al.*, 2001; Thomson *et al.*, 1995, 1996) and eventually from human blastocysts (Thomson *et al.*, 1998). Accumulating knowledge shows that human embryonic stem cells (hESCs) meet most of the acceptable criteria for ESCs (Smith, 2000). To date, there are several established and well-characterized hESC lines in several laboratories around the world (Amit and Itskovitz-Eldor, 2004; Cowan *et al.*, 2004; Verlinsky *et al.*, 2005). The availability of these lines provides a unique new tool with widespread potential for research and for clinical applications.

The possible future use of hESCs in the clinical and industrial arena will require a reproducible, well-defined, and animal-free culture system for their routine culture. The traditional culture and derivation methods for hESCs, however, include mouse embryonic fibroblasts (MEFs) as feeder layers and medium supplemented with fetal bovine or calf serum (FBS) (Thomson *et al.*, 1998). When cultured in these conditions, hESCs grow as flat colonies with typical spaces between the cells, high nucleus/cytoplasm ratio, and with at least two nucleoli (illustrated in Fig. 1A). Culture of hESCs requires meticulous care that includes daily medium change, routine passaging every 4–6 days, and occasionally mechanical removal of differentiated colonies from the culture. Nevertheless, hESCs can be cultured in high quantities and frozen and thawed with reasonable survival rates (Amit and Itskovitz-Eldor, 2002; Reubinoff *et al.*, 2000, 2001; Thomson *et al.*, 1998).

The traditional culture method for hESCs exhibits several major disadvantages: (1) the use of MEFs as feeder layers and FBS may expose the cells to animal photogenes, (2) batch-to-batch variations of the MEFs and serum in supporting undifferentiated hESC culture, and (3) undefined culture

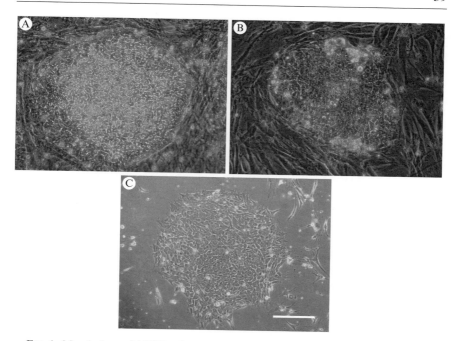

FIG. 1. Morphology of hESC colony cultured in different culture conditions. (A) With mouse embryonic fibroblasts (MEFs), (B) With foreskin fibroblast, and (C) in animal-, serum- and feeder-free conditions. Bar = 100 μM.

conditions. These three drawbacks reduce the reproducibility of the method. To obtain a reproducible, well-defined, and animal-free culture system requires that substitutes for the serum and for the feeder layer be developed. In recent years, broad research into developing these substitutes has yielded four main progresses: (1) the ability to grow cells in serum-free culture conditions (Amit *et al.*, 2000); (2) feeder-free culture method on the basis of the maintenance of the cells in an undifferentiated state on Matrigel matrix with 100% MEF-conditioned medium (Xu *et al.*, 2001). (3) the use of human substitutes for MEFs such as fetal fibroblasts, fallopian tube epithelium (Richards *et al.*, 2002) or foreskin fibroblasts (Amit *et al.*, 2003; Hovatta *et al.*, 2003) as feeder layers, and (4) prolonged culture of hESCs in feeder-layer–free conditions while using selected growth factors and substitute matrices (Amit *et al.*, 2004; Ludwig *et al.*, 2006; Xu *et al.*, 2005a,b).

The simplest alternative to the culture method on the basis of the use of MEF and FBS is the use of human supportive line and human serum or serum replacement. Among the cells proven to support continuous culture of undifferentiated hESCs, one can find human fetal–derived fibroblasts

(Richards *et al.*, 2002), foreskin fibroblasts (Amit *et al.*, 2003; Hovatta *et al.*, 2003), and adult marrow cells (Cheng *et al.*, 2003). Characterizations of hESCs cultured continuously with those cell lines demonstrate that the cells sustained all ESC features. Human fetal–derived fibroblasts and foreskin fibroblasts were also found to support the derivation of new hESC lines under animal-free or serum-free conditions (Hovatta *et al.*, 2003; Inzunza *et al.*, 2005; Richards *et al.*, 2002). In our experience, foreskin fibroblasts used as feeders enable hESCs to be cultured for more than 1 year (124 passages, more than 300 doublings) while exhibiting all stem cells features including (1) expression of typical surface markers such as stage specific embryonic antigen (SSEA)3, SSEA4, tumor recognition antigen (TRA)-1–60, and TRA-1–81; (2) expression of transcription factors as Oct 4, Nanog, and Rex 1; (3) differentiation into representative tissues of the three embryonic germ layers, both in embryoid bodies (EBs) and in teratomas; (4) high telomerase activity; and (5) maintenance of normal karyotype (Amit and Itskovitz-Eldor, unpublished data). The morphology of an hESC colony grown with foreskin fibroblast feeder layers, using an animal-free and serum-free medium, is illustrated in Fig. 1B.

A unique source of supportive cells was offered by Xu *et al.* (2004) on the basis of feeders derived from human EBs. These fibroblast-like cells, immortalized by vectors containing the hTERT gene, were shown to support the culture of hESCs for more than 14 passages. The major disadvantage of this method, however, is the use of FBS for the isolation and culture of the feeder cells from EBs, because it does not provide an animal-free environment (Yoo *et al.*, 2005; Xu *et al.*, 2004).

Although human supportive cell lines were shown to maintain hESCs for prolonged cultures while preserving ESC features, the method has some disadvantages: first, the need for culture of the feeders themselves, which will limit the large-scale culture of hESCs, and second, the culture system cannot be precisely defined because of differences between batches of feeder-layer cells and the used human serum. Ideally, the culture method for hESCs should, therefore, be a combination of an animal-free, serum-free, and feeder-free culture system.

When developing a feeder–free culture method for hESCs, one should consider their differences from mouse ESCs. Although mouse ESCs maintained their stem cell features and remained undifferentiated when grown on gelatin without an MEF feeder layer and medium supplemented with leukemia inhibitory factor (LIF) (Smith *et al.*, 1988; Williams *et al.*, 1988), LIF failed to support a feeder-free culture of hESCs (Thomson *et al.*, 1998). In fact, it had been demonstrated that the phosphorylation of proteins involved in LIF cellular pathway, such as STAT3, is weak or absent in hESCs (Daheron *et al.*, 2004; Humphrey *et al.*, 2004; Sato *et al.*, 2004). Thus, the mechanism underlining hESC self-maintenance is still unrevealed, and new candidate growth factors, cytokines, and matrices should be examined.

The first supportive layer–free culture method for hESCs was reported in a study by Xu and colleagues (2001). The culture method relies on Matrigel, laminin, or fibronectin as matrix and 100% MEF-conditioned medium, supplemented with serum replacement (Xu et al., 2001). When cultured under these conditions, hESCs can be stably maintained for more than 1 year of continuous culture while maintaining their ESC features. The growth and background differentiation rates were found to be similar to those of the traditional culture method, but several significant disadvantages still exist: (1) exposure to animal pathogens through the MEF-conditioned medium or Matrigel matrix; (2) the culture system cannot be accurately defined because of variations between batches of MEFs used for the production of the conditioned medium and the Matrigel matrix; (3) under these culture conditions, hESCs form "auto feeders" that most probably contribute to the cells' maintenance on the one hand but results in the loss of cells to differentiation on the other, and (4) the simultaneous culture of MEFs and hESCs limits the use of this culture system to scale-up the growth of hESCs for future clinical and industrial purposes.

Recent developments have eliminated the major disadvantage of the Xu et al. culture system—the use of MEF–conditioned medium. The same group proposed an improved system on the basis of Matrigel matrix and medium supplemented with serum replacement and 40 ng/ml bFGF (Xu et al., 2005b). The removal of the conditioned-medium increased the background differentiation rate up to 28%, but this rate can be decreased to 20% by adding 75 ng/ml Flt-3 ligand to the culture medium (Xu et al., 2005b). Further improvement was achieved by a different group through the addition of high amount of Noggin (Xu et al., 2005a). The addition of inhibitor to the bone morphogenic protein (BMP) signal pathway, Noggin, allowed a further decrease in the differentiation rate to 10%, which equals that achieved by culturing the cells with Matrigel and MEF-conditioned medium (Xu et al., 2005a). The same efficiency was reported when bFGF was added at a concentration of 100 ng/ml, without Noggin. Thus the importance of Noggin or other inhibitors of the BMP signal transduction pathway is still unclear.

The method described in this chapter is based on fibronectin as matrix, medium supplemented with 20% serum replacement, TGFβ1, and bFGF (Amit and Itskovitz-Eldor, 2004). Under these culture conditions, hESCs were maintained for more than 1 year while maintaining stem cell characteristics. An example of the morphology of a colony cultured in these conditions is illustrated in Fig. 1C. The background differentiation, however, reached a level of 15%. The role of the components of the system is still unrevealed.

TGFβ, a multipotent growth factor, is known to have either a positive or a negative effect on cellular proliferation, differentiation, migration, matrix deposition, or apoptosis in the hematopoietic system, depending on the culture environment and stage of development of the cells, or in cases of response to injury or disease (Fortunel *et al.*, 2000; Massague, 1990). The first clue as to the possible role of TGFβ1 in maintaining undifferentiated hESCs came from a study by Schuldiner and colleagues, who examined the effects of eight different growth factors on hESC differentiation by evaluating cell-specific gene expression (Schuldiner *et al.*, 2000). In that study, TGFβ1 was assumed to repress cell differentiation because it led to the production of relatively reduced cell-specific gene expression (Schuldiner *et al.*, 2000). In addition, TGFβ1 is one of the components in Matrigel matrix, which is the most used matrix found to support hESC cell growth in feeder-free conditions (Xu *et al.*, 2001).

Recently, the involvement of another member of the TGFβ supper family in the self-renewal mechanism of hESCs was put forth. Increasing evidence indicates that TGFβ1, activin, and nodal pathway might be involved in hESC self-maintenance through transcription factor SMAD2/3 (Besser, 2004; James *et al.*, 2005; Valdimarsdottir and Mummery, 2005). SMAD2/3 signaling enhances in undifferentiated cells and reduces at early stages of differentiation, and its activation is required for the expression of markers of undifferentiated cells (Besser, 2004; James *et al.*, 2005). In contrast, SMAD 1/5 signaling, induced by BMP/GDF branch, decreases in undifferentiated cells and increases when differentiation processes begin (James *et al.*, 2005). The signal transduction pathways of TGFβ1/activin/nodal and Wnt were suggested to have a positive effect through SMAD2/3 on Nanog or Oct 4 activity in the nucleus and thus take part in hESC self-renewal mechanism (Valdimarsdottir and Mummery, 2005). Indeed, the supplement of TGFβ1, activin, or Bio (activator of the Wnt signaling, GSK3β inhibitor) to the culture medium contributes to the maintenance of hESCs as undifferentiated cells in supportive cell–free culture systems (Amit *et al.*, 2004; Beattie *et al.*, 2005; Sato *et al.*, 2004; Vallier *et al.*, 2005). However, none of the proposed factors, TGFβ1, activin, nodal, or Wnt were proven to be directly involved in the hESC mechanism of self-maintenance, and in some cases, they failed to maintain prolonged culture of undifferentiated hESCs in a feeder-free environment (Dravid *et al.*, 2005). Thus, extensive research is needed to clarify the mechanism underlining hESC self-renewal, including the possibility that more than one pathway is involved, the existence of alternative pathways, and the factors' synergistic effect.

Another component of the described culture system is fibronectin, which is used as a substitute matrix. Fibronectin, a basal lamina component, is frequently used to increase cell adhesion to the culture dishes. It acts through the integrin receptors, which, in addition to their role as mediators of cell adhesion to extracellular matrix proteins, activate a variety of intracellular signal transduction pathways that may be involved in the cells' proliferation, apoptosis, shape, polarity, motility, gene expression profiles, and differentiation (Hynes, 2002). The fibronectin-specific integrin receptor, $\alpha_5\beta_1$, was demonstrated to be expressed in undifferentiated hESCs (Amit et al., 2004). Further complementary research is required to explain the possible role of extracellular proteins such as fibronectin in the self-renewal of hESCs.

Most of the existing hESCs were derived with MEF as a feeder layer (Amit and Itskovitz-Eldor, 2004; Cowan et al., 2004; Reubinoff et al., 2000; Thomson et al., 1998; Verlinsky et al., 2005). Klimanskaya and colleagues were the first to report the isolation of hESCs in a supportive cell–free culture condition (Klimanskaya et al., 2005). The reported culture system includes MEF-produced matrix and medium supplemented with a high dose of bFGF (16 ng/ml) and LIF, serum replacement, and Plasmanate (Klimanskaya et al., 2005). A new hESC line was successfully derived using this method, in which hESC characteristics are retained, including stable and normal karyotypes, after more than 30 passages of continuous culture. Although the culture system includes some undefined materials (MEF matrix and knockout serum replacement), it proves the feasibility of a supportive feeder layer–less derivation of hESCs. A recent publication by Ludwig and colleagues demonstrates a defined serum-free and animal-free medium that not only supports a culture of undifferentiated hESCs for prolonged periods but is also suitable for hESC isolation under feeder-free culture conditions (Ludwig et al., 2006). Interestingly, the medium combination requires the addition of both bFGF and TGFβ1 in addition to Licl, GABA, and pipeolic acid. The matrix consisted of human collagen, fibronectin, and laminin. After their continuous culture for several months, the newly derived cells sustained most hESC features. Thus for the first time defined, animal-free, serum-free, and feeder-free culture conditions for hESCs are presented. However, one disturbing difficulty of the new method is the karyotype stability. In the study, two new hESC lines were derived: one was reported to harbor 47,XXY after 4 months of continuous culture (it is unclear whether the embryo was originally defected), and the second exhibited trisomy 12 after 7 months of continuous culture. It is yet to be determined whether these are exceptional events of karyotype abnormalities that occurred during the prolonged culture and that may also occur while using feeder layers or whether the culture method does not actually sustain karyotype stability.

Methods for Feeder-Free Culture of hESCs

Fibronectin Coating of Plates

The recommended concentration of fibronectin is 50 μg/10 cm^2. Both human cellular or plasma fibronectin were tested and found suitable for hESC culture (Sigma human foreskin fibroblast cellular fibronectin F6277; Sigma human plasma fibronectin F2006; Chemicon human plasma fibronectin FC010-10) (Amit *et al.*, 2004). All plates should be covered with fibronectin 30 min before plating of cells.

1. Dilute fibronectin to desired concentration. Recommended concentration for the stock solution is 1 mg/10 ml of sterile water (Sigma W1503).
2. Filter the fibronectin through a 22-μm filter. The stock solution can be stored up to 2 weeks at 4°.
3. Cover the dish with fibronectin solution to reach a concentration of 50 μg/10 cm^2. Examples of recommended amounts are listed in Table I.
4. Leave at room temperature or in incubator for at least 30 min. If desired, plates covered with fibronectin can be prepared in advance (overnight).

If water was used to dissolve the fibronectin, there is no need to collect the fibronectin residues before plating the cells. It is recommended to plate the cells directly onto the fibronectin residues.

If desired, Matrigel matrix can replace the fibronectin. The recommended dilution is 1:40 (with plain medium). The matrix should be prepared according to the manufacturer's instructions.

Culture Medium

The medium consists of the following materials: 85% knockout–Dulbecco's modified Eagle medium (ko–DMEM), supplemented with 15% knockout

TABLE I
RECOMMENDED AMOUNT OF FIBRONECTIN STOCK SOLUTION PER WELL

Plate/dish	Volume of fibronectin stock solution per well
4 wells (2.5 cm^2)	0.3 ml
6 wells (10 cm^2)	0.5 ml
35 mm	0.5 ml

serum replacement, 2 mM L-glutamine, 0.1 mM β-mercaptoethanol, 1% nonessential amino acid stock, 0.12 ng/ml TGFβ1, and 4 ng/ml bFGF (all Invitrogen Corporation products, Grand Island, NY, with the exception of the TGFβ1, which is from R&D Systems, Minneapolis, MN).

1. Pour all materials into a 22-μm filter unit, and filter.
2. Store at 4° for up to 5 days. Do not expose to light.

An example for the preparation of 500 ml of medium is described in Table II. Two milliliters of medium should be added to each 10 cm^2 surface area of culture dish and should be replaced daily by fresh medium.

Cell Splitting

The most used splitting medium for hESCs is collagenase-type IV. The splitting medium consists of 1 mg/ml collagenase-type IV (Worthington, CN 17104019) diluted with DMEM (Invitrogen Grand Island, NY, CN 41965–039) and should be filtered through a 0.22-μm filter.

1. Remove medium from well. Add 0.5 ml collagenase splitting medium, and incubate for 30 min. Most colonies will float at the end of the incubation time. If needed, the incubation period can be increased up to 1 h. Do not exceed the recommended incubation time because of possible damage to the cells, which may include increasing incidence of karyotype abnormalities and decreased survival rates.
2. Add 1 ml of culture medium and gently collect cells with a 5-ml pipette.
3. Collect cell suspension and put into conical tube.

TABLE II

EXAMPLES OF RECOMMENDED CONCENTRATIONS AND AMOUNTS OF CULTURE
MEDIUM INGREDIENTS

Material	Final concentrations	For 500 ml medium
Ko-DMEM	85%	414 ml
Ko-Serum replacement	15%	75 ml
Nonessential amino acid	1%	5 ml
L-Glutamine	2 mM	5 ml
β-Mercaptoethanol 50 mM	0.1 mM	1 ml
bFGF	4 ng/ml	2000 ng
TGFβ1	0.12 ng/ml	60 ng

4. Centrifuge 3 min at 300*g* at a recommended temperature of 4°.
5. Resuspend cells in culture media and plate directly on previously fibronectin-covered plate.

Cells should be split at a recommended ratio of 1:2 every 4–5 days.

Freezing Cells

The cells should be frozen at a freezing solution consisting of 20% dimethyl sulfide (DMSO, Sigma D2652), 30% FBS, serum replacement or human serum, and 50% DMEM. The recommended freezing ratio is cells from 10-cm^2 culture surface area or 2 million cells in one Cryovial (volume of 250–500 μl).

1. First, harvest the cells as you would when splitting; add splitting medium (collagenase), and incubate for 30 min.
2. Add 1 ml culture medium, then gently scrape the cells using a 5-ml pipette and transfer cells into conical tube.
3. Centrifuge 3 min at 300*g* at a recommended temperature of 4°.
4. Resuspend cells in the culture medium. Do not fracture the cells into small clumps.
5. Add an equivalent volume of freezing medium drop by drop and mix gently.
6. Transfer 0.5 ml into a 1-ml cryogenic vial.
7. Freeze overnight at −80° (the use of freezing boxes, from Nalgene C.N, increases the survival rates).
8. Transfer to liquid nitrogen on the following day.

Thawing Cells

The freezing process should be conducted as efficiently as possible; delays in the procedure may lead to increased cell death.

1. Remove vial from liquid nitrogen.
2. Gently swirl vial in 37° water bath.
3. When a small pellet of frozen cells remains, wash vial in 70% ethanol.
4. Pipette the content of the vial up and down once to mix.
5. Place contents of vial into conical tube and add, drop by drop, 2 ml of culture medium.
6. Centrifuge 3 min at 300*g* at a recommended temperature of 4°.
7. Remove supernatant and resuspend cells in 3 ml fresh culture medium.
8. Place cell suspension on one well of a 6-well plate or on a 4-well plate previously covered with fibronectin.

Acknowledgments

We thank Mrs. Hadas O'Neill for editing the manuscript. The research conducted by the authors was partly supported by NIH grant R24RR18405. J. I.-E. holds the Sylvia and Stanley Shirvan Chair in Cell and Tissue Regeneration at the Technion–Israel Institute of Technology.

References

Amit, M., Carpenter, M. K., Inokuma, M. S., Chiu, C-P., Harris, C. P., Waknitz, M. A., Itskovitz-Eldor, J., and Thomson, J. A. (2000). Clonally derived human embryonic stem cell lines maintain pluripotency and proliferative potential for prolonged periods of culture. *Dev. Biol.* **227,** 271–278.

Amit, M., and Itskovitz-Eldor, J. (2002). Derivation and spontaneous differentiation of human embryonic stem cells. *J. Anat.* **200,** 225.

Amit, M., Margulets, V., Segev, H., Shariki, C., Laevsky, I., Coleman, R., and Itskovitz-Eldor, J. (2003). Human feeder layers for human embryonic stem cells. *Biol. Reprod.* **68,** 2150–2156.

Amit, M., and Itskovitz-Eldor, J. (2004). Isolation, characterization and maintenance of primate ES cells. *In* "Handbook of Stem Cells" (R. P. Lanza, ed.), pp. 419–436. Elsevier Science, New York.

Amit, M., Shariki, K., Margulets, V., and Itskovitz-Eldor, J. (2004). Feeder and serum-free culture system for human embryonic stem cells. *Biol. Reprod.* **70,** 837–845.

Beattie, G. M., Lopez, A. D., Bucay, N., Hinton, A., Firpo, M. T., King, C. C., and Hayek, A. (2005). Activin A maintains pluripotency of human embryonic stem cells in the absence of feeder layers. *Stem Cells* **23,** 489–495.

Besser, D. (2004). Expression of nodal, lefty-a, and lefty-B in undifferentiated human embryonic stem cells requires activation of Smad2/3. *J. Biol. Chem.* **279,** 45076–45084.

Cheng, L., Hammond, H., Ye, Z., Zhan, X., and Dravid, G. (2003). Human adult marrow cells support prolonged expansion of human embryonic stem cells in culture. *Stem Cells* **21,** 131–142.

Cowan, C. A., Klimanskaya, I., McMahon, J., Atienza, J., Witmyer, J., Zucker, J. P., Wang, S., Morton, C. C., McMahon, A. P., Powers, D., and Melton, D. A. (2004). Derivation of embryonic stem-cell lines from human blastocysts. *N. Engl. J. Med.* **350,** 1353–1356.

Daheron, L., Opitz, S. L., Zaehres, H., Lensch, W. M., Andrews, P. W., Itskovitz-Eldor, J., and Daley, G. Q. (2004). LIF/STAT3 signaling fails to maintain self-renewal of human embryonic stem cells. *Stem Cells* **22,** 770–778.

Dravid, G., Ye, Z., Hammond, H., Chen, G., Pyle, A., Donovan, P., Yu, X., and Cheng, L. (2005). Defining the role of Wnt/beta-catenin signaling in the survival, proliferation, and self-renewal of human embryonic stem cells. *Stem Cells* **23,** 1489–1501.

Evans, M. J., and Kaufman, M. H. (1981). Establishment in culture of pluripotential cells from mouse embryos. *Nature* **292,** 154–156.

Fortunel, N. O., Hatzfeld, A., and Hatzfeld, J. A. (2000). Transforming growth factor-β: Pleiotropic role in the regulation of hematopoiesis. *Blood* **96,** 2022–2036.

Hovatta, O., Mikkola, M., Gertow, K., Stromberg, A. M., Inzunza, J., Hreinsson, J., Rozell, B., Blennow, E., Andang, M., and Ahrlund-Richter, L. (2003). A culture system using human foreskin fibroblasts as feeder cells allows production of human embryonic stem cells. *Hum. Reprod.* **18,** 1404–1409.

Humphrey, R. K., Beattie, G. M., Lopez, A. D., Bucay, N., King, C. C., Firpo, M. T., Rose-John, S., and Hayek, A. (2004). Maintenance of pluripotency in human embryonic stem cells is STAT3 independent. *Stem Cells* **22,** 522–530.

Hynes, R. O. (2002). Integrins: Bidirectional, allosteric signaling machines. *Cell* **110,** 673–687.

James, D., Levine, A. J., Besser, D., and Hemmati-Brivanlou, A. (2005). TGF β/activin/nodal signaling is necessary for the maintenance of pluripotency in human embryonic stem cells. *Development* **132,** 1273–1282.

Klimanskaya, I., Chung, Y., Meisner, L., Johnson, J., West, M. D., and Lanza, R. (2005). Human embryonic stem cells derived without feeder cells. *Lancet* **365,** 1636–1641.

Inzunza, J., Gertow, K., Stromberg, M. A., Matilainen, E., Blennow, E., Skottman, H., Wolbank, S., Ahrlund-Richter, L., and Hovatta, O. (2005). Derivation of human embryonic stem cell lines in serum replacement medium using postnatal human fibroblasts as feeder cells. *Stem Cells* **23,** 544–549.

Ludwig, T. E., Levenstein, M. E., Jones, J. M., Berggren, W. T., Mitchen, E. R., Frane, J. L., Crandall, L. J., Daigh, C. A., Conard, K. R., Piekarczyk, M. S., Llanas, R. A., and Thomson, J. A. (2006). Derivation of human embryonic stem cells in defined conditions. *Nat Biotechnol.* **24,** 185–187.

Massague, J. (1990). The transforming growth factor-beta family. *Ann. Rev. Cell Biol.* **6,** 597–641.

Martin, G. R. (1981). Isolation of a pluripotent cell line from early mouse embryos cultured in medium conditioned by teratocarcinoma stem cells. *Proc. Natl. Acad. Sci. USA* **78,** 7634–7638.

Reubinoff, B. E., Pera, M. F., Fong, C., Trounson, A., and Bongso, A. (2000). Embryonic stem cell lines from human blastocysts: Somatic differentiation *in vitro.* *Nat. Biotechnol.* **18,** 399–404.

Reubinoff, B. E., Pera, M. F., Vajta, G., and Trounson, A. O. (2001). Effective cryopreservation of human embryonic stem cells by the open pulled straw vitrification method. *Hum. Reprod.* **16,** 2187–2194.

Richards, M., Fong, C. Y., Chan, W. K., Wong, P. C., and Bongso, A. (2002). Human feeders support prolonged undifferentiated growth of human inner cell masses and embryonic stem cells. *Nat. Biotechnol.* **20,** 933–936.

Sato, N., Meijer, L., Skaltsounis, L., Greengard, P., and Brivanlou, A. H. (2004). Maintenance of pluripotency in human and mouse embryonic stem cells through activation of Wnt signaling by a pharmacological GSK-3–specific inhibitor. *Nat. Med.* **10,** 55–63.

Schuldiner, M., Yanuka, O., Itskovitz-Eldor, J., Melton, D. A., and Benvenisty, N. (2000). Effect of eight-growth factors on the differentiation of cells derived from human ES cells. *Proc. Natl. Acad. Sci. USA* **97,** 11307–11312.

Smith, A. G., Heath, J. K., Donaldson, D. D., Wong, G. G., Moreau, J., Stahl, M., and Rogers, D. (1988). Inhibition of pluripotential embryonic stem cell differentiation by purified polypeptides. *Nature* **336,** 688–690.

Smith, A. G. (2000). Embryonic stem cells. *In* "Stem Cell Biology" (D. R. Marshak, R. L. Gardner, and D. Gottlieb, eds.), pp. 205–230. Cold Spring Harbor Laboratory Press, Cold Spring Harbor, New York.

Suemori, H., Tada, T., Torii, R., Hosoi, Y., Kobayashi, K., Imahie, H., Kondo, Y., Iritani, A., and Nakatsuji, N. (2001). Establishment of embryonic stem cell lines from cynomolgus monkey blastocysts produced by IVF or ICSI. *Dev. Dyn.* **222,** 273–279.

Thomson, J. A., Kalishman, J., Golos, T. G., Durning, M., Harris, C. P., Becker, R. A., and Hearn, J. P. (1995). Isolation of a primate embryonic stem cell line. *Proc. Natl. Acad. Sci. USA* **92,** 7844–7848.

Thomson, J. A., Kalishman, J., Golos, T. G., Durning, M., Harris, C. P., and Hearn, J. P. (1996). Pluripotent cell lines derived from common marmoset *(Callithrix jacchus)* blastocysts. *Biol. Reprod.* **55,** 254–259.

Thomson, J. A., Itskovitz-Eldor, J., Shapiro, S. S., Waknitz, M. A., Swiergiel, J. J., Marshall, V. S., and Jones, J. M. (1998). Embryonic stem cell lines derived from human blastocysts. *Science* **282,** 1145–1147; [erratum in *Science* (1998) 282, 1827].

Vallier, L., Alexander, M., and Pedersen, R. A. (2005). Activin/Nodal and FGF pathways cooperate to maintain pluripotency of human embryonic stem cells. *J. Cell Sci.* **118,** 4495–4509.

Valdimarsdottir, G., and Mummery, C. (2005). Functions of the TGFbeta superfamily in human embryonic stem cells. *APMIS* **113,** 773–789.

Verlinsky, Y., Strelchenko, N., Kukharenko, V., Rechitsky, S., Verlinsky, O., Galat, V., and Kuliev, A. (2005). Human embryonic stem cell lines with genetic disorders. *Reprod. Biomed. Online* **10,** 105–110.

Williams, R., Hilton, D., Pease, S., Wilson, T., Stewart, C., Gearing, D., Wagner, E., Metcalf, D., Nicola, N., and Gough, N. (1988). Myeloid leukemia inhibitory factor maintains the developmental potential of embryonic stem cells. *Nature* **336,** 684–687.

Xu, C., Inokuma, M. S., Denham, J., Golds, K., Kundu, P., Gold, J. D., and Carpenter, M. K. (2001). Feeder-free growth of undifferentiated human embryonic stem cells. *Nat. Biotechnol.* **19,** 971–974.

Xu, C., Jiang, J., Sottile, V., McWhir, J., Lebkowski, J., and Carpenter, M. K. (2004). Immortalized fibroblast-like cells derived from human embryonic stem cells support undifferentiated cell growth. *Stem Cells* **22,** 972–980.

Xu, R. H., Peck, R. M., Li, D. S., Feng, X, Ludwig, T., and Thomson, J. A. (2005a). Basic FGF and suppression of BMP signaling sustain undifferentiated proliferation of human ES cells. *Nat. Methods.* **2,** 185–190.

Xu, C., Rosler, E., Jiang, J., Lebkowski, J. S., Gold, J. D., O'Sullivan, C., Delavan-Boorsma, K., Mok, M., Bronstein, A., and Carpenter, M. K. (2005b). Basic fibroblast growth factor supports undifferentiated human embryonic stem cell growth without conditioned medium. *Stem Cells* **23,** 315–323.

Yoo, S. J., Yoon, B. S., Kim, J. M., Song, J. M., Roh, S., You, S., and Yoon, H. S. (2005). Efficient culture system for human embryonic stem cells using autologous human embryonic stem cell-derived feeder cells. *Exp. Mol. Med.* **37,** 399–407.

[4] Transgene Expression and RNA Interference in Embryonic Stem Cells

By Holm Zaehres and George Q. Daley

Abstract

Over the last 30 years of biomedical research, technologies for transgene expression and gene loss of function have been developed from animal model systems to human gene therapy, and, increasingly, embryonic stem cells are a key target for these genetic engineering strategies. In this chapter, we describe how retrovirus/lentivirus vectors can be used to transfer and stably express genes or small interfering RNAs in mouse and human embryonic stem cells and their progeny, thereby allowing genetic gain-of-function or loss-of-function analysis and cell lineage selection in a multitude of experimental settings.

METHODS IN ENZYMOLOGY, VOL. 420   0076-6879/06 $35.00
Copyright 2006, Elsevier Inc. All rights reserved.   DOI: 10.1016/S0076-6879(06)20004-1

Retrovirus Expression Vectors and Embryonic Stem Cells

The first transgenic mouse strain was developed 30 years ago when mouse embryos were exposed to infectious Moloney murine leukemia retrovirus (MoMuLV), and germ line integration and Mendelian transmission of the foreign DNA was demonstrated (Jaenisch, 1976). Recombinant DNA technology has been used to redesign retroviruses as vector systems for efficient gene transfer and stable expression of genomically integrated transgenes in a broad range of mammalian cells (Cepko *et al.*, 1984; Mann *et al.*, 1983; Shimotohno and Temin, 1981). Retroviral vector expression in mouse embryonic stem cells (mESCs) has been studied since their derivation (Evans and Kaufman, 1981) but has proven problematic, because the provirus can be transcriptionally inactivated through a process termed *silencing* (Cherry *et al.*, 2000; Laker *et al.*, 1998). Initial transcriptional repression of the proviruses is attributed to the effect of trans-acting repressors or the lack of transactivators to start transcription from the regulatory elements in the retroviral long terminal repeat (LTR) and leader region. DNA methylation is the main mechanism of silencing of the retroviral control elements in mESC undergoing differentiation. This mechanism has been described in particular for murine leukemia virus (MLV)/gammaretrovirus-based vectors. The mESC virus MESV (Grez *et al.*, 1990), also termed MSCV (Hawley *et al.*, 1992), allows efficient initial expression in mESC; however, this provirus is also subject to long-term methylation-dependent silencing during embryogenesis. Additional LTR/leader modifications increased the expression levels in mESC (Robbins *et al.*, 1997). The LTR/leader configuration of MESV with improved expression in embryonic stem cells also predicted vector design for efficient expression profiles in hematopoietic stem and progenitor cells (Baum *et al.*, 1995). MLV-derived vectors have been used for a significant number of clinical human gene therapy applications, in which transgene expression has been reported for several years. In most studies, transgene modification of cells of the blood-forming lineages allowed these cells to have competitive growth advantages, thereby enforcing *in vivo* selection of highly expressing subclones. The lack of significant provirus transcription under nonselective conditions has hampered the use of simple retroviral vectors in transgenic *in vivo* experiments.

The advent of more complex vectors based on lentivirus (e.g., human immunodeficiency virus (HIV [Naldini *et al.*, 1996; Poznansky *et al.*, 1991]) has improved the prospect of retroviral gene transfer considerably. Lentiviral vectors derived from HIV-1 with the internal phosphoglycerate kinase (PGK) promoter (Hamaguchi *et al.*, 2000), the chicken beta actin/cytomegalovirus enhancer (CAG) promoter (Pfeifer *et al.*, 2002), and the ubiquitin-C promoter (Lois *et al.*, 2002) have all been used successfully to express transgenes in mESC and *in vitro* differentiated progeny. Transfer of lentivector-transduced ES cells into blastocysts can generate chimeric mice that express the transgene in multiple tissues. Thus, germ line transmission of lentiviral vector–driven transgenes has allowed efficient generation of novel transgenic mouse models.

Human embryonic stem cells (hESCs) have the ability to differentiate along all embryonic and adult developmental lineages, which makes them a valuable model to study early developmental processes and potentially a source of cells for gene and cell therapies (Thomson *et al.*, 1998). Genetic modification of hESCs is playing a key role in driving the directed differentiation and selection of particular cell lineages, thereby exploiting their potential for basic research and regenerative medicine applications. Lentivirus-mediated gene transfer and expression of the green fluorescent protein (GFP) in hESCs have been described with vectors incorporating the elongation factor 1 alpha (EF1α), the phosphoglycerate kinase (PGK), and cytomegalovirus (CMV) promoters (Gropp *et al.*, 2003; Ma *et al.*, 2003; Zaehres *et al.*, 2005).

RNA Interference and ESCs

RNA interference (RNAi) is an evolutionary conserved cellular pathway of sequence-specific gene silencing at the messenger RNA level. The basic mechanism behind RNAi is the cleavage of a double-stranded RNA (dsRNA) matching a specific gene sequence into short pieces called *short interfering RNA* (siRNA), which triggers the degradation of mRNA that matches its sequence (Fire *et al.*, 1998; McManus and Sharp, 2002). Knockout of the Dicer endonuclease that processes endogenous small RNAs, including siRNAs, results in lethality early in mouse development, with Dicer1-null embryos depleted of ESCs (Bernstein *et al.*, 2003). Transfection of chemically synthesized siRNA duplexes has been successfully used to suppress different genes in mammalian cells (Elbashir *et al.*, 2001). siRNAs can be expressed from different promoters as fold-back stem-loop structures (small hairpin RNAs [shRNAs]) that give rise to siRNAs after intracellular processing. Several groups have reported RNA polymerase III promoter–based vectors for transient and stable expression of siRNAs in mammalian cells (Brummelkamp *et al.*, 2002). An increasing number of reports describe the use of shRNA expression cassettes to generate transgenic RNAi in mESCs and thereby derived mice with knockdown and knockout phenotypes (Kunath *et al.*, 2003). Several lentiviral vector systems have been developed for the stable expression of small interfering RNAs in mouse ESCs and mice (Rubinson *et al.*, 2003; Tiscornia *et al.*, 2003; Ventura *et al.*, 2004).

We and others have demonstrated efficient gene knockdowns in hESCs (H9/WA09) using siRNA transfection (Vallier *et al.*, 2004) and siRNA expression delivered by retroviral and lentiviral vectors (Zaehres *et al.*, 2005). In this chapter, we introduce detailed protocols to stably express transgenes or small interfering RNAs in mouse and hESCs and their progeny, thereby allowing genetic gain-of-function or loss-of-function analysis and cell lineage selection.

siRNA Expression Vector Design

Recent chapters of *Methods in Enzymology* have described the design of siRNA and shRNA expression vector systems in detail (Li and Rossi, 2005; Sano *et al.*, 2005). Background material is available for the lentiviral *Lentilox* vector system (Rubinson *et al.*, 2003) and *Lentihair* vector system (Stewart *et al.*, 2003) that we are using for siRNA expression in mouse and hESCs. A strategy is presented in the following:

- Search for sequences targeting your gene of interest using the siRNA Selection Program at the Whitehead Institute for Biomedical Research, Cambridge, MA (http://jura.wi.mit.edu/siRNAext/), or refer to other published siRNA prediction schemes. The consensus sequence should correspond to: $AAGN_{18}TT$. Test three targets for each gene of interest.
- Design two oligonucleotides that will form the shRNA structure on expression from the U6 promoter:
    Sense oligonucleotide: 5′ T-(GN_{18})-(TTCAAGAGA)-(^{81}NC)-TT TTTT
    Antisense oligonucleotide: Complement of sense
    Additional nucleotides can be added to create restriction sites for cloning into the lentiviral vector.
- Anneal sense and antisense oligonucleotide (60 pmol/μl) in annealing buffer (100 mM K-acetate, 30 mM HEPES–KOH, pH 7.4, 2 mM Mg acetate) by slowly decreasing the temperature from 70–4°.
- Clone sequences into your lentiviral vector under the control of the U6 promoter.
- Verify the presence of the oligonucleotide in your vector by sequencing.

The RNAi consortium at the BROAD Institute, Cambridge, MA, is creating up to 150,000 custom-designed lentiviral vectors that express short hairpin RNAs targeting 15,000 human genes and 15,000 mouse genes. This fundamental resource is made available to scientists worldwide through commercial and academic distributors. All constructs are based on the lentiviral *Lentihair* vector system (Stewart *et al.*, 2003) that we have validated for use in hESCs.

- Search for lentiviral vectors targeting your gene of interest using the RNAi Consortium shRNA Library at the BROAD Institute (http://www.broad.mit.edu/genome_bio/trc/).

Retrovirus Production

Retroviral and lentiviral vectors pseudotyped with the vesicular stomatitis virus (VSV-G) surface protein (Burns *et al.*, 1993) can infect all mammalian cells, and the titers produced by ultracentrifugation are of the same order as virus stocks used in human gene therapy applications (10^8–10^9 infectious particles/ml). Therefore, refer to the local biosafety guidelines of your institution and always handle virus production under BL2/BL2+ conditions. Bleach and autoclave all used plastic materials that have been in contact with virus.

- Plate 293T cells (maintained in Dulbecco's modified Eagle's medium [DMEM] supplemented with 10% fetal bovine serum [FBS]) in ten 100-mm tissue culture dishes 24 h before transfection so that they are 80% confluent for transfection.
- Cotransfect 293T cells with 3 μg retroviral/lentiviral vector, 2 μg packaging plasmid, 1 μg VSV-G expression vector (for a three-plasmid system), and 18 μl *FuGENE 6* (Roche) per plate according to the suppliers conditions. *FuGENE 6* is non toxic to the 293T, so there is no need for further medium changes.
- Collect virus supernatant from all plates 48 h or 72 h after transfection with plastic pipettes and filter supernatant through a 0.45-μm filter.
- Transfer filtered supernatants (35 ml each) to centrifuge tubes (Beckman Polyallomer, 25 × 89 mm) and spin at 23,000 rpm for 90 min at 4° in a Beckman SW28 swinging bucket rotor.
- Remove supernatant carefully. You normally see a pellet that is opaque and at the bottom center of the tube. Add 1 ml DMEM to the tube and keep the paraffin-wrapped tubes at 4° overnight.
- Resuspend and mix all tubes containing the same virus, aliquot into 10 freeze vials, and store virus stocks at −80° until use. Avoid multiple freeze–thaws.
- For titer determination, plate 1 × 10^5 293T cells/well in a 6-well plate and add 1 μl, 10 μl, and 100 μl concentrated virus 6 h later; 24 h later, wash twice with PBS and supplement with fresh media. Analyze cells for GFP expression 48 h after infection by fluorescence activated cell sorter (FACS).

The titer can be calculated as follows: (percentage of GFP+ cells) $\times 10^5 \times$ (dilution factor) and is represented as IU (infectious units)/ml concentrated vector; $100\times$ concentrated stocks of the Lentilox vector have titers between 1×10^8 and 1×10^9 IU/ml. For vectors without a reporter gene, quantitative real-time PCR can determine the number of vector DNA molecules/ml. Use 0.4% paraformaldehyde in your transduced cell solutions to inactivate remaining virus during titer determination.

• Each virus stock should be assayed for replication-competent retrovirus (RCR). Supernatant collected from infected cells (e.g., 293T) should itself be tested for presence of virus 48 h after infection (by transferring supernatant onto another dish of 293T cells). This supernatant should be virus free. The retrovirus literature describes more detailed protocols for ruling out the generation of RCR during viral passage.

Retroviral and Lentiviral Gene Transfer into Mouse and Human ESCs

We cultivate our hESCs cell cultures on mouse embryo fibroblast feeder layers (MEFs) (Specialty Media) (Thomson *et al.*, 1998) or on Matrigel in basic fibroblast growth factor (bFGF)–supplemented MEF conditioned medium (Xu *et al.*, 2001). Please refer to the many described protocols for human ES cell culture.

• Dissociate your human embryonic stem cell culture by trypsinization (0.25% trypsin/5 mM ethylenediaminetetraacetic acid/phosphate-buffered saline (EDTA/PBS) for 2–3 min) to a single cell suspension or alternately disperse cells by collagenase treatment into small cell clumps.

• Plate 1×10^5 cells on a tissue culture 6-well plate pretreated with Matrigel basement membrane matrix (BD). Use MEF conditioned medium supplemented with bFGF (4 ng/ml) to keep the hESCs cells undifferentiated.

• Add virus supernatant 6 h later with a calculated multiplicity of infection (MOI). The MOI is defined as the number of infectious units used per cell to be infected. For most high-efficiency gene transfer applications into hESCs use a MOI of 50 (5×10^6 IU on 1×10^5 cells). Evaluate different transduction efficiencies by infecting with different MOIs. For your RNAi knockdown experiments, use the nontargeting vector and/or a vector–targeting GFP, luciferase, or an other irrelevant gene as a control.

• Add 6 μg/ml protamine sulfate (Sigma) to your culture to enhance virus binding to the cells. Because of our highly efficient gene transfer rates, we have not tried to improve retroviral transduction further by spin infection.

- Culture cells with the virus for 24 h, wash three times with PBS, and then add fresh media.
- On day 3 after infection, measure for transgene activity and continue the culture on MEFs or Matrigel. To evaluate the knockdown efficiency, use quantitative real-time (QRT) PCR analysis of RNA/cDNA extracts and Western blotting of protein extracts from the transduced cells.
- Optional: Determine the provirus copy number by Southern blot or QRT-PCR analysis of genomic DNA from the transduced cells.

We also infected hESC cultures grown on mouse embryo fibroblast feeder layers during the transduction process. As expected, the gene transfer rates are reduced in comparison to transductions under feeder-free conditions, because virus also transduces the feeder cells.

ESCs cultivated in suspension and in the absence of differentiation inhibitors form proliferating and differentiating multicellular clusters known as *embryoid bodies* (EBs) consisting of ectoderm-derived, endoderm-derived, and mesoderm-derived lineages. The EB culture system has proven to be very valuable to recapitulate hematopoiesis *in vitro* and to generate repopulating hematopoietic stem cells (HSCs) from ESCs in the mouse system (Kyba *et al.*, 2003). These protocols can be adapted for human ES cell cultures:

- To initiate embryoid body (EB) hanging drop cultures from genetically modified human ESCs, plate drops of 200 hESCs in 30 μl EB differentiation medium (human ESC medium without bFGF) on 150-mm non-tissue culture–treated dishes.
- Invert the dishes and incubate for 4 days at 37° in 5% CO_2.
- Collect EBs in 10 ml of fresh differentiation medium and transfer to 100-mm bacterial-grade dishes. Culture under slow swirling conditions on a rotating shaker inside of an incubator. Initiate your differentiation conditions of interest.

For lentiviral gene transfer into mouse ESCs, the procedures are similar:

- Dissociate your mouse ESC culture by trypsinization.
- Plate 1×10^5 cells on a tissue culture 6-well plate pretreated with Matrigel basement membrane matrix (BD) or gelatin under described feeder-free conditions (Mouse ES cell medium supplemented with LIF (leukemia inhibitory factor [1000 U/ml]).
- Add virus supernatant 6 h later with a calculated MOI.
- Add 6 μg/ml protamine sulfate (Sigma) to your culture to enhance virus binding.
- Culture cells with the virus for 24 h, wash three times with PBS, and then add fresh media.

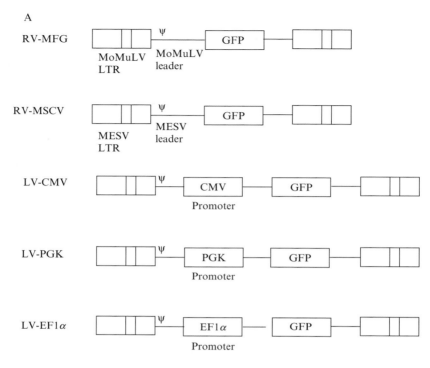

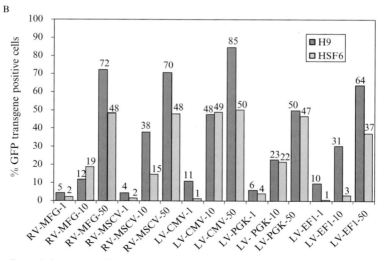

Retroviral vectors: MFG MoMuLV–LTR   Lentiviral vectors: CMV promoter

                     MSCV MESV–LTR   PGK promoter

                     1, 10, 50: MOI (multiplicity of infection) EF1α promoter

- On day 3 after infection, measure for transgene activity or gene knockdown efficiency.
- To initiate EB hanging drop cultures from genetically modified mouse ES cells plate drops of 100 hESCs in 10 μl EB differentiation medium (Mouse ESC medium lacking supplemental LIF) on 150-mm non-tissue culture–treated dishes.
- Invert the dishes and incubate for 2 days at 37° in 5% CO_2.
- Collect EBs in 10 ml of fresh differentiation medium and transfer to 100-mm bacterial-grade dishes. Culture under slow swirling conditions on a rotating shaker inside of an incubator. Initiate your differentiation conditions of interest.

Transgene and siRNA Expression in Mouse and Human ESCs

We have compared expression from a set of VSV-G pseudotyped and concentrated retroviral and lentiviral vectors in the human ESC lines H9/WA09 and HSF6/UC06 (Fig. 1). All vectors tested allowed efficient transgene expression in undifferentiated human embryonic stem cells, and the amount of transduced cells was virus dose dependent. The percentage of enhanced GFP expression in the hESC populations correlates with the MOI for all vectors tested in both human ESC lines. At a MOI of 1, we can achieve transgene expression in the range of 1–15% of cells; at a MOI of 10 in the range of 10–60%; and at a MOI of 50 in the range of 40–85%, depending on the retrovirus/lentivirus used. The retroviral vector MFG drives expression from the MoMuLV–LTR and leader region, and the retroviral vector MSCV from the MESV–LTR and leader (Cherry et al., 2000). The MESV–LTR/leader region has point mutations that allow expression in mouse ESCs (Grez et al., 1990). MSCV, but not MFG, permits expression in mouse ESCs before and throughout in vitro differentiation; however, MSCV is also subject to methylation-dependent silencing (Cherry et al., 2000). In contrast to mouse ESCs, both retroviral vector types allowed efficient transgene

Fig. 1. Retroviral and lentiviral vectors allow viral dose-dependent transgene expression in human ESCs. (A) Retroviral (RV) and lentiviral (LV) vectors for transgene expression in human embryonic stem cells. The retroviral vectors express transgenes from the MoMuLV–LTR (long terminal repeat) or the MESV–LTR; the lentiviral vectors express transgenes from the internal CMV cytomegalovirus (CMV) promoter, the PGK phosphoglycerate kinase (PGK) promoter, or the EF1α (elongation factor 1 alpha) promoter. (B) Human embryonic stem cells (H9/WA09 and HSF6/UC06) were transduced with the retroviral and lentiviral vectors at multiplicities of infection (MOIs) of 1, 10, and 50. Enhanced green fluorescent protein (GFP) transgene positivity was measured 72 h after transduction by fluorescence activated cell sorter (FACS).

expression in human ESCs (up to 70% GFP positive H9/WA09 at MOI 50 [Fig. 1]; see also Daheron *et al.* [2004]). This is of practical importance, because many available MoMuLV-based vectors can be directly exploited to transduce hESCs in the described manner. To analyze for long-term expression during differentiation of human ESCs, we injected MFG vector (MoMuLV–LTR)–driven GFP transgenic H9/WA09 in NOD/SCID mice (2×10^6 cells by subcutaneous injection). Teratomas developed within 6 weeks and were found to be GFP fluorescence positive.

The evaluated lentiviral vectors driving transgene expression from the CMV promoter (*Lentilox* vector [Rubinson *et al.*, 2003], the PGK promoter (*RRL* vector [Zufferey *et al.*, 1998], and the EF1α (elongation factor 1 alpha) promoter [*HPV* vector, Philippe Leboulch, Harvard Medical School]) allowed a similar virus dose-dependent expression in human ESCs, like their gammaretroviral counterparts (Fig. 1). In addition to the reported lentiviral vectors incorporating the EF1α promoter (Ma *et al.*, 2003) and the PGK promoter (Gropp *et al.*, 2003), these vectors are suitable for efficient transgene expression in human ESCs (hESC cell lines H9/WA09 and HSF6/UC06). We could not detect any changes in the differentiation status of the human ESCs by lentiviral transductions itself, as measured by TRA1–60 surface marker staining (Zaehres *et al.*, 2005).

Whether lentiviral vectors are less prone to silencing then their gammaretroviral counterparts when examined at the single–copy provirus level still remains controversial (Ellis, 2005). On the basis of our data, gammaretrovirus-based vectors can be used for efficient *in vitro* genetic modification of human embryonic stem cells. Cellular defense mechanisms directed against foreign DNA regulatory structures (e.g., DNA methylation-dependent silencing of the LTR of murine oncoretroviruses in murine ESCs) may not be similarly effective in human ESCs. Retroviral/lentiviral vector-driven transgene expression in ESCs is affected by position-effect-variegation (PEV), depending on the proviral integration side. To reduce PEV and silencing chromatin insulators and scaffold/matrix-attachment-regions can be incorporated into the vector backbones (Ma *et al.*, 2003; Rivella *et al.*, 2000; Schubeler *et al.*, 1996; Stief *et al.*, 1989). The performance of these genomic bordering modules in ESCs has yet to be evaluated in detail.

We have demonstrated high-efficiency silencing of a GFP transgene and the stem cell–specific transcription factors Oct4/POU5F1 and Nanog using lentiviral siRNA expression in human ESCs (Zaehres *et al.*, 2005). As expected, gene knockdown of Oct4 and Nanog but not of GFP promoted differentiation into cells expressing trophectodermal and endodermal markers, thereby demonstrating a conserved role for these factors in human ESC self-renewal. Our data demonstrated that the mouse, as well as the human, U6 promoter can be used to drive efficient expression of siRNAs/shRNAs in human ESCs (Fig. 2A). An expression vector with the RNA polymerase III H1 promoter has proven to work as well to express siRNAs in human ESCs (Vallier *et al.*, 2004). We also evaluated potential apoptotic effects of lentiviral transduction and siRNA expression on the human ESC cell cultures; Annexin V staining was only slightly increased in the RNAi lentivector–modified cells with MOIs up to 50, suggesting that RNAi is well tolerated.

Expression cassettes for small interfering RNAs can also be incorporated for stable expression in ESCs by site-specific or homologous recombination. Episomal expression of siRNAs/shRNAs using adenovirus vectors might increase the efficiency of delivery but does not seem to be advantageous over direct delivery of chemically synthesized siRNAs for applications that entail transient genetic modification.

RNA interference has been reported to vary in efficiency in different developmental stages derived from mouse ESCs with the same siRNA expression cassette (Oberdoerffer *et al.*, 2005). Variable knockdown efficiency might also be observed when deriving specified lineages from human ESCs.

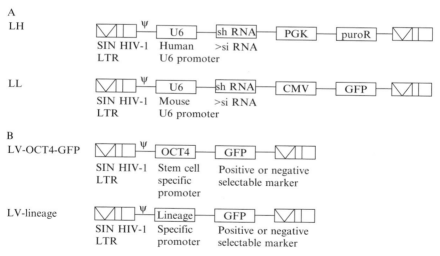

Fig. 2. (A) Lentiviral vectors for expression of small interfering RNAs to mediate gene silencing in ESCs. The lentiviral vectors express small hairpin RNAs (shRNAs) from the mouse or human U6 promoter that are processed to small interfering RNAs (siRNAs) and further contain a selection marker to monitor vector presence. (B) Lentiviral vectors for lineage selection in ESCs and their progeny. Lentiviral vectors for lineage selection incorporate positive or negative selectable markers whose expression is directed by stem cell–specific (e.g., Oct4 promoter) or lineage-specific promoter/enhancer elements.

In our current experiments, U6 promoter-driven knockdowns are maintained during embryoid body differentiation of ESCs.

To derive specified cell lineages and to produce and propagate pure populations of specific cell types from a complex culture of differentiating ESCs, lineage selection methods must be applied to the culture systems. Essentially, all strategies use vectors with positive or negative selectable markers whose expression is directed by stem cell or lineage-specific promoter/enhancer elements (Klug *et al.*, 1996). We have developed a lentiviral vector expressing enhanced GFP under the control of 3.2 kb of the upstream promoter sequences of the human POU5F1/Oct4 gene (Fig. 2B). We transduced ESCs (WA09/H9) with this vector at a low MOI, isolated single cell clones using FACS, and expanded them in culture. We identified clones in which GFP expression correlated with the differentiation status of the stem cells, as measured by surface marker expression (TRA1-60). Low MOI infections seem to be necessary to conserve the lineage specificity of the promoter element in the lentiviral vector because multiple proviral integrations increase the potential for positional influences on promoter fidelity. The lentiviral vector itself has a self-inactivating (SIN) LTR configuration. It does not incorporate any further promoter/enhancer elements from its HIV parent that could lead to promoter interference and derangement of lineage specificity of the internal promoter. This concept of lineage selection using lentiviral vector technology should be widely applicable to human ESCs. Our strategy is as follows:

- Clone a positive or negative selectable marker under the control of a lineage-specific promoter/enhancer element in a (SIN-) lentiviral vector backbone (Fig. 2B).
- Transduce human ESCs with lentivirus at a low MOI.
- Sort single cell clones and expand the undifferentiated stem cell population.
- Evaluate the cell population for the selectable marker during differentiation.

Biotechnological and Medical Applications

Our laboratory is now routinely using retroviral/lentiviral vector technology for transgene and siRNA expression in mouse and human ESCs and their differentiated progeny. We are especially interested in gain-of-function and loss-of-function analysis of transcription factors involved in self-renewal and the developmental transitions of ESCs to hematopoietic stem cells and to germ cells. Retroviral/lentiviral expression and RNAi libraries can be used to carry out genome-wide screening experiments in ESCs to identify new factors involved in self-renewal and directed differentiation.

Engineering of cardiomyocytes, blood, neurons, pancreatic cells, or a multitude of other lineages from ESCs depends on defined *in vitro* differentiation protocols and a pristine starting population of undifferentiated ESCs. Transgene expression and gene knockdown technologies are crucial to the development of these *in vitro* differentiation protocols, and lineage selection methods will be a requirement for clinical applications. Vectors designed for transgene expression in ESCs might also be suitable for efficient expression in adult stem cells, thereby facilitating human gene therapy applications. Transgenic mice with constitutive, inducible, conditional, and cell type–specific gain-of-function or loss-of-function phenotypes have proven invaluable as advanced models for human diseases and for the evaluation of drug, protein, gene, and cell therapies. Transgenic human ESCs and their *in vitro* differentiation into defined cell lineages will have a similar impact as model systems for human diseases, including the study of cancer stem cells. This immediate impact is independent of the long-term goal of providing allogeneic or autologous cell grafts, which may not have clinical impact for a decade or longer. The lessons learned from transgenic ESC systems and their self-renewal properties might be productively applied to discover and modulate endogenous regenerative cell programs in the human body and to reprogram somatic cells.

Acknowledgments

We thank Sheila Stewart and Philippe Leboulch for providing us with viral vectors and virus production protocols, variations of which are described herein. Joseph Itskovitz-Eldor was instrumental in launching our efforts to culture human embryonic stem cells. This work was supported by grants from the National Institutes of Health, the NIH Director's Pioneer Award of the NIH Roadmap for Medical Research, the Burroughs Wellcome Fund, and philanthropic funds from the Bekenstein Family and the Thomas Anthony Pappas Charitable Foundation.

References

Baum, C., Hegewisch-Becker, S., Eckert, H. G., Stocking, C., and Ostertag, W. (1995). Novel retroviral vectors for efficient expression of the multidrug resistance (mdr-1) gene in early hematopoietic cells. *J. Virol.* **69,** 7541–7547.

Bernstein, E., Kim, S. Y., Carmell, M. A., Murchison, E. P., Alcorn, H., Li, M. Z., Mills, A. A., Elledge, S. J., Anderson, K. V., and Hannon, G. J. (2003). Dicer is essential for mouse development. *Nat. Genet.* **35,** 215–217.

Brummelkamp, T. R., Bernards, R., and Agami, R. (2002). A system for stable expression of short interfering RNAs in mammalian cells. *Science* **296,** 550–553.

Burns, J. C., Friedmann, T., Driever, W., Burrascano, M., and Yee, J. K. (1993). Vesicular stomatitis virus G glycoprotein pseudotyped retroviral vectors: Concentration to very high titer and efficient gene transfer into mammalian and nonmammalian cells. *Proc. Natl. Acad. Sci. USA* **90,** 8033–8037.

Cepko, C. L., Roberts, B. E., and Mulligan, R. C. (1984). Construction and applications of a highly transmissible murine retrovirus shuttle vector. *Cell* **37,** 1053–1062.

Cherry, S. R., Biniszkiewicz, D., van Parijs, L., Baltimore, D., and Jaenisch, R. (2000). Retroviral expression in embryonic stem cells and hematopoietic stem cells. *Mol. Cell Biol.* **20,** 7419–7426.

Daheron, L., Opitz, S. L., Zaehres, H., Lensch, W. M., Andrews, P. W., Itskovitz-Eldor, J., and Daley, G. Q. (2004). LIF/STAT3 signaling fails to maintain self-renewal of human embryonic stem cells. *Stem Cells* **22,** 770–778.

Elbashir, S. M., Harborth, J., Lendeckel, W., Yalcin, A., Weber, K., and Tuschl, T. (2001). Duplexes of 21-nucleotide RNAs mediate RNA interference in cultured mammalian cells. *Nature* **411,** 494–498.

Ellis, J. (2005). Silencing and variegation of gammaretrovirus and lentivirus vectors. *Hum. Gene Ther.* **16,** 1241–1246.

Evans, M. J., and Kaufman, M. H. (1981). Establishment in culture of pluripotential cells from mouse embryos. *Nature* **292,** 154–156.

Fire, A., Xu, S., Montgomery, M. K., Kostas, S. A., Driver, S. E., and Mello, C. C. (1998). Potent and specific genetic interference by double-stranded RNA in *Caenorhabditis elegans. Nature* **391,** 806–811.

Grez, M., Akgun, E., Hilberg, F., and Ostertag, W. (1990). Embryonic stem cell virus, a recombinant murine retrovirus with expression in embryonic stem cells. *Proc. Natl. Acad. Sci. USA* **87,** 9202–9206.

Gropp, M., Itsykson, P., Singer, O., Ben-Hur, T., Reinhartz, E., Galun, E., and Reubinoff, B. E. (2003). Stable genetic modification of human embryonic stem cells by lentiviral vectors. *Mol. Ther.* **7,** 281–287.

Hamaguchi, I., Woods, N. B., Panagopoulos, I., Andersson, E., Mikkola, H., Fahlman, C., Zufferey, R., Carlsson, L., Trono, D., and Karlsson, S. (2000). Lentivirus vector gene expression during ES cell-derived hematopoietic development *in vitro. J. Virol.* **74,** 10778–10784.

Hawley, R. G., Fong, A. Z., Burns, B. F., and Hawley, T. S. (1992). Transplantable myeloproliferative disease induced in mice by an interleukin 6 retrovirus. *J. Exp. Med.* **176,** 1149–1163.

Jaenisch, R. (1976). Germ line integration and Mendelian transmission of the exogenous Moloney leukemia virus. *Proc. Natl. Acad. Sci. USA* **73,** 1260–1264.

Klug, M. G., Soonpaa, M. H., Koh, G. Y., and Field, L. J. (1996). Genetically selected cardiomyocytes from differentiating embryonic stem cells form stable intracardiac grafts. *J. Clin. Invest.* **98,** 216–224.

Kunath, T., Gish, G., Lickert, H., Jones, N., Pawson, T., and Rossant, J. (2003). Transgenic RNA interference in ES cell-derived embryos recapitulates a genetic null phenotype. *Nat. Biotechnol.* **21,** 559–561.

Kyba, M., Perlingeiro, R. C., and Daley, G. Q. (2003). Development of hematopoietic repopulating cells from embryonic stem cells. *Methods Enzymol.* **365,** 114–129.

Laker, C., Meyer, J., Schopen, A., Friel, J., Heberlein, C., Ostertag, W., and Stocking, C. (1998). Host cis-mediated extinction of a retrovirus permissive for expression in embryonal stem cells during differentiation. *J. Virol.* **72,** 339–348.

Li, M. J., and Rossi, J. J. (2005). Lentiviral vector delivery of recombinant small interfering RNA expression cassettes. *Methods Enzymol.* **392,** 218–226.

Lois, C., Hong, E. J., Pease, S., Brown, E. J., and Baltimore, D. (2002). Germline transmission and tissue-specific expression of transgenes delivered by lentiviral vectors. *Science* **295,** 868–872.

Ma, Y., Ramezani, A., Lewis, R., Hawley, R. G., and Thomson, J. A. (2003). High-level sustained transgene expression in human embryonic stem cells using lentiviral vectors. *Stem Cells* **21,** 111–117.

Mann, R., Mulligan, R. C., and Baltimore, D. (1983). Construction of a retrovirus packaging mutant and its use to produce helper-free defective retrovirus. *Cell* **33,** 153–159.

McManus, M. T., and Sharp, P. A. (2002). Gene silencing in mammals by small interfering RNAs. *Nat. Rev. Genet.* **3,** 737–747.

Naldini, L., Blomer, U., Gallay, P., Ory, D., Mulligan, R., Gage, F. H., Verma, I. M., and Trono, D. (1996). *In vivo* gene delivery and stable transduction of nondividing cells by a lentiviral vector. *Science* **272,** 263–267.

Oberdoerffer, P., Kanellopoulou, C., Heissmeyer, V., Paeper, C., Borowski, C., Aifantis, I., Rao, A., and Rajewsky, K. (2005). Efficiency of RNA interference in the mouse hematopoietic system varies between cell types and developmental stages. *Mol. Cell Biol.* **25,** 3896–3905.

Pfeifer, A., Ikawa, M., Dayn, Y., and Verma, I. M. (2002). Transgenesis by lentiviral vectors: lack of gene silencing in mammalian embryonic stem cells and preimplantation embryos. *Proc. Natl. Acad. Sci. USA* **99,** 2140–2145.

Poznansky, M., Lever, A., Bergeron, L., Haseltine, W., and Sodroski, J. (1991). Gene transfer into human lymphocytes by a defective human immunodeficiency virus type 1 vector. *J. Virol.* **65,** 532–536.

Rivella, S., Callegari, J. A., May, C., Tan, C. W., and Sadelain, M. (2000). The cHS4 insulator increases the probability of retroviral expression at random chromosomal integration sites. *J. Virol.* **74,** 4679–4687.

Robbins, P. B., Yu, X. J., Skelton, D. M., Pepper, K. A., Wasserman, R. M., Zhu, L., and Kohn, D. B. (1997). Increased probability of expression from modified retroviral vectors in embryonal stem cells and embryonal carcinoma cells. *J. Virol.* **71,** 9466–9474.

Rubinson, D. A., Dillon, C. P., Kwiatkowski, A. V., Sievers, C., Yang, L., Kopinja, J., Zhang, M., McManus, M. T., Gertler, F. B., Scott, M. L., and Van Parijs, L. (2003). A lentivirus-based system to functionally silence genes in primary mammalian cells, stem cells and transgenic mice by RNA interference. *Nat. Genet.* **33,** 401–406.

Sano, M., Kato, Y., Akashi, H., Miyagishi, M., and Taira, K. (2005). Novel methods for expressing RNA interference in human cells. *Methods Enzymol.* **392,** 97–112.

Schubeler, D., Mielke, C., Maass, K., and Bode, J. (1996). Scaffold/matrix-attached regions act upon transcription in a context-dependent manner. *Biochemistry* **35,** 11160–11169.

Shimotohno, K., and Temin, H. M. (1981). Formation of infectious progeny virus after insertion of herpes simplex thymidine kinase gene into DNA of an avian retrovirus. *Cell* **26,** 67–77.

Stewart, S. A., Dykxhoorn, D. M., Palliser, D., Mizuno, H., Yu, E. Y., An, D. S., Sabatini, D. M., Chen, I. S., Hahn, W. C., Sharp, P. A., Weinberg, R. A., and Novina, C. D. (2003). Lentivirus-delivered stable gene silencing by RNAi in primary cells. *RNA* **9,** 493–501.

Stief, A., Winter, D. M., Stratling, W. H., and Sippel, A. E. (1989). A nuclear DNA attachment element mediates elevated and position-independent gene activity. *Nature* **341,** 343–345.

Thomson, J. A., Itskovitz-Eldor, J., Shapiro, S. S., Waknitz, M. A., Swiergiel, J. J., Marshall, V. S., and Jones, J. M. (1998). Embryonic stem cell lines derived from human blastocysts. *Science* **282,** 1145–1147.

Tiscornia, G., Singer, O., Ikawa, M., and Verma, I. M. (2003). A general method for gene knockdown in mice by using lentiviral vectors expressing small interfering RNA. *Proc. Natl. Acad. Sci. USA* **100**, 1844–1848.

Vallier, L., Rugg-Gunn, P. J., Bouhon, I. A., Andersson, F. K., Sadler, A. J., and Pedersen, R. A. (2004). Enhancing and diminishing gene function in human embryonic stem cells. *Stem Cells* **22**, 2–11.

Ventura, A., Meissner, A., Dillon, C. P., McManus, M., Sharp, P. A., Van Parijs, L., Jaenisch, R., and Jacks, T. (2004). Cre-lox-regulated conditional RNA interference from transgenes. *Proc. Natl. Acad. Sci. USA* **101**, 10380–10385.

Xu, C., Inokuma, M. S., Denham, J., Golds, K., Kundu, P., Gold, J. D., and Carpenter, M. K. (2001). Feeder-free growth of undifferentiated human embryonic stem cells. *Nat. Biotechnol.* **19**, 971–974.

Zaehres, H., Lensch, M. W., Daheron, L., Stewart, S. A., Itskovitz-Eldor, J., and Daley, G. Q. (2005). High-efficiency RNA interference in human embryonic stem cells. *Stem Cells* **23**, 299–305.

Zufferey, R., Dull, T., Mandel, R. J., Bukovsky, A., Quiroz, D., Naldini, L., and Trono, D. (1998). Self-inactivating lentivirus vector for safe and efficient *in vivo* gene delivery. *J. Virol.* **72**, 9873–9880.

[5] Lentiviral Vector–Mediated Gene Delivery into Human Embryonic Stem Cells

By Michal Gropp and Benjamin Reubinoff

Abstract

Human embryonic stem cells (hESCs) are pluripotent cells derived from the inner cell mass of preimplantation embryos. These cells can be cultured for long periods as undifferentiated cells and still retain their potential to give rise to cell types representing all three germinal layers. Given their unique properties, hESCs are expected to serve as an invaluable tool for basic and applied research. However, to exploit their remarkable potentials, the development of effective strategies for genetic modification of hESCs is required. Lentiviral-based vectors offer an attractive system for efficient gene delivery into hESCs. These vectors are derived from lentiviruses, a group of complex retroviruses that cause slow chronic immunodeficiency diseases in humans and animals. Gene delivery into hESCs by vectors derived from lentiviruses has the following advantages: (1) lentiviral vectors efficiently transduce hESCs; (2) they integrate into the host-cell genome, thus promoting stable transgene expression; (3) transgene expression is not significantly silenced in hESCs; and (4) transduced hESCs retain their self-renewal and pluripotent potential. In recent years, we and others have developed protocols for efficient transduction of hESCs by advanced

METHODS IN ENZYMOLOGY, VOL. 420
0076-6879/06 $35.00
DOI: 10.1016/S0076-6879(06)20005-3

modified replication-defective lentiviral-based vectors. Transduction of hESCs by these vectors resulted in high and stable transgene expression that was maintained over long periods of undifferentiated cultivation and after differentiation. This chapter focuses on methods for the use of lentiviral-based vectors for gene delivery into hESCs.

Introduction

Human embryonic stem cells (hESCs) are pluripotent cells derived from the inner cell mass of preimplantation embryos (Reubinoff et al., 2000; Thomson et al., 1998). These cells can self-renew for prolonged periods in culture, and yet retain their potential to differentiate into cells representing all three germinal layers both in vivo and in vitro. Given their unique properties, hESCs are expected to serve as an invaluable tool for the study of early human development. Moreover, these cells could be potentially used as an unlimited source of transplantable cells for cell replacement therapies.

However, to exploit the potential of hESCs, the development of effective methods for genetic modification of these cells is required. Several strategies have been used to introduce exogenous genes into hESCs. These strategies included the use of nonviral delivery methods such as transfection or electroporation and viral vectors such as lentiviruses. Although nonviral systems are considered safer than viral systems, they mostly promote gene transfer at low efficiencies and with transient gene expression. In contrast, lentiviral-based vectors were reported to promote highly efficient stable gene transfer into hESC (see review by Menendez and colleagues [2005]).

In this chapter, we will focus on the use of lentiviral-based vectors as gene delivery tools into hESCs. More specifically, we will concentrate on the design of lentiviral-based vectors suitable for transduction of hESCs and on the methods for production and delivery of recombinant virus particles into hESCs.

Development of Lentiviral-Based Vectors

Since the first report 10 years ago on the development of gene delivery system based on the human immunodeficiency virus type I (HIV-1) (Naldini et al., 1996b), vectors derived from lentiviruses have proved to be efficient gene delivery tools into a variety of cell types both in vitro and in vivo.

Lentiviral-based vectors are derived from lentiviruses, a group of complex retroviruses that cause slow chronic diseases in humans and animals. This group includes the human immunodeficiency virus type I (HIV-1), which causes acquired immunodeficiency syndrome (AIDS) in humans, and lentiviruses, which are nonpathogenic to humans, such as the simian immunodeficiency virus (SIV), and the feline immunodeficiency virus (FIV). All lentiviruses share a common infection mechanism: The virus binds to specific receptors on the host-cell membrane and enters the cell. In the cytoplasm, the viral RNA is uncoated and reverse transcribed by its own reverse transcriptase into double-stranded proviral DNA. The proviral DNA then enters the nucleus and integrates into the host cell genome. The virus remains permanently integrated and uses the host-cell cellular machinery for its replication and expression. A detailed description of the biology of lentiviruses can be found elsewhere (Buchschacher, 2001; Goff, 2001; Palu *et al.*, 2000).

Lentiviral-based vectors were designed to take advantage of the unique characteristics of lentiviruses: (1) efficient infection of both dividing and nondividing cells; (2) integration of the virus into the genome of the infected cell, enabling stable expression and germline transmission of the transgene; (3) lack of immunogenicity; and (4) the unique sequence arrangement of the viral genome, which allows easy genetic manipulation of the regulatory and the coding sequences.

Design of HIV-1–Based Vectors

The current advanced HIV-1–based vectors were designed to improve viral performance. Moreover, because HIV-1 causes a severe disease in humans, great effort was invested in the design of safer HIV-1–based vectors. Accordingly, several steps were carried out to improve vector biosafety and performance. First, all pathogenic coding sequences were deleted from the vector, resulting in a replication-defective vector containing only the transgene and several essential regulatory viral sequences, such as the encapsidation signal and the viral LTR. Second, the proteins necessary for the early steps of viral infection (entering into the host cell, reverse transcription, and integration) were provided *in trans* by two additional plasmids: a packaging plasmid expressing the *gag*, *pol*, and *rev* genes, and an envelope plasmid expressing a heterologous envelope glycoprotein of the vesicular stomatitis virus (VSV-G). The use of the heterologous envelope prevented generation of wild-type virus. It was also beneficial because it broadened the viral host range and increased the stability of the viral particles (Naldini *et al.*, 1996a). Third, a large deletion was introduced into the U3 region of the viral LTR abolishing the viral promoter/enhancer activity. The self-inactivating (SIN) vector that was generated contained a heterologous internal promoter driving the expression of the transgene (Miyoshi *et al.*, 1998; Zufferey *et al.*, 1998). These steps resulted in a vector that could only undergo one round of infection and integration, a process termed *transduction*. Moreover, they minimized the risk of generation of wild-type HIV-1 by recombination.

The HIV-1–based vector was further improved by the addition of two regulatory sequences: First, the central polypurine tract (cPPT) sequence, which is found within the *pol* gene of HIV-1, was reinserted into the vector upstream of the internal promoter. cPPT is necessary for the nuclear import of HIV-1 into the nucleus of the host cell. Insertion of this element into the vector greatly increased transduction efficiencies (Follenzi *et al.*, 2000), Second, the posttranscriptional regulatory element of the woodchuck hepatitis virus (WPRE) was introduced into the vector downstream of the transgene. WPRE was shown to increase transgene expression by a mechanism that is still unclear and might involve increasing the number of nuclear RNA transcripts or enhancing mRNA export into the cytoplasm (Zufferey *et al.*, 1999).

To date, the advanced recombinant viral particles are generated by transient cotransfection into producer cells of three plasmids: (1) the advanced modified replication-defective, SIN transfer vector, expressing the transgene from an internal promoter; (2) a packaging plasmid expressing the *gag*, *pol*, and *env* genes; and (3) an envelope plasmid expressing VSV-G (see Fig. 1).

Transduction of hESCs by Lentiviral-Based Vectors

Vectors based on retroviruses such as the Moloney murine leukemia virus (MoMLV) were used for transduction of mouse ESCs. However, it was found that the expression of the transgene was silenced over time (Niwa *et al.*, 1983; Pannell and Ellis, 2001). The recent reports on the development of advanced HIV-1–based vectors, which could efficiently transduce a variety of cell types, promoted the study of these vectors as potential gene transfer vectors into ESCs. Several groups have reported that advanced lentiviral-based vectors pseudotyped with VSV-G could efficiently transduce mouse (Hamaguchi *et al.*, 2000; Pfeifer *et al.*, 2002) and cynomolgus monkey (Asano *et al.*, 2002) ESCs. Furthermore, transgene expression was not silenced throughout undifferentiated proliferation, as well as after differentiation *in vivo* and *in vitro*. These results indicated that lentiviral-based vectors might prove advantageous over MoMLV vectors for transduction of ESCs, thus encouraging the use of these vectors for genetic modifications of hESCs.

In recent years, we and others have developed protocols for efficient transduction of hESCs by advanced modified HIV-1–based vectors pseudotyped with VSV-G (Gropp *et al.*, 2003; Ma *et al.*, 2003; Pfeifer *et al.*, 2002; Suter *et al.*, 2006; Xiong *et al.*, 2005; Zaehres *et al.*, 2005). Transduction of

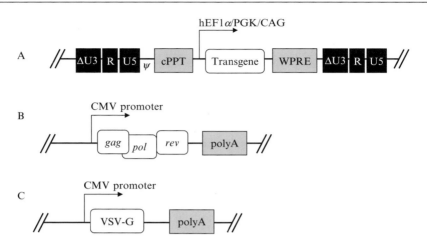

FIG. 1. The advanced modified HIV-1–based vector system. The figure depicts a schematic representation of the three plasmids used to generate the recombinant HIV-1–based viral particles. (A) The transfer vector is a replication-defective advanced HIV-1–based vector, expressing the transgene from an internal constitutive promoter such as the human elongation factor 1α (hEF1α) promoter, the human phosphoglycerate (hPGK) promoter, or the hybrid CAG promoter composed of the cytomegalovirus (CMV) immediate early enhancer, chicken β-actin promoter and a rabbit β-globin intron. This vector is self-inactivating because of a large deletion in the 3′UTR region of its LTR, which abolishes the viral promoter/enhancer activity. The performance of the transfer vector is increased by the addition of two regulatory elements: the central polypurine tract (cPPT) sequence that is found within the *pol* gene of HIV-1, which increases viral integration, and the posttranscriptional regulatory element of the woodchuck hepatitis virus (WPRE), which increases transgene expression. (B) The packaging plasmid expresses the three viral genes, *gag, pol*, and *rev*, from a constitutive CMV promoter. The proteins provided by this plasmid are essential for the early steps of viral infection (entry into the host cell, reverse transcription, and viral integration into the genome of the host cell). (C) The envelope plasmid expresses the heterologous envelope glycoprotein of the vesicular stomatitis virus (VSV-G) from the CMV promoter. The use of the heterologous envelope prevents generation of wild-type virus, broadens the viral host range, and increases the stability of the viral particles.

hESCs by these vectors resulted in high and stable transgene expression that was maintained over long periods of undifferentiated cultivation, as well as after differentiation (Gropp *et al.*, 2003).

Thus, HIV-1–based vectors have proved to be efficient gene delivery tools into hESCs. Moreover, these vectors confer stable transgene expression within hESCs that is sustained throughout prolonged proliferation of undifferentiated hESCs, as well as after differentiation of the cells *in vitro* and *in vivo*. Most importantly, the transduced hESCs retain their potential for self-renewal and their pluripotency.

Potential Applications of Gene Delivery into hESCs
    by Lentiviral-Based Vectors

Transduction of hESCs by lentiviral-based vectors could be used for various applications, both in regenerative medicine and basic research.

Lentiviral-based vectors overexpressing specific transcription factors could direct the differentiation of hESCs toward a desired cell lineage or cell type. In addition, lentiviral-based vectors expressing a reporter or a selectable marker under the control of a tissue-specific or cell type–specific promoter will enable us to select and thus enrich a specific cell type. The ability to direct the differentiation of hESCs or to derive enriched populations of specific types of differentiated cells may allow the exploitation of hESCs as an unlimited source of cells for transplantation.

Transduced hESCs could be used not only for cell therapy but also for gene therapy. For this purpose, hESC transduced by lentiviral-based vectors expressing genes that are defective in specific genetic diseases will be transplanted and could potentially correct these diseases.

Transduction of hESCs by lentiviral-based vectors expressing a reporter gene (GFP, RFP, or luciferase) will generate reporter hESC cell lines, allowing easy detection and monitoring the fate of transplanted hESCS within the animals.

Finally, lentiviral-based vectors could be used to silence genes of interest in hESCS. Thus, they might prove invaluable for studying the role of specific genes involved in early human development.

Design of HIV-1–Based Vectors for Transduction of hESCs

Choice of HIV-1–Based Vector

Thus far, only HIV-1–based vectors have been reported to transduce hESCs. We will, therefore, concentrate on the design and production of these vectors. Most groups have used the safer advanced SIN transfer HIV-1–based vectors, containing cPPT and WPRE, for transduction of hESCs.

The simple monocistronic HIV-1–based vectors express a single transgene from an internal promoter. However, for various applications, it is desired to coexpress two genes. In vectors coexpressing two genes, usually the first gene is the gene of interest, whereas the second gene is the reporter/selection gene. This design allows monitoring of transduction efficiencies and transgene expression or selection for cells expressing the transgene.

Monocistronic Lentiviral-Based Vectors

These vectors are suitable for generation of reporter hESC lines. For example, we transduced hESCs with an HIV-1–based vector expressing the reporter gene eGFP from a constitutive internal promoter. After further mechanical selection of colonies expressing eGFP, a hESC line expressing high levels of eGFP was generated (Gropp *et al.*, 2003). This eGFP-hESC line is valuable for monitoring the fate of hESCs after transplantation into animals.

Lentiviral-Based Vectors Coexpressing Two Genes

Two strategies have been used thus far to coexpress two genes in hESCs.

Bicistronic Vectors

In these vectors, the two genes are transcribed from a single promoter but are translated separately. This is achieved by insertion of an internal ribosome entry site (IRES) between the two genes (Fig. 2A). This strategy ensures a coordinated expression of the two genes. Bicistronic vectors coexpressing GFP and the puromycin resistance gene were recently used by Xiong and colleagues for successful transduction of hESCs (Xiong *et al.*, 2005). However, a major drawback of bicistronic vectors is that the expression of the gene downstream to the IRES may be low and inconsistently dependent on the first gene sequence in an unpredictable manner (Yu *et al.*, 2003). In addition, IRESs do not allow uncoupled expression of the two genes.

Dual-Promoter Vectors

Dual-promoter vectors contain two separate expression cassettes; thus, each gene is expressed from its own promoter (Fig. 2B). The uncoupled expression of transgenes is required for a variety of applications, such as the development of genetically modified hESCs that allow tracing of differentiated cells of a specific lineage. For this purpose constitutive expression of a selectable marker is required in combination with the expression of a reporter gene under a tissue-specific promoter. The potential of dual-promoter lentiviral vectors for the transduction of hESCs was recently reported by Suter and colleagues (2006). The major disadvantage of this strategy is that the expression driven by one promoter may be disrupted by interference from the other promoter.

Dual-promoter vectors are very efficient tools for silencing specific genes by means of RNA interference (RNAi). In this case, the silencing cassette contains a specific short hairpin RNA (shRNA) under the control of a pol III promoter (H1 or U6), whereas the second cassette harbors a reporter/selection gene expressed from a constitutive pol II promoter (Fig. 2C). Because the expression of the shRNA is directed from a pol III promoter and the silencing cassette includes a unique transcription termination signal, these dual-promoter vectors do not encounter promoter interference. Several

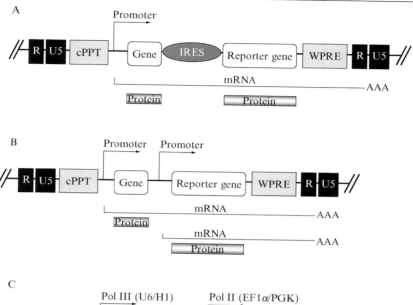

FIG. 2. HIV-1 transfer vectors coexpressing two genes. The figure depicts a schematic representation of two types of advanced HIV-1–based vectors coexpressing two genes. These vectors enable the expression of a gene of interest together with a reporter/selection gene. (A) Bicistronic vectors. In these vectors, the coordinated expression of the two genes is achieved by transcription of the two genes from a single promoter. An internal ribosome entry site (IRES) inserted between the two genes allows separate translation of their transcripts. (B) Dual promoter vectors. These vectors contain two separate expression cassettes, each harboring a gene under the control of its own promoter, thus enabling an uncoupled expression of transgenes. (C) Dual promoter vectors for silencing specific genes by means of RNA interference (RNAi). These vectors contain two cassettes, each harboring a different type of promoter: (1) a silencing cassette expressing a specific short hairpin RNA (shRNA) from a pol III promoter (H1 or U6) and harboring a unique transcription termination signal (ttttt), and (2) a second cassette harboring a reporter/selection gene expressed from a constitutive pol II promoter.

groups have recently used dual-promoter vectors to silence specific genes in hESCs (Suter *et al.*, 2006; Xiong *et al.*, 2005; Zaehres *et al.*, 2005).

To summarize, various lentiviral vector types can be used for transduction of hESCs. The choice of which vector to use depends on the desired application. It should be noted that the efficiency of various lentiviral vectors might vary, depending on the vector construct, the specific promoters, and the transgenes that are expressed.

Choice of Internal Promoter

Constitutive expression of the transgene in hESCs requires the use of promoters active in undifferentiated hESCs and their differentiated derivatives. So far, several constitutive promoters have been used to drive lentiviral-mediated transgene expression in hESCs. We and others have found that the human elongation factor 1α (hEF1α) promoter promoted high transgene expression in hESCs that was not silenced over time or after differentiation (Gropp *et al.*, 2003; Ma *et al.*, 2003; Suter *et al.*, 2006; Xiong *et al.*, 2005). Several other promoters that have been used are the human phosphoglycerate (hPGK) promoter (Zaehres *et al.*, 2005), the SV40 promoter (Suter *et al.*, 2006), and the hybrid CAG promoter composed of the cytomegalovirus (CMV) immediate early enhancer, chicken β-actin promoter and a rabbit β-globin intron (Pfeifer *et al.*, 2002). A regulated expression of the transgene has not yet been reported for hESCs, although there are several reports on the development of conditional lentiviral-mediated gene expression systems (Vigna *et al.*, 2005; Wiznerowicz and Trono, 2003).

Generation of Recombinant Viral Particles

In general, recombinant viral particles are generated by transient cotransfection of the transfer vector, the packaging plasmid, and the envelope plasmid into the highly transfectable human embryonic kidney (HEK) 293T cell line. The supernatant containing the viral particles is collected, concentrated, and used to transduce hESCs.

Plasmid Constructs

The transfer vectors used by most groups are advanced modified HIV-1–based vectors, expressing the transgene from an internal promoter (Gropp *et al.*, 2003). The envelope plasmid expressing the heterologous envelope protein is pMDG (Naldini *et al.*, 1996a), and the packaging plasmid expressing the *gag*, *pol*, and *rev* genes is pCMVΔR8.91 (Zufferey *et al.*, 1997). Note that some groups use a more advanced packaging system, in which the *rev* gene is expressed from a separate promoter (Follenzi and Naldini, 2002). Plasmid DNA should be pure and can be purified by commercial kits.

Production of Viral Particles

Viral particles are produced by transient cotransfection into 293T cells. We routinely use FuGene-6 transfection reagent (Roche Molecular Biochemicals, Mannheim, Germany) or TransIT-LT1 transfection reagent

(Mirus, Madison, WI). These reagents yield high reproducible transfection efficiencies, which lead to high viral titers. An alternate economical strategy is the calcium-phosphate transfection method (Follenzi and Naldini, 2002). In general, for production of high viral titers, the transfection method chosen should be very efficient. The transfection protocol described in the following is suitable for both FuGene-6 and TransIT-LT1 transfection reagents. The components of the transfection are calculated for 10-cm tissue culture dishes. However, transfection can be performed in larger or smaller tissue culture dishes, provided that all the other components of the transfection (DNA, transfection reagent, and medium) are scaled proportionally.

FuGene-6/TransIT-LT1 Transfection Protocol

1. 293T cells are routinely cultured in 90% Dulbecco's modified Eagle's medium (DMEM, Gibco-BRL, Gaithersburg, MD) supplemented with 10% fetal calf serum (FCS, Biological Industries, Beit Haemek, Israel), 1 mM L-glutamine, 100 U/ml penicillin, and 50 μg/ml streptomycin. Note that 293T cells are highly susceptible to mycoplasma infection, which leads to low viral titers. Therefore, it is recommended to ascertain before transfection that the cells are mycoplasma free.

2. Twenty-four hours before transfection, plate 1.4–2 × 10^6 293T cells on a 10-cm tissue culture dish, in 10 ml 293T tissue culture medium. The confluence of the cells on the day of transfection should be approximately 70%.

3. Incubate the cells overnight at 37°.

4. The next day, perform the transfection in a total volume of 600 μl.

5. Prepare the plasmid mixture: in a sterile Eppendorf tube, combine 10 μg of the transfer vector, 6.5 μg of the packaging plasmid, and 3.5 μg of the envelope plasmid (a total of 20 μg plasmid DNA).

6. In a second Eppendorf tube, prepare the transfection reagent solution: place a serum-free medium (Optimem, Gibco) in the tube. The volume of the Optimem medium is determined according to the volumes of the other components of the transfection (transfection reagent and plasmid DNA). Add 55 μl of the FuGene-6/TransIT-LT1 transfection reagent (a ratio of 2.7 μl reagent per 1 μg DNA) directly to the Optimem medium in a dropwise manner. Mix completely by gently flicking the tube. Incubate at room temperature for approximately 5 min.

7. Add the reagent solution to the plasmid mixture in a dropwise manner. Mix by gently flicking the tube. Incubate at room temperature for 15–45 min to enable reagent/DNA complex formation.

8. Add the reagent/DNA complex mixture dropwise to the 293T cells. Gently rock the tissue culture dish to ensure even distribution of the mixture. Incubate for 16–20 h at 37°.

Collection of Recombinant Viral Particles

1. Sixteen–20 hours after transfection, replace the medium with 10 ml fresh 293T culture medium.
2. After additional incubation for 24 h at 37°, collect the supernatant containing the viral particles. Store the supernatant in the dark at 4°.
3. Add 10 ml fresh medium and incubate the transfected cells further for 24 h. Collect the supernatant.
4. Combine the supernatants that were collected 48 and 72 h after transfection (a total of 20 ml). Filter them through a 0.45-μm filter (we use Sartorius, Goettingen, Germany). Proceed directly to concentration of the virus. Save a small volume for determination of viral titer.

Concentration of Viral Particles

High viral titers (10^7–10^8 TU/ml) are vital for efficient transduction of hESCs. Therefore, the collected viral particles should be concentrated. The use of the VSV-G envelope generates a stable virus that can be concentrated by ultracentrifugation without a significant loss of viral titer.

1. Concentrate the virus by centrifugation at 50,000g at 4° for 2 h. We use a Sorvall ultracentrifuge model Discovery 100, with a Surespin 630 swinging bucket rotor.
2. After centrifugation, resuspend the pellet containing the viral particles immediately in 0.1 volume of the collected supernatant (2 ml from each 10-cm tissue culture dish) in the desired hESC culture medium. Proceed directly to transduction of hESCs. Save a small volume for determination of viral titer. Note that the viral pellet is very loose and mostly invisible. Therefore, mark the centrifugation tubes in advance and aspirate the supernatant carefully using a pipette.
3. Optionally, the concentrated viral pellet can be resuspended in a minimal volume of freezing buffer and stored in small aliquots at −80°. The freezing buffer is composed of 19.75 mM Tris-HCl buffer pH7, 40 mg/ml lactose, 37.5 mM sodium chloride, 1 mg/ml human or bovine serum albumin, and 5 μg/ml protamine sulfate. Avoid freeze–thaw cycles.

Transduction of hESCs

Transduction of hESCs can be performed using several strategies. The strategy chosen depends on the culture method of the hESCs. Each of the three protocols described in the following section is suitable for a different culture method.

Transduction of hESCs Cultured in Serum-Containing Medium and Passaged as Cell Clusters

hESCs are routinely cultured in 80% high glucose DMEM (Gibco) supplemented with 20% fetal bovine serum (FBS, Hyclone, Logan, UT), 1 mM L-glutamine, 50 U/ml penicillin, 50 μg/ml streptomycin, 1% nonessential amino-acids, and 0.1 mM β-mercaptoethanol. The cells grow on mouse embryonic fibroblasts (MEF) feeders and are passaged weekly as clusters of 100–200 cells (Reubinoff et al., 2000).

1. At the time of routine passage, isolate small clusters of undifferentiated hESCs by mechanical slicing of undifferentiated sections of the hES colonies, followed by treatment with 10 mg/ml Dispase (Gibco).
2. Resuspend the viral pellet in 2 ml hESC culture medium (described previously). Incubate the hESC clusters with 1 ml of the concentrated virus in the presence of 5 μg/ml polybrene (Sigma, St. Louis, MO) in a 35-mm petri dish (BD Falcon, Franklin Lakes, NJ) at 37° for 2 h. At time intervals, gently rock the dish to prevent adherence of the clusters and increase exposure of the clusters to the virus.
3. Add 1 ml fresh concentrated virus and continue the incubation for 1–2 h.
4. Wash the transduced hESC clusters with PBS and plate them on fresh MEF feeders on a 35-mm tissue culture dish.
5. After 1 week, determine transduction efficiency. This method generally promotes maximal transduction efficiencies of 30%. However, transduced hESC populations can be further enriched.

Transduction of hESCs Cultured in Serum-Free Medium on Feeders and Passaged as Single Cells

hESCs are routinely cultured in 85% knockout (KO) DMEM medium (Gibco) supplemented with 15% KO-serum replacement (SR, Gibco), 1 mM L-glutamine, 50 U/ml penicillin, 50 μg/ml streptomycin, 1% nonessential amino acids, and 4 ng/ml basic fibroblast growth factor (bFGF, Cytolab, Rehovot, Israel). The cells grow on human foreskin feeders and are passaged weekly as single cells. Note that because of the high frequency of chromosomal abnormalities observed after extended passaging of hESCs as single cells, it is recommended that the cells be cultured in this method for not more than 12–15 passages (Mitalipova et al., 2005).

1. At the time of routine passage, dissociate the cells into a single cell suspension by digestion with 0.05% trypsin/0.53 mM ethylenediaminetetraacetic acid (EDTA) (Gibco).

2. Resuspend the viral pellet in 2 ml hESCs culture medium (described previously).
3. Combine 1×10^5 trypsinized hESCs with the virus containing culture medium in the presence of 5 μg/ml polybrene.
4. Plate the cells in the virus-containing culture medium on fresh foreskin feeders on 35-mm tissue culture dishes. Incubate overnight at 37°.
5. The next day, replace the medium with fresh hESCs culture medium.
6. Because this method promotes transduction of not only the hESCs but also the feeders, one or two passages are required to eliminate the transduced feeders.
7. Determine transduction efficiency 2 weeks after transduction. This method generally promotes high efficiencies of more than 90%.

Transduction of hESCs Cultured in Serum-Free Medium without Feeders and Passaged Enzymatically as Small Clusters

hESCs are grown in a feeder-free culture system. In this system, the cells are routinely cultured on Matrigel-coated plates in MEF-conditioned medium. The cells are passaged weekly as small clusters using collagenase type IV (a detailed culture protocol is described by Xu *et al.* [2001]).

1. At the time of routine passage, dissociate the cells into small clusters by digestion with 200 U/mg collagenase type IV (Gibco).
2. Resuspend the viral pellet in 2 ml MEF-conditioned medium containing 5 μg/ml polybrene.
3. Combine the hESC clumps with the virus-containing medium.
4. Plate the cells in the virus-containing medium on fresh Matrigel–coated 35-mm tissue culture dishes. Incubate overnight at 37°.
5. The next day, replace the medium with fresh conditioned medium.
6. Determine transduction efficiency 1 week after transduction. This method enables transduction of pure populations of hESCs (no feeders). Therefore, high efficiencies can be obtained, even though the cells are transduced as small clusters.

Measurement of Transduction Efficiency

The method described in the following for determining transduction efficiency is based on fluorescence-activated cell sorter (FACS) analysis of the expression of a reporter gene (GFP or RFP) by the transduced cells. The percentage of undifferentiated cells among the transduced hESCs is determined by the analysis of the percentage of transduced cells that are also immunoreactive with antibodies against stem cell–specific markers, such as GCTM2 (Pera *et al.*, 1988), SSEA-4 or TRA-1–60 (both are available commercially).

1. Depending on the method of hESC culture, separate the transduced hESCs from the feeders.
2. Dissociate the transduced hESCs cells into a single-cell suspension using 0.05% trypsin/0.53 mM EDTA.
3. Wash with cold PBS and spin for 5 min at 1500 rpm.
4. Incubate 1×10^5 cells with the stem cell–specific antibody on ice for 30 min.
5. As a control, incubate 1×10^5 cells with the appropriate isotype control.
6. Wash the cells with cold PBS and spin again for 5 min at 1500 rpm.
7. Incubate the cells with the secondary fluorescent antibody on ice for 30 min.
8. Wash the cells with cold PBS and spin for 5 min at 1500 rpm. Resuspend the pellet in cold FACS buffer ($1\times$ PBS supplemented with 1% BSA, and 0.1% sodium azide) containing propidium iodide (PI) to gate out dead cells.
9. Analyze the percentage of GFP-expressing cells by FACS. Determine the percentage of the undifferentiated transduced hESCs by analyzing the percentage of GFP-expressing cells that are immunoreactive with the stem cell–specific antibody.

Enrichment for Transduced hESCs Expressing High Levels of the Transgene

Transduction of hESCs by lentiviral-based vectors without selection leads to a population of cells with varied transgene expression levels. However, high and homogenous transgene expression is preferred for many applications. Here we describe several strategies to obtain homogenous and high expression levels of transgenes within hESCs transduced by lentiviral-based vectors.

Enrichment of Transduced hESC Colonies Expressing High Levels of a Reporter Gene

This method is suitable for enrichment of hESCs transduced with a lentiviral-based vector expressing a reporter gene that is maintained on feeders and passaged mechanically as small clusters.

1. At the time of routine passage, examine the transduced hESC colonies by fluorescence microscopy and mark colonies expressing high levels of the reporter gene.

2. Selectively passage the marked colonies by mechanical slicing of undifferentiated sections of the hESCs colonies, followed by treatment with 10 mg/ml Dispase (Gibco).
3. Continue propagating the transduced colonies. Repeat the enrichment protocol for three to four additional passages, until the most of the transduced hESC population expresses high levels of the transgene.
4. Determine transgene expression levels in the enriched transduced hESCs population by FACS.

Isolation of Transduced hESC Clones Expressing High Levels of a Reporter Gene

This method can be used to obtain transduced hESC clones with high and relatively homogenous expression of a reporter gene. It is suitable for hESCs maintained and transduced as single cells.

1. At the time of routine passage, dissociate the transduced hESCs into a single cell suspension using 0.05% trypsin/0.53 mM EDTA (Gibco), and plate them at low density on feeders (2–3×10^3 hESCs per 35-mm tissue culture dish).
2. Culture the cells for 1 week.
3. After 1 week, pick single colonies using a micropipette, and replate them on fresh feeders in separate wells, in a 48-well tissue culture dish. Because each transduced hES cell colony evolved from a single transduced cell, the clones should express homogenous transgene levels.
4. One week after cloning, examine reporter gene expression by fluorescence microscopy and select clones expressing high levels of the reporter gene.
5. Continue propagation of the selected clones.
6. Determine transgene expression levels in individual clones by FACS.

Enrichment of Transduced hESC Cells Expressing High Levels of the Transgene Using Antibiotic Selection

This enrichment protocol can be used for hESCs transduced by lentiviral vectors coexpressing a gene of interest, together with an antibiotic resistance gene. It allows robust and simple development of nonclonal transduced hESC populations, with high levels of transgene expression.

1. Before transduction, test the sensitivity of the hESCs to the specific antibiotic. We found that different hESC lines exhibit varied sensitivities to specific antibiotics.

2. Three days after transduction, start antibiotic selection. Antibiotic selection can be performed on hESCs transduced on Matrigel or on feeders. For cells maintained on feeders, the feeders should be resistant to the specific antibiotic used.

3. Continue antibiotic selection until the most of the transduced hESCs express high homogenous levels of the gene of interest.

Determination of Viral Titer

Because efficient transduction of hESCs depends on high viral titers, it is important to determine viral titers before transduction. The method described in the following is based on measurement of the expression of the reporter gene (GFP or RFP). However, if the lentiviral construct does not contain a reporter gene, other methods can be used to determine viral titers (see Follenzi and Naldini [2002]).

1. One day before transduction, plate 5×10^4 293T cells per well in a 12-well tissue culture dish, in 2 ml 293T culture medium. The number of cells per well at the time of transduction should be 1×10^5. Incubate overnight at 37°.

2. The next day, transduce the 293T cells with dilutions of the virus samples that were collected before and after concentration. Use dilutions that will promote transduction efficiencies of less than 15% to avoid transductions with multiple integration sites. We usually transduce the cells with 200 μl, 100 μl, and 50 μl of the nonconcentrated virus, and 20 μl, 10 μl, and 5 μl of the concentrated virus. The transduction is performed in a total volume of 1 ml in the presence of 5 μg/ml polybrene. Incubate the transduced cells overnight at 37°.

3. The next day, replace the medium with fresh 293T culture medium and continue growing the cells for 2–3 days, until they reach 80–90% confluence.

4. Dissociate the cells into a single-cell suspension using 0.25% trypsin/ 1 mM EDTA.

5. For each dilution, analyze the percentage of GFP/RFP expressing cells by FACS.

6. The viral titer is represented as transducing units per ml (TU/ml). Calculate the titer as follows: the number of cells at the time of transduction (1×10^5) multiplied by the percentage divided by 100 of the GFP/RFP-expressing cells, multiplied by the fraction of 1 ml of the virus used for transduction, and multiplied by the final dilution in the culture medium. For example, if you use 200 μl of 1 ml virus for transduction in a total volume

of 1 ml culture medium, and the percentage of GFP expressing cells is 15%, then the viral titer is $10^5 \times 15/100 \times 5 \times 5 = 3.75 \times 10^5$ TU/ml.

7. Average the titers from the three dilutions and determine the viral titer.

References

Asano, T., Hanazono, Y., Ueda, Y., Muramatsu, S., Kume, A., Suemori, H., Suzuki, Y., Kondo, Y., Harii, K., Hasegawa, M., Nakatsuji, N., and Ozawa, K. (2002). Highly efficient gene transfer into primate embryonic stem cells with a simian lentivirus vector. *Mol. Ther.* **6,** 162–168.

Buchschacher, G. L., Jr. (2001). Introduction to retroviruses and retroviral vectors. *Somat. Cell Mol. Genet.* **26,** 1–11.

Follenzi, A., Ailles, L. E., Bakovic, S., Geuna, M., and Naldini, L. (2000). Gene transfer by lentiviral vectors is limited by nuclear translocation and rescued by HIV-1 pol sequences. *Nat. Genet.* **25,** 217–222.

Follenzi, A., and Naldini, L. (2002). Generation of HIV-1 derived lentiviral vectors. *Methods Enzymol.* **346,** 454–465.

Goff, S. P. (2001). Retroviridae; The retroviruses and their replication. *In* Fields Virology, Vol. 2, pp. 1871–1939. Lippincott Williams and Wilkins, Phildelphia.

Gropp, M., Itsykson, P., Singer, O., Ben-Hur, T., Reinhartz, E., Galun, E., and Reubinoff, B. E. (2003). Stable genetic modification of human embryonic stem cells by lentiviral vectors. *Mol. Ther.* **7,** 281–287.

Hamaguchi, I., Woods, N. B., Panagopoulos, I., Andersson, E., Mikkola, H., Fahlman, C., Zufferey, R., Carlsson, L., Trono, D., and Karlsson, S. (2000). Lentivirus vector gene expression during ES cell-derived hematopoietic development *in vitro. J. Virol.* **74,** 10778–10784.

Ma, Y., Ramezani, A., Lewis, R., Hawley, R. G., and Thomson, J. A. (2003). High-level sustained transgene expression in human embryonic stem cells using lentiviral vectors. *Stem Cells* **21,** 111–117.

Menendez, P., Wang, L., and Bhatia, M. (2005). Genetic manipulation of human embryonic stem cells: A system to study early human development and potential therapeutic applications. *Curr. Gene Ther.* **5,** 375–385.

Mitalipova, M. M., Rao, R. R., Hoyer, D. M., Johnson, J. A., Meisner, L. F., Jones, K. L., Dalton, S., and Stice, S. L. (2005). Preserving the genetic integrity of human embryonic stem cells. *Nat. Biotechnol.* **23,** 19–20.

Miyoshi, H., Blomer, U., Takahashi, M., Gage, F. H., and Verma, I. M. (1998). Development of a self-inactivating lentivirus vector. *J. Virol.* **72,** 8150–8157.

Naldini, L., Blomer, U., Gage, F. H., Trono, D., and Verma, I. M. (1996a). Efficient transfer, integration, and sustained long-term expression of the transgene in adult rat brains injected with a lentiviral vector. *Proc. Natl. Acad. Sci. USA* **93,** 11382–11388.

Naldini, L., Blomer, U., Gallay, P., Ory, D., Mulligan, R., Gage, F. H., Verma, I. M., and Trono, D. (1996b). *In vivo* gene delivery and stable transduction of nondividing cells by a lentiviral vector. *Science* **272,** 263–267.

Niwa, O., Yokota, Y., Ishida, H., and Sugahara, T. (1983). Independent mechanisms involved in suppression of the Moloney leukemia virus genome during differentiation of murine teratocarcinoma cells. *Cell* **32,** 1105–1113.

Palu, G., Parolin, C., Takeuchi, Y., and Pizzato, M. (2000). Progress with retroviral gene vectors. *Rev. Med. Virol.* **10**, 185–202.

Pannell, D., and Ellis, J. (2001). Silencing of gene expression: Implications for design of retrovirus vectors. *Rev. Med. Virol.* **11**, 205–217.

Pera, M. F., Blasco-Lafita, M. J., Cooper, S., Mason, M., Mills, J., and Monaghan, P. (1988). Analysis of cell-differentiation lineage in human teratomas using new monoclonal antibodies to cytostructural antigens of embryonal carcinoma cells. *Differentiation* **39**, 139–149.

Pfeifer, A., Ikawa, M., Dayn, Y., and Verma, I. M. (2002). Transgenesis by lentiviral vectors: Lack of gene silencing in mammalian embryonic stem cells and preimplantation embryos. *Proc. Natl. Acad. Sci. USA* **99**, 2140–2145.

Reubinoff, B. E., Pera, M. F., Fong, C. Y., Trounson, A., and Bongso, A. (2000). Embryonic stem cell lines from human blastocysts: Somatic differentiation *in vitro*. *Nat. Biotechnol.* **18**, 399–404.

Suter, D. M., Cartier, L., Bettiol, E., Tirefort, D., Jaconi, M. E., Dubois-Dauphin, M., and Krause, K. H. (2006). Rapid generation of stable transgenic embryonic stem cell lines using modular lentivectors. *Stem Cells* **24**, 615–623.

Thomson, J. A., Itskovitz-Eldor, J., Shapiro, S. S., Waknitz, M. A., Swiergiel, J. J., Marshall, V. S., and Jones, J. M. (1998). Embryonic stem cell lines derived from human blastocysts. *Science* **282**, 1145–1147.

Vigna, E., Amendola, M., Benedicenti, F., Simmons, A. D., Follenzi, A., and Naldini, L. (2005). Efficient Tet-dependent expression of human factor IX *in vivo* by a new self-regulating lentiviral vector. *Mol. Ther.* **11**, 763–775.

Wiznerowicz, M., and Trono, D. (2003). Conditional suppression of cellular genes: Lentivirus vector-mediated drug-inducible RNA interference. *J. Virol.* **77**, 8957–861.

Xiong, C., Tang, D. Q., Xie, C. Q., Zhang, L., Xu, K. F., Thompson, W. E., Chou, W., Gibbons, G. H., Chang, L. J., Yang, L. J., and Chen, Y. E. (2005). Genetic engineering of human embryonic stem cells with lentiviral vectors. *Stem Cells Dev.* **14**, 367–377.

Xu, C., Inokuma, M. S., Denham, J., Golds, K., Kundu, P., Gold, J. D., and Carpenter, M. K. (2001). Feeder-free growth of undifferentiated human embryonic stem cells. *Nat. Biotechnol.* **19**, 971–974.

Yu, X., Zhan, X., D'Costa, J., Tanavde, V. M., Ye, Z., Peng, T., Malehorn, M. T., Yang, X., Civin, C. I., and Cheng, L. (2003). Lentiviral vectors with two independent internal promoters transfer high-level expression of multiple transgenes to human hematopoietic stem-progenitor cells. *Mol. Ther.* **7**, 827–838.

Zaehres, H., Lensch, M. W., Daheron, L., Stewart, S. A., Itskovitz-Eldor, J., and Daley, G. Q. (2005). High-efficiency RNA interference in human embryonic stem cells. *Stem Cells* **23**, 299–305.

Zufferey, R., Donello, J. E., Trono, D., and Hope, T. J. (1999). Woodchuck hepatitis virus posttranscriptional regulatory element enhances expression of transgenes delivered by retroviral vectors. *J. Virol.* **73**, 2886–2892.

Zufferey, R., Dull, T., Mandel, R. J., Bukovsky, A., Quiroz, D., Naldini, L., and Trono, D. (1998). Self-inactivating lentivirus vector for safe and efficient *in vivo* gene delivery. *J. Virol.* **72**, 9873–9880.

Zufferey, R., Nagy, D., Mandel, R. J., Naldini, L., and Trono, D. (1997). Multiply attenuated lentiviral vector achieves efficient gene delivery *in vivo*. *Nat. Biotechnol.* **15**, 871–875.

[6] The Use of Retroviral Vectors for Gene Transfer into Hematopoietic Stem Cells

By JEFF HOLST and JOHN E. J. RASKO

Introduction

Effective gene transfer requires the efficient incorporation of new genetic material into a specific target cell, with consequent gene expression. Retroviral vector systems offer the opportunity to permanently modify gene expression of target cells, after DNA integration into the genome, and, as such, have been used for diverse gene transfer and gene therapy applications. Currently, approximately a quarter of clinical gene therapy trials make use of retrovirus-based vectors, with all virus-based vectors comprising approximately two thirds of trials (http://www.wiley.co.uk/genetherapy/clinical, 2006). The most common retroviral vectors in use have been derived from the gammaretrovirus genus, such as murine leukemia virus (MLV), and lentivirus genus and human immunodeficiency virus (HIV). Although most early retroviral gene transfer studies used MLV-based vectors, the ability of lentivirus vectors to enter nondividing cells has led to a substantial increase in their use both *in vitro* and in animal models (Naldini *et al.*, 1996).

Viral Pseudotype

The term *pseudotype,* by analogy with *serotype*, refers to the use of an alternate virus coat protein (envelope) for a given retroviral vector. Pseudotyping of retroviral vectors with heterologous viral glycoproteins and receptor-specific ligands permits the selective introduction of genes into specific target cells, thus making them ideally suited for gene therapy applications. For murine-restricted expression, the ecotropic MLV envelope can be used (Miller and Rosman, 1989). Other commonly used envelopes include those encoded by the feline type C virus (RD114) (Battini *et al.*, 1999; Rasko *et al.*, 1999), gibbon ape leukemia virus (GALV) (Miller *et al.*, 1991), amphotropic MLV (Miller and Buttimore, 1986; Miller *et al.*, 1994), xenotropic and polytropic MLV (Battini *et al.*, 1999), and vesicular stomatitis virus G protein (VSV-G) (Emi *et al.*, 1991).

VSV-G pseudotyped vectors permit the expression of genes in a wide variety of cell types and organisms, including nonmammalian cells, because of the wide biodistribution of its receptor (Gonin and Gaillard, 2004;

METHODS IN ENZYMOLOGY, VOL. 420
0076-6879/06 $35.00
DOI: 10.1016/S0076-6879(06)20006-5

Naldini *et al.*, 1996). Since the VSV-G–pseudotyped viral particles can be concentrated by ultracentrifugation, very high titers of greater than 10^9 transducing units per milliliter can be obtained (Burns *et al.*, 1993). However, the creation of stable VSV-G packaging cell lines has been problematical, because VSV-G is toxic to most cells (Burns *et al.*, 1993). Typically, retroviral vector production using the VSV-G envelope has required either transient transfection or the use of stable inducible expression systems. Thus, the investigator is often faced with resolving the dilemma between targeted versus broad-range cell transduction and the convenience of stable versus transient packaging systems.

Chimeric receptor-specific envelopes have been developed by fusing a cognate ligand to an existing envelope, which targets specific cell surface receptors. Recombinant proteins that bind the epidermal growth factor (EGF), CD117 (c-Kit), von Willebrand factor, and interleukin-2 (IL-2) cell surface molecules, as well as different single-chain variable fragmented antibodies, have been constructed (Yi *et al.*, 2005). Although these chimeric envelopes target the correct receptor, transduction efficiency is often lower or nonexistent; for example, an EGF envelope did not allow entry into the target cells that express the EGF receptor (Cosset *et al.*, 1995a). An IL-2 chimeric envelope, on the other hand, not only targeted T cells and cancer cells but it also provided increased transduction efficiency because of enhanced proliferation of the cells resulting from IL-2R activation (Maurice *et al.*, 1999).

Vector Design

A number of important advances in vector design have increased their usefulness and safety. During the early years of vector development, Moloney murine leukemia virus (MoMLV)–based vectors were widely used to achieve efficient gene transfer in some cell lines and rodents. Self-inactivating vectors were created with a deletion in their $3'$ long terminal repeat (LTR) so that on reverse transcription, the deletion is transferred to the $5'$ LTR, abolishing the ability of the LTR to act as a promoter and thus improving safety (Zufferey *et al.*, 1998; Modlich *et al.*, 2006). The use of different promoters and inducible systems has provided greater control over expression of genes within target cells. The use of autofluorescent proteins as convenient reporter systems has further expanded the usefulness of retroviral vector systems (Rasko, 1999). The addition of an internal ribosome entry site (IRES) and, more recently, the picornavirus 2A sequence, has facilitated simultaneous expression of multiple genes (Ghattas *et al.*, 1991; Holst *et al.*, 2006; Szymczak *et al.*, 2004). As our understanding of the important factors involved in viral transduction and expression increases, and as viral vectors become more complex, their usefulness for achieving increasingly diverse gene transfer applications will continue to expand.

Packaging Cell Lines

Numerous systems are available for simple and safe one-step production of high titer, replication-incompetent virus (Table I). PA317 is an amphotropic packaging cell line based on NIH-3T3 cells, which was used in early gene therapy clinical trials (Kun *et al.*, 1995). Other NIH-3T3 systems that stably express the ecotropic envelope, such as GP+E-86 (Markowitz *et al.*, 1988) and PE501 (Miller and Rosman, 1989) cells, have been widely used to transduce murine hematopoietic stem cells (HSCs) (Holst *et al.*, 2006; Szymczak *et al.*, 2004). The NIH-3T3 packaging cell lines were developed by expressing one or two integrated plasmid(s), which encode the viral envelope and structural proteins *in trans*. The vectors used in these systems have multiple deletions in the viral genome that are required for autonomous replication, thereby reducing the potential for production of replication-competent virus. The risk of recombination

TABLE I
COMMONLY USED RETROVIRAL PACKAGING CELL LINES

Name	Cell type	Host range	Availability/reference
PA317	NIH-3T3	Amphotropic	Miller and Buttimore, 1986
Phoenix	HEK 293 T	Ecotropic	ATCC 3444
		Amphotropic	ATCC 3443
		GP	ATCC 3514
BOSC 23	HEK 293 T	Ecotropic	Pear *et al.*, 1993
PG13	TK-NIH-3T3	GALV	Miller *et al.*, 1991
GP+E-86	NIH-3T3	Ecotropic	Markowitz *et al.*, 1988
PE501	HEK 293T	Ecotropic	Miller and Rosman, 1989
FLYRD18	HT1080	RD114	Cosset *et al.*, 1995a
FLYA13	HT1080	Amphotropic	Cosset *et al.*, 1995b
AmphoPack	HEK 293T	Amphotropic	Clontech Cat. No. 631505
EcoPack2	HEK 293T	Ecotropic	Clontech Cat. No. 631507
RetroPack	HEK 293T	Dual-tropic	Clontech Cat. No. 631510

Phoenix: http://www.stanford.edu/group/nolan/MTAs/mtas.html.
Clontech: http://www.clontech.com/clontech/expression/retro/retro17.shtml

between plasmids is reduced by separating essential viral genes and by minimizing homologous sequences.

The Phoenix cell system is based on HEK 293T cells (Achacoso and Nolan, unpublished work), which can easily be transfected. They contain two plasmids: the envelope gene (specified later) driven by the cytomegalovirus promoter, and the *gag* and *pol* genes driven by the respiratory syncytial virus promoter. The use of two heterologous promoters further reduces the possibility of producing replication-competent virus through recombination. These stable packaging cells are available with either the ecotropic pseudotype (Phoenix-Eco that only transduces rodent cells) or the amphotropic pseudotype (Phoenix-Ampho transduces a wide range of mammalian cells). In addition, the Phoenix-GP cell line, which lacks expression of an envelope, permits pseudotyping with an envelope introduced by the investigator and thus control over target receptor specificity. Currently, numerous packaging cell lines are available from companies such as Clontech, Orbigen, and ATCC, some of which are detailed in Table I.

Clinical Applications

The choice of vector, pseudotype, and packaging cells is important in achieving safe and efficacious clinical gene therapy. Gene therapy trials in X-linked severe combined immunodeficiency (SCID) using retrovirus-mediated gene transfer into bone marrow stem cells have shown long-term benefits in most patients (Cavazzana-Calvo et al., 2000, 2005; Fischer et al., 2005; Hacein-Bey-Abina et al., 2002). However, three patients who had originally benefited developed leukemia 3 years after the treatment, caused in part by insertional activation of the LMO2 transcription factor (Cavazzana-Calvo et al., 2005; Fischer et al., 2005; Hacein-Bey-Abina et al., 2003; Woods et al., 2006). As such, there is concern that the random integration of retrovirus into the genome may cause insertional mutagenesis or deregulation of other nearby genes, even though this may sometimes be advantageous, as observed in one clinical trial (Kustikova et al., 2005; Ott et al., 2006). In addition to self-inactivating modifications, vectors have been designed to avoid these potential problems, for example, by inserting a chromatin insulator into the U3 region of the 5′ untranslated region (UTR) (Emery et al., 2000). This has two benefits: it reduces the possibility of silencing of the inserted promoter by nearby regulatory elements, and it blocks effects of the U3 enhancer on downstream genes.

The coexpression of a drug resistance or susceptibility gene in vectors containing a therapeutic gene has also been studied for clinical applications.

By incorporating these genes into a vector, either selection of bone marrow cells that are transduced (e.g., O^6-methylguanine-DNA methyltransferase; MGMT) or deletion of transduced cells (e.g., herpes simplex virus thymidine kinase; HSV-tk) can be achieved. MGMT has been used for *in vivo* selection of transduced HSCs in both canine and human/NOD-SCID models using O^6-benzylguanine (O^6BG) or 1,3-bis-(2 chloroethyl)-1-nitrosourea (BCNU) to deplete nontransduced cells (Neff *et al.*, 2003; Zielske *et al.*, 2003). In future studies, HSV-tk, which confers ganciclovir susceptibility to transduced cells, may be used to alleviate some concerns about genetic modification because these cells can be selectively targeted (albeit with killing of bystander cells) if problems are observed (Bonini *et al.*, 1997; Yi *et al.*, 2005). The feasibility of this approach has been demonstrated *in vitro* for B cell lines from patients with SCID, which were transduced with a retroviral vector containing both the common gamma chain and HSV-tk (Uchiyama *et al.*, 2006). This reconstituted B cell function and allowed selective killing of transduced cells (Uchiyama *et al.*, 2006). HSV-tk has already been used in gene therapy clinical trials for an alternate use: to kill bystander cells by injection of HSV-tk–expressing cells into tumors (Barzon *et al.*, 2003).

Generation of Retrovirus Packaging Cell Lines

Efficient gene transfer requires the use of high-titer retroviral vector. Typically, established stable packaging cells such as those detailed previously can be directly transfected once using a retroviral vector. However, the method described herein is a two-step process involving transfection of HEK 293T cells with a three-plasmid system (Fig. 1). The transfected

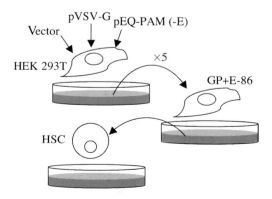

FIG. 1. Schematic of transduction process for murine hematopoietic stem cells.

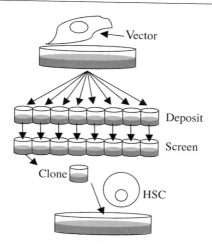

Fɪɢ. 2. Schematic of transduction process for human hematopoietic stem cells.

HEK 293T cell supernatant is then used to achieve high-level transduction of the ecotropic packaging cell line GP+E-86. We have found this method to consistently produce high-titer stable packaging cells. However, this method is not suitable for human clinical applications because the virus vector only transduces murine cells and relies on coculture of retroviral packaging cell lines and stem cells. As such, a second method involving RD114 pseudotyped envelope is provided, which is suitable for creating high-titer viral packaging cells for clinical applications (Fig. 2). For this method, transfection of FLYRD18 packaging cells (Cosset *et al.*, 2003) is performed, although the transfection is followed by selection of high-titer clones using a high-throughput method. Each protocol will be detailed separately, with the GP+E-86 protocol used for the production of virus to transduce murine stem cells and the FLYRD18 protocol for the transduction of human cells. For both methods, it is assumed that the investigator would first obtain a retroviral vector modified to express a transgene of interest, in addition to the autofluorescent protein already present.

Reagents

   pMIGII (mouse stem cell virus vector, containing an IRES-GFP) (Szymczak *et al.*, 2004), pEQ-Pam3(-E) (Szymczak *et al.*, 2004), pVSV-G (Szymczak *et al.*, 2004), and pLNCG (Green and Rasko, 2002)

HEK 293T cell (American Type Culture Collection, Manassas, VA; CRL-11268)

NIH-3T3 cell (American Type Culture Collection; CRL-1658)

GP+E-86 cell (American Type Culture Collection; CRL-9642)

FLYRD18 cell (Cosset *et al.*, 1995b)

*Trans*IT (Mirus through Fisher Scientific Co., Pittsburgh, PA)

Dulbecco's modified Eagle's medium (DMEM) and other tissue culture solutions, plastic ware, and Corning 0.45-μm syringe tip filters (Fisher Scientific Co.)

Fetal bovine serum (Biomedicals, Irvine, CA or Hyclone, Logan, UT)

Cipro (Ciprofloxacin, Bayer HealthCare, Tarrytown, NY)

Mycoplasma PCR Elisa Test Kit (Roche Molecular Biochemicals, Indianapolis, IN)

Polybrene (Hexadimethrine bromide; Sigma, St. Louis, MO) 6 mg/ml stock in filter sterilized deionized water

Adrucil 5-fluorouracil (5-FU) (Sicor Pharmaceuticals, Inc., Irvine, CA)

mIL-3, recombinant, 1 mg (Biosource International, Camarillo, CA)

hIL-6, recombinant, 1 mg (Biosource International)

mSCF, recombinant, 1 mg (Biosource International)

Sulfatrim Pediatric Suspension (sulfamethoxazole and trimethoprim oral suspension; Alpharma, Fort Lee, NJ)

Other chemicals including heparin were obtained from Sigma and mice from The Jackson Laboratory (Bar Harbor, ME).

Cell Culture Conditions

Cell lines used, including HEK 293T, FLYRD18, GP+E-86, and NIH-3T3 cells, are grown in Dulbecco's modified Eagle's medium (DMEM) supplemented with L-glutamine (2 mM), sodium pyruvate (1 mM), MEM nonessential amino acids (100 μM), HEPES (5 mM), 2-mercaptoethanol (5.5×10^{-5} U/ml), penicillin (100 U/ml), and streptomycin (100 μg/ml). For routine culture, 10% fetal bovine serum (FBS) is added to supplemented DMEM (10% DMEM). For culture of murine bone marrow cells, 20% FBS is added (20% DMEM). Cells are grown in sterile plastic ware maintained in a 5% CO_2 humidified 37° incubator.

Generation of Stable Retrovirus Packaging Cells for Transduction of Murine HSCs

Day −1: 1 million HEK 293T cells are plated out in the afternoon in a 100-mm plastic dish or flask in 10 ml 10% DMEM.

Day 0: For transfection of cells, combine room temperature DMEM (480 μl; without supplements) and lipid-based transfection reagent (20 μl; e.g. TransIT, Lipofectamine), vortex, and incubate at room temperature for 15 min. It is vital that the manufacturers' instructions be strictly adhered to for each step in this procedure to ensure efficient transfection because mixing and incubation times may vary. Alternately, a calcium phosphate chemical transfection can be performed according to well-established protocols (Anonymous, 2005). In a separate 1.5-ml tube, add the retroviral vector containing a reporter gene (4 μg; e.g., pMIGII), packaging plasmid (4 μg; pEQ.PAM-E), and envelope-encoding plasmid (2 μg; pVSV-G). Dropwise add the transfection mixture to DNA, gently mix, and incubate at room temperature for 15 min. Dropwise add the transfection/DNA mixture to HEK 293T cells, gently rocking the plate before returning it to the incubator at 37° for 24 h.

Day 1: Aspirate media from the HEK 293T cells and continue incubation for 12 h in 10 ml fresh 10% DMEM. Plate out packaging cell line (10^5 GP+E-86 cells) in 10 ml 10% DMEM in a 100-mm plate and incubate at 37° in parallel with the HEK 293T cells for 12 h.

Days 2–4: By use of a 10-ml syringe, remove supernatant media from HEK 293T cells, and pass through a 0.45-μm syringe filter into a sterile plastic tube. Aspirate media from packaging cells and add filtered supernatant from HEK 293T cells. Add polybrene (6 μg/ml final concentration) to packaging cells. Working quickly, add 10 ml of fresh 10% DMEM to HEK 293T cells. Incubate HEK 293T and packaging cells at 37° for a further 12 h. The transduction step must be repeated every 12 h for a minimum of five cycles to achieve high-titer vector production from the packaging cells.

Days 5–6: Allow packaging cells to become confluent, trypsinize, and collect the top 50% GFP$^+$ cells using a fluorescence-activated cell sorter. Packaging cells are grown to confluence and frozen in liquid nitrogen.

Determining the Vector Titer Yield of Retrovirus Packaging Cells for Murine Transductions

Day 0: For retroviral vector titer determination, 2×10^6 packaging cells are plated out in 2 ml 10% DMEM in a 6 well plate and incubated for 24 h at 37°.

Day 1: Incubate NIH-3T3 cells (1×10^4 cells per well, 4 wells per titer) in 1 ml 10% DMEM in a 12-well plate, at least 4–8 h before adding viral supernatant. After the packaging cell incubation is complete, filter supernatant from cells through a 0.45-μm syringe filter into a sterile plastic tube. Add filtered supernatant to NIH-3T3 cells to obtain final dilutions of 0, 1/10, 1/33, and 1/100. Add polybrene (6 μg/ml final concentration) and top up the volume of each well to 2 ml using 10% DMEM. Incubate a further 48–72 h at 37° to allow retroviral vector to transduce NIH-3T3 cells.

Days 3–4: Harvest transduced NIH-3T3 cells by trypsinizing and analyze by flow cytometry to determine the percentage of GFP cells. Titer is taken from the well where the percentage of GFP cells is closest to 50% to ensure it is in the linear range.

Formula for calculation of titer: (% gated GFP) $\times$ (0.01) $\times$ (dilution factor) $\times$ (10^4) with results expressed as transducing units per milliliter. For example, if the well in which 55% of cells are shown to be GFP was from the 1:33 dilution, then the titer would be $55 \times 0.01 \times 33 \times 10^4 = 1.8 \times 10^5$ TU/ml. An adequate titer resulting from this protocol would range between 1 and 2×10^5 based on more than 50 such procedures performed by the authors.

Retrovirus-Mediated Murine HSC Gene Transfer

Day −3: Plate out the retrovirus packaging cell line on 150-mm plates. Allow enough time to culture the packaging cell line to obtain two confluent 150-mm plates (approximately 8×10^6 packaging cells per plate) per five recipient mice by Day 3. All steps throughout the protocol assume the investigator wishes to transduce stem cells for the repopulation of five recipient mice.

Day 0: Weigh the donor mice (5–12 weeks old) to determine the amount of 5-flurouracil (5-FU) required. Make a working solution of 5-FU (10 mg/ml in sterile PBS), with each mouse receiving 0.15 mg/g of body weight. Deliver the appropriate volume of 5-FU by intraperitoneal injection with a 25-gauge needle 48 h before harvest of bone marrow. Because 5-FU is a myelotoxic agent, extreme care must be taken to prevent inadvertent exposure to the operator.

Day 2: Donor bone marrow is obtained by the following protocol: dissect out the femurs and tibiae and remove all surrounding tissue using scissors and paper towel to obtain clean bones. Sterile procedure must be maintained throughout, and tissues should remain moist by dipping in sterile PBS + 2% FBS. Cut both ends off each bone, and insert a 10-ml syringe containing PBS + 2% FBS, with a 21-gauge needle for the femur or a 23-gauge needle for the tibia, into one end of the bone.

Flush bone marrow directly into a 50-ml tube, until the red plug of bone marrow is removed. Repeat until all bone marrow is released from the bones, and resuspend the bone marrow plugs with a 21-gauge needle and a 10-ml syringe.

Day 3: Centrifuge cells at 300g for 10 min at room temperature (RT), decant supernatant, and resuspend thoroughly in 10 ml of 20% DMEM. Remove a 10-μl sample and lyse red blood cells briefly using 10 μl 2% acetic acid solution. Estimate the cell concentration using a Neubauer counting chamber. The total yield of bone marrow cells should be approximately 1–2 × 10^7 per mouse; however, different strains may vary. Plate out bone marrow cells at 6 × 10^7 cells per 150-mm plate, in 30 ml of 20% DMEM, supplemented with IL-3 (20 ng/ml), IL-6 (50 ng/ml), and SCF (50 ng/ml) for 48 h in a 37° incubator.

Day 4: Trypsinize the packaging cell lines and resuspend in 20–50 ml 10% DMEM. Gamma-irradiate the packaging cells at 1200 cGy, wash with 10 ml 20% DMEM, centrifuge, and plate out at 8 × 10^6 cells per 150-mm plate, with two plates per five recipient mice. Plate cells in 19 ml 20% DMEM for 24 h in a 37° incubator.

Day 5: Harvest bone marrow cells from plates by decanting media into sterile 50-ml tubes, then wash and scrape plates using a cell scraper with 15 ml sterile PBS. Ensure the entire surface of the plate has been scraped, decant PBS into the same 50 ml tubes, and wash 5 ml PBS over plates to recover remaining cells. Centrifuge cells at 300g for 10 min at RT, decant supernatant, and resuspend cells in approximately 1 ml of 20% DMEM per five donor mice. Remove a 10-μl sample, lyse red blood cells briefly using 10 μl 2% acetic acid solution, and estimate cell concentration using a Neubauer counting chamber. Resuspend to approximately 2 × 10^7 cells/ml in 20% DMEM. Supplement cell suspension with IL-3 (400 ng/ml), IL-6 (1000 ng/ml), SCF (1000 ng/ml), and protamine sulfate (80 μg/ml), and add 1 ml of mixture to each viral packaging cell plate for 48 h in a 37° incubator. The final volume of 20 ml/plate will contain final concentrations of IL-3 (20 ng/ml), IL-6 (50 ng/ml), SCF (50 ng/ml), and protamine sulfate (4 μg/ml).

Day 7: After 48 h, bone marrow cells are gently harvested from packaging cell plates by washing media over cells and decanting supernatant into a sterile 50-ml tube. Once the media is removed, wash plate with 15 ml sterile PBS, working from top to bottom three times, from different angles, before adding to the media in the 50-ml tube. Centrifuge cells at 300g for 10 min at RT, and decant supernatant. For reconstitution of five mice, add 2.75 ml PBS + 2% FBS supplemented with heparin (20 units/ml) per group, which will allow injection of 0.5 ml per mouse. Remove a 10-μl sample, lyse red blood cells briefly using 10 μl 2% acetic acid solution, and estimate cell concentration using a Neubauer counting chamber. Yield should be at least 4×10^6 cells per recipient mouse. Remove a further 10-μl sample to analyze by flow cytometry for GFP$^+$ cells. The percentage of GFP cells at this stage may be quite low, often only 2–5%, although in some cases, it can be significantly higher. Irradiate mice to achieve myeloablation before injection of gene-modified HSCs. For example, RAG-1$^{-/-}$ achieves myeloablation at 450 cGy, C57BL/6 at 900 cGy, and NOD-SCID at 400 cGy (Holst *et al.*, 2006; Larsen *et al.*, 2006). If mice are not in an SPF/*Helicobacter*–free facility, they should be placed on Sulfatrim water before irradiation and injection for the duration of the experiment. Sulfatrim antibiotic is administered in the drinking water, 7 ml of Sulfatrim per 500 ml H_2O, changed once a week. For injection, cells are drawn up into 3-ml syringes using blunt needles and injected using 27-gauge needles. Each mouse is heated using a lamp, and 0.5 ml is injected through the tail vein.

Generation of Stable Retrovirus Packaging Cells for Transduction of Human HSCs

Day −1: 1 million FLYRD18 cells are plated out overnight in a 100-mm plastic dish or flask in 10 ml 10% DMEM.

Day 0: To prepare the transfection mixture, combine room temperature DMEM (480 μl; without supplements) and lipid-based transfection reagent (20 μl; e.g., Lipofectamine), mix well, and incubate at room temperature for 15 min. It is vital that the manufacturers' instructions be strictly adhered to for each step in this procedure to ensure efficient transfection because mixing and incubation times may vary. Alternately, a calcium phosphate chemical transfection can be performed according to well-established protocols (Anonymous, 2005). In a separate 1.5-ml tube, add retroviral vector (4 μg; e.g., pLNCG). Dropwise add the transfection mixture to DNA, gently mix, and incubate at room temperature for 15 min. Dropwise add the transfection/DNA solution to FLYRD18 cells, gently rocking the plate before returning to the incubator at 37° for 24 h.

Day 1: Aspirate media from FLYRD18 cells and replace with 10 ml 10% DMEM. Incubate cells at 37° for a further 48 h to allow for GFP expression.

Day 3: Individual cells are then sorted using the automated cell deposition unit of a fluorescence-activated cell sorter to deposit high-expressing GFP$^+$ cells into single wells of a 96-well plate. Each well of the 96-well plate contains 5×10^3 untransfected, irradiated FLYRD18 cells (3500 cGy) in 100 μl 10% DMEM to improve clonogenicity. Alternatively single cell clones may be obtained using limited dilation. Incubate plates until wells are approximately 80% confluent.

Days 10–18: When the cells have reached approximately 80% confluence, replace 10% DMEM with 200 μl 10% alamar blue–containing media and incubate for 4 h at 37°. Alamar-blue is a nontoxic fluorometric compound that can be detected using a filter set of 550/590 nm on a Wallac Victor^2 1420 Multilabel Counter. After washing cells with PBS, GFP cells can then be detected with a 485/535-nm filter set.

High-Throughput Analysis of High-Titer Retrovirus Packaging Cells for Human Transductions

Day 0: After analysis of alamarBlue and GFP on days 10–18 previously, the cells are incubated a further 12–24 h in 100 μl 10% DMEM. Plate out 2×10^4 HEK 293T cells per well, in 96-well plates, and incubate for 12–24 h to obtain a confluence of 80% before transduction.

Day 1: Remove (and then replace with fresh 10% DMEM) a 60-μl sample from each well using a multichannel pipette, and place into a 96-well MultiScreen-FL FilterPlate that has been prewashed with PBS (Millipore, Bedford MA). Vacuum-filter the supernatant directly onto HEK 293T target cells and add polybrene (4 μg/ml final concentration).

Day 2: Supernatant is removed from the transduced HEK 293T cells after 12–24 h, and cells are incubated a further 48–72 h before analysis using the Wallac Victor^2 1420 Multilabel Counter to identify wells containing the greatest amount of GFP$^+$ cells. FLYRD18 clones producing the highest titer (having achieved the highest transduction of target HEK 293T cells) are subsequently expanded into 6-well plates before long-term storage in liquid nitrogen.

Determining the Vector Titer Yield of Retrovirus Packaging Cells for Human Transductions

The protocol for the titer of retrovirus packaging cell lines for human transductions is identical to that used for murine transductions, with the single difference being that HT-1080 cells, and not NIH-3T3 cells, are used. Alternately, if an antibiotic-resistance cassette is incorporated in the vector, such as G418 resistance encoded by a neomycin cassette, the following colony forming assay protocol can be followed.

Day 0: Target HT-1080 cells (10^5 cells per 60-mm dish) are incubated for 24 h.

Day 1: The media is removed from the HT-1080 cells, and serial dilutions of the test virus are added together with polybrene (8 μg/ml final concentration) in fresh 10% DMEM. HT-1080 cells are incubated for 24 h.

Day 2: Cells are replated at a density of 2000 cells/100-mm dish in 10% DMEM containing G418 (750 μg/ml).

Day 10: Colonies are stained with Giemsa and scored. Viral titer (colony-forming units [CFU]/ml) is calculated by the following formula:

No. colonies $\times$ virus volume added (ml) $\times$ dilution factor from original HT-1080 cell supernatant.

Summary and Future Directions

The transduction of stem cells using GP+E-86 packaging cells and hematopoietic repopulation of irradiated recipient mice has been used to examine T-cell development in different knockout mouse models, as well as in the study of diabetes, cancer, and stem cell biology. For such experiments, the method described herein using GP+E-86 packaging cells was sufficient, although a number of alterations to the procedure may be required to optimize the transduction and purification of HSCs. The purification of HSCs can be facilitated by magnetic bead depletion of lineage-positive cells, enrichment of Sca1$^+$/cKit$^+$ or CD34$^+$ cells by magnetic- and/ or fluorescence-activated cell sorting (FACS), or sorting of side population cells by Hoechst 33342 staining. When this is combined with FACS purification of GFP cells, repopulation of mice would be restricted to purified transduced cells, resulting in easier interpretation of results. However, preenrichment of transduced cells before reinfusion does not seem to improve rates of gene marking in long-term repopulating studies of non-human primate HSCs (Kiem *et al.*, 2002). Single gene–marked HSCs should be able to repopulate the entire hematopoietic compartment of a mouse provided the animal does not succumb during the period (Camargo *et al.*, 2006; Szilvassy and Cory, 1994). Protection can be afforded during this period by the use of irradiated "compromised" hematopoietic cells to provide short-term support of the blood (Innes *et al.*, 1999). The transduction of stem cells using the FLYRD18 cells could also use these purification methods for human HSCs (Goerner et al., 2001). Furthermore, FLYRD18 supernatants could be collected, filtered, and concentrated by ultracentrifugation, allowing for transduction of stem cells using purified supernatant, rather than coculture.

As alluded to in the introduction, the use of lentiviral vectors, which can enter nondividing cells, and self-inactivating vectors may provide an advantage for many gene therapeutic applications. Self-inactivating lentiviral vectors that use tissue-specific promotors have been tested in mouse HSCs, demonstrating successful long-term expression of human β^A-globin in HSC transplanted mice (Pawliuk et al., 2001). HIV-1–based lentiviral vectors have also been used to correct hemophilia B in mice (Bigger et al., 2006; Waddington et al., 2004). In a nonhuman primate model, hepatocytes have been transduced with HIV-based lentiviral vectors and successfully transplanted into newborn mice, contributing to liver development (Parouchev et al., 2006). In addition to these HIV-derived lentiviral vectors, equine infectious anemia virus (EIAV) lentiviral vectors have been used to transduce both murine and human HSCs (Siapati et al., 2005) to treat Parkinson's disease in rats (Azzouz et al., 2004), as well as to target the nervous system in mice (Mazarakis et al., 2001; Mitrophanous et al., 1999). At present, however, safety and regulatory concerns make it difficult to generate large volumes of lentiviral vector. Lentiviral vectors have now been safely used in the first human clinical studies, but they will continue to be carefully regulated during the foreseeable future.

Injection of stem cells intravenously into mice or humans requires the HSCs to circulate in the blood and migrate through the bone marrow vasculature before engrafting within the marrow environment. Although the natural homing ability of HSCs facilitates this, the frequency of HSCs moving from the blood into the bone marrow is very low. Injection of HSCs directly into the bone marrow has been shown to require approximately 10–15 times fewer HSCs than using intravenous injection, as well as reconstituting mice more rapidly than intravenous techniques (Mazurier et al., 2003; Yahata et al., 2003). Because HSCs numbers are often limiting, this may be a useful technique for HSC repopulation.

As discussed in the introduction, the generation of leukemia in three patients in the X-SCID gene therapy trials is believed to be caused in part by the integration of retroviral DNA into the genome and subsequent increase of the LMO2 transcription factor. Over the past few years, mapping of chromosomal integration sites in vivo for HIV, MLV, and avian sarcoma-leukosis virus has shown different patterns of integrations, suggesting this process is semitargeted rather than exclusively random as had been assumed (Mitchell *et al.*, 2004; Schroder *et al.*, 2002; Wu *et al.*, 2003). Although the integration of viral DNA into the genome can cause detrimental effects, it has also been shown to offer possible selective advantage to HSCs, possibly because of integration at sites with roles in self-renewal or survival (Kustikova *et al.*, 2005). Indeed, it seems that promoter trapping by MLV, whereby the DNA integrates near an active promoter, can occur as frequently as one of every five integrations (De Palma *et al.*, 2005). This process may lead to abnormal and unwanted proliferation of transduced cells. Further understanding of virus biology will enable advances in the safety of retroviral vectors, as well as the potential for targeting integration to specific sites in the genome.

Acknowledgments

We thank Dario Vignali and Bronwyn Green for assistance with the development of these protocols, as well as Marcus Hayward for critical review of this manuscript.

References

Anonymous (2005). Calcium phosphate-mediated transfection of eukaryotic cells. *Nat. Meth.* **2,** 319–320.

Azzouz, M., Ralph, S., Wong, L. F., Day, D., Askham, Z., Barber, R. D., Mitrophanous, K. A., Kingsman, S. M., and Mazarakis, N. D. (2004). Neuroprotection in a rat Parkinson model by GDNF gene therapy using EIAV vector. *Neuroreport* **15,** 985–990.

Barzon, L., Bonaguro, R., Castagliuolo, I., Chilosi, M., Franchin, E., Del Vecchio, C., Giaretta, I., Boscaro, M., and Palu, G. (2003). Gene therapy of thyroid cancer via retrovirally-driven combined expression of human interleukin-2 and herpes simplex virus thymidine kinase. *Eur. J. Endocrinol.* **148,** 73–80.

Battini, J. L., Rasko, J. E., and Miller, A. D. (1999). A human cell-surface receptor for xenotropic and polytropic murine leukemia viruses: Possible role in G protein-coupled signal transduction. *Proc. Natl. Acad. Sci. USA* **96,** 1385–1390.

Bigger, B. W., Siapati, E. K., Mistry, A., Waddington, S. N., Nivsarkar, M. S., Jacobs, L., Perrett, R., Holder, M. V., Ridler, C., Kemball-Cook, G., Ali, R. R., Forbes, S. J., Coutelle, C., Wright, N., Alison, M., Thrasher, A. J., Bonnet, D., and Themis, M. (2006). Permanent partial phenotypic correction and tolerance in a mouse model of hemophilia B by stem cell gene delivery of human factor IX. *Gene. Ther.* **13,** 117–126.

Bonini, C., Ferrari, G., Verzeletti, S., Servida, P., Zappone, E., Ruggieri, L., Ponzoni, M., Rossini, S., Mavilio, F., Traversari, C., and Bordignon, C. (1997). HSV-TK gene transfer into donor lymphocytes for control of allogeneic graft-versus-leukemia. *Science* **276,** 1719–1724.

Burns, J. C., Friedmann, T., Driever, W., Burrascano, M., and Yee, J. K. (1993). Vesicular stomatitis virus G glycoprotein pseudotyped retroviral vectors: Concentration to very high titer and efficient gene transfer into mammalian and nonmammalian cells. *Proc. Natl. Acad. Sci. USA* **90,** 8033–8037.

Camargo, F. D., Chambers, S. M., Drew, E., McNagny, K. M., and Goodell, M. A. (2006). Hematopoietic stem cells do not engraft with absolute efficiencies. *Blood* **107,** 501–7.

Cavazzana-Calvo, M., Hacein-Bey, S., de Saint Basile, G., Gross, F., Yvon, E., Nusbaum, P., Selz, F., Hue, C., Certain, S., Casanova, J. L., Bousso, P., Deist, F. L., and Fischer, A. (2000). Gene therapy of human severe combined immunodeficiency (SCID)-X1 disease. *Science* **288,** 669–672.

Cavazzana-Calvo, M., Lagresle, C., Hacein-Bey-Abina, S., and Fischer, A. (2005). Gene therapy for severe combined immunodeficiency. *Annu. Rev. Med.* **56,** 585–602.

Cosset, F. L., Morling, F. J., Takeuchi, Y., Weiss, R. A., Collins, M. K., and Russell, S. J. (1995a). Retroviral retargeting by envelopes expressing an N-terminal binding domain. *J. Virol.* **69,** 6314–6322.

Cosset, F. L., Takeuchi, Y., Battini, J. L., Weiss, R. A., and Collins, M. K. (1995b). High-titer packaging cells producing recombinant retroviruses resistant to human serum. *J. Virol.* **69,** 7430–7436.

De Palma, M., Montini, E., de Sio, F. R., Benedicenti, F., Gentile, A., Medico, E., and Naldini, L. (2005). Promotor trapping reveals significant differences in integration site selection between MLV and HIV vectors in primary hematopoietic cells. *Blood* **105,** 2307–2315.

Emery, D. W., Yannaki, E., Tubb, J., and Stamatoyannopoulos, G. (2000). A chromatin insulator protects retrovirus vectors from chromosomal position effects. *Proc. Natl. Acad. Sci. USA* **97,** 9150–9155.

Emi, N., Friedmann, T., and Yee, J. K. (1991). Pseudotype formation of murine leukemia virus with the G protein of vesicular stomatitis virus. *J. Virol.* **65,** 1202–1207.

Fischer, A., Hacein-Bey-Abina, S., Lagresle, C., Garrigue, A., and Cavazana-Calvo, M. (2005). [Gene therapy of severe combined immunodeficiency disease: Proof of principle of efficiency and safety issues. Gene therapy, primary immunodeficiencies, retrovirus, lentivirus, genome]. *Bull. Acad. Natl. Med.* **189,** 779–785; discussion 86–88.

Ghattas, I. R., Sanes, J. R., and Majors, J. E. (1991). The encephalomyocarditis virus internal ribosome entry site allows efficient coexpression of two genes from a recombinant provirus in cultured cells and in embryos. *Mol. Cell. Biol.* **11,** 5848–5859.

Goerner, M., Horn, P. A., Peterson, L., Kurre, P., Storb, R., Rasko, J. E., and Kiem, H. P. (2001). Sustained multilineage gene persistence and expression in dogs transplanted with CD34(+) marrow cells transduced by RD114-pseudotype oncoretrovirus vectors. *Blood* **98,** 2065–2070.

Gonin, P., and Gaillard, C. (2004). Gene transfer vector biodistribution: pivotal safety studies in clinical gene therapy development. *Gene. Ther.* **11** (Suppl. 1), S98–S108.

Green, B. J., and Rasko, J. E. (2002). Rapid screening for high-titer retroviral packaging cell lines using an *in situ* fluorescence assay. *Hum. Gene. Ther.* **13,** 1005–1013.

Hacein-Bey-Abina, S., Fischer, A., and Cavazzana-Calvo, M. (2002). Gene therapy of X-linked severe combined immunodeficiency. *Int. J. Hematol.* **76,** 295–298.

Hacein-Bey-Abina, S., Von Kalle, C., Schmidt, M., McCormack, M. P., Wulffraat, N., Leboulch, P., Lim, A., Osborne, C. S., Pawliuk, R., Morillon, E., Sorensen, R., Forster, A., Fraser, P., Cohen, J. I., de Saint Basile, G., Alexander, I., Wintergerst, U., Frebourg, T., Aurias, A., Stoppa-Lyonnet, D., Romana, S., Radford-Weiss, I., Gross, F., Valensi, F.,

Delabesse, E., Macintyre, E., Sigaux, F., Soulier, J., Leiva, L. E., Wissler, M., Prinz, C., Rabbitts, T. H., Le Deist, F., Fischer, A., and Cavazzana-Calvo, M. (2003). LMO2-associated clonal T cell proliferation in two patients after gene therapy for SCID-X1. *Science* **302**, 415–419.

Holst, J., Vignali, K. M., Burton, A. R., and Vignali, D. A. (2006). Rapid analysis of T-cell selection *in vivo* using T cell-receptor retrogenic mice. *Nat. Methods* **3**, 191–197.

Innes, K. M., Szilvassy, S. J., Davidson, H. E., Gibson, L., Adams, J. M., and Cory, S. (1999). Retroviral transduction of enriched hematopoietic stem cells allows lifelong Bcl-2 expression in multiple lineages but does not perturb hematopoiesis. *Exp. Hematol.* **27**, 75–87.

Kiem, H. P., Rasko, J. E., Morris, J., Peterson, L., Kurre, P., and Andrews, R. G. (2002). *Ex vivo* selection for oncoretrovirally transduced green fluorescent protein-expressing CD34-enriched cells increases short-term engraftment of transduced cells in baboons. *Hum. Gene. Ther.* **13**, 891–899.

Kun, L. E., Gajjar, A., Muhlbauer, M., Heideman, R. L., Sanford, R., Brenner, M., Walter, A., Langston, J., Jenkins, J., and Facchini, S. (1995). Stereotactic injection of herpes simplex thymidine kinase vector producer cells (PA317-G1Tk1SvNa.7) and intravenous ganciclo-vir for the treatment of progressive or recurrent primary supratentorial pediatric malignant brain tumors. *Hum. Gene. Ther.* **6**, 1231–1255.

Kustikova, O., Fehse, B., Modlich, U., Yang, M., Dullmann, J., Kamino, K., von Neuhoff, N., Schlegelberger, B., Li, Z., and Baum, C. (2005). Clonal dominance of hematopoietic stem cells triggered by retroviral gene marking. *Science* **308**, 1171–1174.

Larsen, S. R., Kingham, J. A., Hayward, M. D., and Rasko, J. E. (2006). Damage to incisors after nonmyeloablative total body irradiation may complicate NOD/SCID models of hemopoietic stem cell transplantation. *Comp. Med.* **56**, 209–214.

Markowitz, D., Goff, S., and Bank, A. (1988). A safe packaging line for gene transfer: Separating viral genes on two different plasmids. *J. Virol.* **62**, 1120–1124.

Maurice, M., Mazur, S., Bullough, F. J., Salvetti, A., Collins, M. K., Russell, S. J., and Cosset, F. L. (1999). Efficient gene delivery to quiescent interleukin-2 (IL-2)-dependent cells by murine leukemia virus-derived vectors harboring IL-2 chimeric envelope glycoproteins. *Blood* **94**, 401–410.

Mazarakis, N. D., Azzouz, M., Rohll, J. B., Ellard, F. M., Wilkes, F. J., Olsen, A. L., Carter, E. E., Barber, R. D., Baban, D. F., Kingsman, S. M., Kingsman, A. J., O'Malley, K., and Mitrophanous, K. A. (2001). Rabies virus glycoprotein pseudotyping of lentiviral vectors enables retrograde axonal transport and access to the nervous system after peripheral delivery. *Hum. Mol. Genet.* **10**, 2109–2121.

Mazurier, F., Doedens, M., Gan, O. I., and Dick, J. E. (2003). Rapid myeloerythroid repopulation after intrafemoral transplantation of NOD-SCID mice reveals a new class of human stem cells. *Nat. Med.* **9**, 959–963.

Miller, A. D., and Buttimore, C. (1986). Redesign of retrovirus packaging cell lines to avoid recombination leading to helper virus production. *Mol. Cell. Biol.* **6**, 2895–2902.

Miller, A. D., Garcia, J. V., von Suhr, N., Lynch, C. M., Wilson, C., and Eiden, M. V. (1991). Construction and properties of retrovirus packaging cells based on gibbon ape leukemia virus. *J. Virol.* **65**, 2220–2224.

Miller, A. D., and Rosman, G. J. (1989). Improved retroviral vectors for gene transfer and expression. *Biotechniques* **7**, 980–982, 84–86, 89–90.

Miller, D. G., Edwards, R. H., and Miller, A. D. (1994). Cloning of the cellular receptor for amphotropic murine retroviruses reveals homology to that for gibbon ape leukemia virus. *Proc. Natl. Acad. Sci. USA* **91**, 78–82.

Mitchell, R. S., Beitzel, B. F., Schroder, A. R., Shinn, P., Chen, H., Berry, C. C., Ecker, J. R., and Bushman, F. D. (2004). Retroviral DNA integration: ASLV, HIV, and MLV show distinct target site preferences. *PLoS Biol.* **2,** E234.

Mitrophanous, K., Yoon, S., Rohll, J., Patil, D., Wilkes, F., Kim, V., Kingsman, S., Kingsman, A., and Mazarakis, N. (1999). Stable gene transfer to the nervous system using a non-primate lentiviral vector. *Gene. Ther.* **6,** 1808–1818.

Modlich, U., Bohne, J., Schmidt, M., von Kalle, C., Knoss, S., Schambach, A., and Baum, C. (2006). Cell-culture assays reveal the importance of retroviral vector design for insertional genotoxicity. *Blood* **108,** 2545–2553.

Naldini, L., Blomer, U., Gallay, P., Ory, D., Mulligan, R., Gage, F. H., Verma, I. M., and Trono, D. (1996). *In vivo* gene delivery and stable transduction of nondividing cells by a lentiviral vector. *Science* **272,** 263–267.

Neff, T., Horn, P. A., Peterson, L. J., Thomasson, B. M., Thompson, J., Williams, D. A., Schmidt, M., Georges, G. E., von Kalle, C., and Kiem, H. P. (2003). Methylguanine methyltransferase-mediated *in vivo* selection and chemoprotection of allogeneic stem cells in a large-animal model. *J. Clin. Invest.* **112,** 1581–1588.

Ott, M. G., Schmidt, M., Schwarzwaelder, K., Stein, S., Siler, U., Koehl, U., Glimm, H., Kuhlcke, K., Schilz, A., Kunkel, H., Naundorf, S., Brinkmann, A., Deichmann, A., Fischer, M., Ball, C., Pilz, I., Dunbar, C., Du, Y., Jenkins, N. A., Copeland, N. G., Luthi, U., Hassan, M., Thrasher, A. J., Hoelzer, D., von Kalle, C., Seger, R., and Grez, M. (2006). Correction of X-linked chronic granulomatous disease by gene therapy, augmented by insertional activation of MDS1-EVI1, PRDM16 or SETBP1. *Nat. Med.* **12,** 401–409.

Parouchev, A., Nguyen, T. H., Dagher, I., Mainot, S., Groyer-Picard, M. T., Branger, J., Gonin, P., Di Santo, J., Franco, D., Gras, G., and Weber, A. (2006). Efficient *ex vivo* gene transfer into non-human primate hepatocytes using HIV-1 derived lentiviral vectors. *J. Hepatol.* **45,** 99–107.

Pawliuk, R., Westerman, K. A., Fabry, M. E., Payen, E., Tighe, R., Bouhassira, E. E., Acharya, S. A., Ellis, J., London, I. M., Eaves, C. J., Humphries, R. K., Beuzard, Y., Nagel, R. L., and Leboulch, P. (2001). Correction of sickle cell disease in transgenic mouse models by gene therapy. *Science* **294,** 2368–2371.

Pear, W. S., Nolan, G. P., Scott, M. L., and Baltimore, D. (1993). Production of high-titer helper-free retroviruses by transient transfection. *Proc. Natl. Acad. Sci. USA* **90,** 8392–8396.

Rasko, J. E., Battini, J. L., Gottschalk, R. J., Mazo, I., and Miller, A. D. (1999). The RD114/simian type D retrovirus receptor is a neutral amino acid transporter. *Proc. Natl. Acad. Sci. USA* **96,** 2129–2134.

Rasko, J. E. J. (1999). Reporters of gene expression: Autofluorescent proteins. John Wiley and Sons.

Schroder, A. R., Shinn, P., Chen, H., Berry, C., Ecker, J. R., and Bushman, F. (2002). HIV-1 integration in the human genome favors active genes and local hotspots. *Cell* **110,** 521–529.

Siapati, E. K., Bigger, B. W., Miskin, J., Chipchase, D., Parsley, K. L., Mitrophanous, K., Themis, M., Thrasher, A. J., and Bonnet, D. (2005). Comparison of HIV- and EIAV-based vectors on their efficiency in transducing murine and human hematopoietic repopulating cells. *Mol. Ther.* **12,** 537–546.

Szilvassy, S. J., and Cory, S. (1994). Efficient retroviral gene transfer to purified long-term repopulating hematopoietic stem cells. *Blood* **84,** 74–83.

Szymczak, A. L., Workman, C. J., Wang, Y., Vignali, K. M., Dilioglou, S., Vanin, E. F., and Vignali, D. A. (2004). Correction of multi-gene deficiency *in vivo* using a single 'self-cleaving' 2A peptide-based retroviral vector. *Nat. Biotechnol.* **22,** 589–594.

Uchiyama, T., Kumaki, S., Ishikawa, Y., Onodera, M., Sato, M., Du, W., Sasahara, Y., Tanaka, N., Sugamura, K., and Tsuchiya, S. (2006). Application of HSVtk suicide gene to X-SCID gene therapy: Ganciclovir treatment offsets gene corrected X-SCID B cells. *Biochem. Biophys. Res. Commun.* **341,** 391–398.

Waddington, S. N., Nivsarkar, M. S., Mistry, A. R., Buckley, S. M., Kemball-Cook, G., Mosley, K. L., Mitrophanous, K., Radcliffe, P., Holder, M. V., Brittan, M., Georgiadis, A., Al-Allaf, F., Bigger, B. W., Gregory, L. G., Cook, H. T., Ali, R. R., Thrasher, A., Tuddenham, E. G., Themis, M., and Coutelle, C. (2004). Permanent phenotypic correction of hemophilia B in immunocompetent mice by prenatal gene therapy. *Blood* **104,** 2714–2721.

Woods, N. B., Bottero, V., Schmidt, M., von Kalle, C., and Verma, I. M. (2006). Gene therapy: Therapeutic gene causing lymphoma. *Nature* **440,** 1123.

Wu, X., Li, Y., Crise, B., and Burgess, S. M. (2003). Transcription start regions in the human genome are favored targets for MLV integration. *Science* **300,** 1749–1751.

Yahata, T., Ando, K., Sato, T., Miyatake, H., Nakamura, Y., Muguruma, Y., Kato, S., and Hotta, T. (2003). A highly sensitive strategy for SCID-repopulating cell assay by direct injection of primitive human hematopoietic cells into NOD/SCID mice bone marrow. *Blood* **101,** 2905–2913.

Yi, Y., Hahm, S. H., and Lee, K. H. (2005). Retroviral gene therapy: safety issues and possible solutions. *Curr. Gene. Ther.* **5,** 25–35.

Zielske, S. P., Reese, J. S., Lingas, K. T., Donze, J. R., and Gerson, S. L. (2003). *In vivo* selection of MGMT(P140K) lentivirus-transduced human NOD/SCID re-populating cells without pretransplant irradiation conditioning. *J. Clin. Invest.* **112,** 1561–1570.

Zufferey, R., Dull, T., Mandel, R. J., Bukovsky, A., Quiroz, D., Naldini, L., and Trono, D. (1998). Self-inactivating lentivirus vector for safe and efficient *in vivo* gene delivery. *J. Virol.* **72,** 9873–9880.

[7] Engineering Embryonic Stem Cells with Recombinase Systems

By Frank Schnütgen, A. Francis Stewart,
Harald von Melchner, and Konstantinos Anastassiadis

Abstract

The combined use of site-specific recombination and gene targeting or trapping in embryonic stem cells (ESCs) has resulted in the emergence of technologies that enable the induction of mouse mutations in a prespecified temporal and spatially restricted manner. Their large-scale implementation by several international mouse mutagenesis programs will lead to the assembly of a library of ES cell lines harboring conditional mutations in every single gene of the mouse genome. In anticipation of this unprecedented

METHODS IN ENZYMOLOGY, VOL. 420
Copyright 2006, Elsevier Inc. All rights reserved.

0076-6879/06 $35.00
DOI: 10.1016/S0076-6879(06)20007-7

resource, this chapter will focus on site-specific recombination strategies and issues pertinent to ESCs and mice. The upcoming ESC resource and the increasing sophistication of site-specific recombination technologies will greatly assist the functional annotation of the human genome and the animal modeling of human disease.

Introduction

The combined use of site-specific recombination and gene targeting or trapping in mouse embryonic stem ESCs has resulted in the emergence of a precise technology to manipulate the mouse genome.

The preeminent application of this technology is conditional mutagenesis, which permits the controlled mutagenesis of specific genes in the mouse or in cells in culture for functional studies. Because conditional mutagenesis presents an unrivalled accuracy for mammalian functional studies, international efforts are underway to generate conditional alleles for every protein-coding gene in the mouse genome. On the basis of the development of high-throughput methods, this task is now feasible, and international cooperation has been initiated to build a complete set of mutated ESC lines as a readily available resource (Austin *et al.*, 2004; Auwerx *et al.*, 2004). Because this resource will contain alleles that can be modified in various ways by site-specific recombination, here we will focus on issues and methods relevant to the generation and use of site-specific recombination strategies in ESCs and mice.

Site-Specific Recombination

Site-specific recombinases (SSRs) mediate DNA rearrangements by breaking and joining DNA molecules at two specific sites, termed *recombination targets* (RTs). These enzymes fall into two main classes termed *tyrosine* or *serine recombinases* according to the amino acid that becomes transiently covalently linked to DNA during recombination. They have been found in diverse prokaryotes and lower eukaryotes; however, only three so far have been shown to work efficiently in ESCs. These are the tyrosine recombinases, Cre and FLPe, and the large serine recombinase, ΦC31 integrase. We will first consider the characteristics of these proteins and their expression for engineering, followed by characteristics of their RTs.

Cre and FLPe

Cre and FLPe are presently the recombinases most widely used in ESCs. Cre recombinase was found in the *E. coli* P1 phage (Sternberg *et al.*, 1986). In contrast to several other prokaryotic enzymes that have been used in mammalian cells, the prokaryotic codon bias present in the original Cre coding region seems to be satisfactory for expression in mammalian cells. Altering the codon bias from prokaryotic to mammalian to create a version termed iCre only slightly improved expression levels and performance (Shimshek *et al.*, 2002). Therefore, most applied studies are still performed with the original prokaryotic coding sequence. For Cre recombination in ESCs, the early expression vector generated by Gu *et al.* (1993), MC1Cre, routinely delivers high levels of recombination (>25%) on transient expression in ESCs. Consequently, it is still widely used. However, for difficult recombination exercises or recombination in mice (see later), more potent expression vectors have been used, such as pOG231 (O'Gorman *et al.*, 1997; Zheng *et al.*, 2000), pBS185 (Li *et al.*, 1996), pBS500 (Schlake *et al.*, 1999), pICCre (Madsen *et al.*, 1999), and pCAGGSCre (Okabe *et al.*, 1997).

FLP recombinase was found in the yeast 2-micron circle. Not surprisingly this enzyme's optimum temperature is 30°, and it is quite inefficient at 37° (Buchholz *et al.*, 1996). Therefore, molecular evolution was applied to develop an enzyme, termed FLPe, with a better optimum temperature (Buchholz *et al.*, 1998). However, FLPe is still significantly less efficient than Cre as evaluated by transient expression in ESCs. It is, therefore, important to use the best FLPe expression vector, pCAGGS-FLPe-IRES-puro (Schaft *et al.*, 2001), for transient expression experiments. Even with this vector, no one has yet achieved more than 10% recombination in ESCs for any allele. Consequently, this vector was designed to also express puromycin resistance, which can be used to enhance recombination frequencies by transient selection pressure (see later) or stable selection in difficult cases. Both Cre and FLPe are relatively small enzymes that seem to be able to enter the mammalian nucleus. Although Cre has its own weak, cryptic, nuclear localization signal (nls) (Le *et al.*, 1999), addition of an nls to FLPe increases the efficiency of recombination about threefold (Schaft *et al.*, 2001).

For experiments in mice, it is usually advisable to establish a mouse line from the engineered ESC as soon as possible because germ-line transmission can be compromised by multiple handling of the cells. This is particularly important for ESCs derived from the C57BL/6 strain, which are less robust in tissue culture than ESCs derived from other strains, such as 129Sv. Consequently, two methods for site-specific recombination in the germ line have been developed, which avoid ESC handling. First, recombination can be induced in the zygote by injection of an expression plasmid. For pCAGGS-FLPe, recombination in one third of surviving zygotes has been reported (Schaft *et al.*, 2001). Second, recombination can be induced by crossing to a "deleter" mouse line, which expresses either Cre or FLPe in the germ line so that the progeny of the cross carry the recombination event. Deleters for both Cre and FLPe work perfectly for small events (<3 kb). Some Cre deleter strains possibly express dangerously high levels of the enzyme, which provoke unwanted mutagenesis by mediating recombination between cryptic RTs in the genome (Loonstra *et al.*, 2001; Schmidt *et al.*, 2000). In the absence of a systematic study of Cre deleters, we can only comment that the numerous reported successes with Cre recombination in mice indicate that the window between adequate and excessive levels of Cre expression is rather wide.

Two FLPe deleter lines have been published thus far, and both work very well (Farley *et al.*, 2000; Rodriguez *et al.*, 2000). The first of these is a β-actin FLPe transgenic (Rodriguez *et al.*, 2000), which seems to express FLPe more strongly than the second, which is a ROSA26 FLPe knock-in (Farley *et al.*, 2000). With the β-actin FLPe deleter, in addition to deletion of small cassettes in all expected progeny, we have observed deletion of a 150-kb interval in nearly all expected progeny (G. Testa, K. Anastassiadis, and A. Francis Stewart, unpublished). It, therefore, seems that the FLPe in the mouse performs better than expected from transient expression experiments in ESCs.

The efficiency difference between Cre and FLPe provokes a simple consequence. Cre is the enzyme of choice for demanding applications, such as conditional mutagenesis or long-distance chromosomal engineering, whereas FLPe is used for simpler tasks, such as removal of selectable cassettes.

For conditional mutagenesis, the recombination event needs to be spatially and/or temporally regulated. Spatial regulation is achieved by expressing Cre recombinase in a cell type–specific manner. Consequently, recombination only occurs in those cells that express Cre. A variety of mice lines have been developed that express Cre in cell type–specific patterns. Information regarding these lines is available from the CreXMice database assembled by Andras Nagy (http://www.mshri.on.ca/nagy/). It is worth mentioning again that the use of Cre recombinase presents some potential risk, which entails careful controls. The interested reader may wish to consider a recent case involving cell type–specific expression of Cre (Lee *et al.*, 2005).

The most popular method for temporal regulation of recombination is based on expression of the SSR fused to a steroid receptor ligand-binding domain (LBD; Logie and Stewart [1995]). In the absence of ligand binding to the LBD, the fusion protein is cytoplasmic. Binding of a ligand triggers recombination, because it permits translocation to the nucleus. Consequently, SSR–LBD constructs should not contain a nuclear localization signal added to the SSR, because this partially circumvents regulation and increases recombination before ligand activation. In addition to temporal control, the SSR–LBD strategy reduces the chances of unwanted mutagenesis by limiting the activity of the SSR to the experimental need. The most popular application of the SSR–LBD strategy in the mouse uses the fusion of a mutated estrogen receptor LBD to Cre, called CreER(T2), because the mutated ER(T2) LBD is insensitive to endogenous estrogens yet activatable by the synthetic estrogen antagonist, 4-hydroxytamoxifen (Feil *et al.*, 1997). The CreER(T2) fusion protein is superior to the earlier version CreERT (Danielian *et al.*, 1998; Feil *et al.*, 1996; Schwenk *et al.*, 1998) because it requires lower concentrations of 4-hydroxytamoxifen for activation (Feil *et al.*, 1997). It should be noted that the actual ligand is 4-hydroxytamoxifen; however, tamoxifen, which is cheaper, can be used *in vivo* because it is rapidly metabolized in the liver to the 4-hydroxy form. Experiments with cells in culture must use 4-hydroxytamoxifen. Commercially available 4-hydroxytamoxifen is an equal mixture of two enantiomers, only one of which is active. Although pure preparations of each enantiomer can be obtained at considerable expense, no benefit to experiments with cultured cells was observed (A. Stewart, unpublished). Several other SSR-mutant LBD fusions have been described, such as Cre-PR (Wunderlich *et al.*, 2001); however, none have yet emerged with good properties to match the CreER(T2).

Conditional mutagenesis has also been reported using tetracycline regulation of Cre transgene expression (Saam and Gordon, 1999). Possibly because the tetracycline system is more complicated to establish, or still entails certain unpredictabilities, this approach for conditional mutagenesis has not found widespread application. However, the fact that synthetic steroids like tamoxifen are not neutral ligands in mammalian cells, whereas tetracycline is, recommends further work with tetracycline and other neutral ligand strategies (Cronin *et al.*, 2001). This point is particularly relevant for conditional mutagenesis during differentiation studies with ESCs in culture. Whereas treatment of ESC with either 4-hydroxytamoxifen, dexamethasone, RU486, or mibolerone for 5 days in normal LIF culture did not noticeably promote differentiation or loss of germ line transmission (K. Vintersten, F. van der Hoeven, and A. Stewart, unpublished), the prominent roles that steroid hormones play in ESC differentiation protocols make it unlikely that these ligands can be used without consequence. Similarly, the use of synthetic steroids to induce conditional mutagenesis *in utero* is possible but problematic (Danielian *et al.*, 1998). Therefore, the development of a tetracycline, or similar, strategy to avoid steroid ligand use will be particularly relevant for studies *in utero* or with ESCs *in vitro* (Mao *et al.*, 2005).

Other Tyrosine Recombinases

Two other tyrosine recombinases, R and Kw, have been examined for eukaryotic genetic engineering applications (Araki *et al.*, 1992; Ringrose *et al.*, 1997). Both originate from variations of the 2-micron circle found in divergent yeasts. Although both recognize distinct sequences, they share several features with FLP, including reduced efficiencies at 37°. Recently a search for Cre-like enzymes among P1 phages uncovered a new candidate, Dre, which could be the long-sought-after tool that works as well as Cre (Sauer and McDermott, 2004).

Large Serine Recombinases

Until the discovery of an unexpected subset of the serine recombinases, termed the large serine recombinases (Smith and Thorpe, 2002), it had been assumed that serine recombinases were unlikely to be useful for genetic engineering. ΦC31 was the first large serine recombinase described (Thorpe and Smith, 1998) and has subsequently been used in mammalian cells (Andreas *et al.*, 2002; Belteki *et al.*, 2003; Olivares *et al.*, 2002). However, it is still not clear how useful the ΦC31 and other large serine recombinases will prove to be nor how best they may be used.

Designing Substrates for Site-Specific Recombination

On expression, the SSR acts on two, or more, recombinase target sites (RTs) that have been introduced into the genome. Designing how the RTs are deployed in the genome is the first step. The design choices are influenced by the objective and also by certain constraints that affect the efficiency of recombination.

For both tyrosine and large serine recombinases, the site of recombination is a short crossover region of hybrid DNA composed of one strand from each of the substrate RTs. Because the recombination product must have complementarity in the crossover regions, and because none of the RTs usually used for genetic engineering are palindromic in the hybrid region, it follows that RTs have a directionality.

Characteristics of loxP and FRTs

In general, tyrosine recombinases have RTs that are centered on a palindromic recombinase–binding site, which flanks the recombination site. For FLP and Cre, these minimal RTs are termed *FRT* and *loxP*, respectively (Fig. 1A). They are both composed of inverted 13-bp binding sites flanking an 8-bp spacer, which includes the 8-bp or 6-bp hybrid region. For FLP and other 2-micron recombinases, the minimal RT is usually accompanied by an additional 13-bp binding site. This extra binding site seems to convey only a very moderate effect for genetic engineering (Ringrose *et al.*, 1999) and is usually

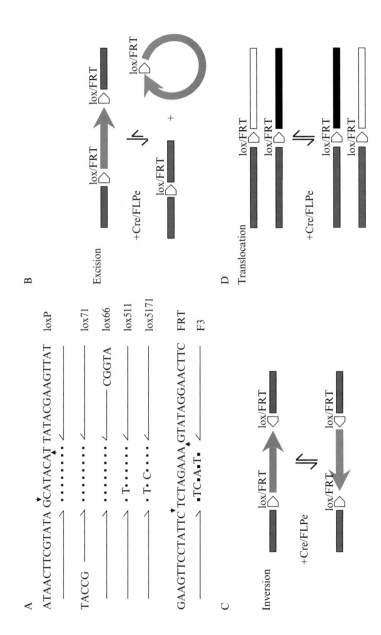

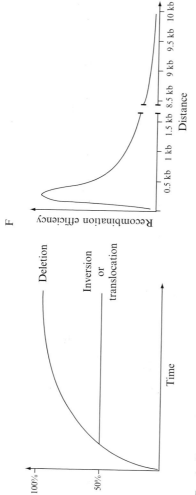

FIG. 1. Characteristics of Cre and FLP site-specific recombination substrates. (A) Cre or FLP recombinations targets (RTs) known as loxP or FRT, respectively, are depicted along with several useful variations. The 13-bp inverted binding sites are illustrated by inverted arrows flanking the spacer sequences, which contain the region of recombination. The recombination region is denoted by arrowheads above and below the sequence at each end of the spacer. For the variant RTs, only the sequence differences are shown. (B) Excision recombination between two directly repeated RTs. The excised DNA is released as a covalent circle. Reintegration is possible but disfavored. (C) Inversions occur when RTs are arranged as indirect repeats. (D) Recombination between RTs on different molecules results in a reciprocal translocation. The orientation of the translocated fragments is dictated by the orientation of the RTs. White pentagons indicate RTs and their orientation. Note that all three reactions approach 50% with equivalent kinetics. Thereafter, excisions approach 100%, whereas inversions and translocations equilibrate at 50%. See Logie and Stewart, 1995, for supporting data. (F) Site-specific recombination frequency as a product of the distance between two RTs, as determined for naked DNA (Ringrose et al., 1999). Note the maximum recombination efficiency at 400 bps.

not used. Recombination is usually occurs between two identical RTs and is inherently reversible (Ennifar *et al.*, 2003; van Duyne, 2001).

Recombination will still occur between RTs that carry limited sequence variations, however, the sequence in the crossover regions must be identical. Consequently, two classes of sequence variations can be defined.

First, the binding sites can be altered, which will reduce the binding affinity of the recombinase for the binding site. Because binding of both FLP and Cre to their palindromic RTs is cooperative (Ringrose *et al.*, 1998), it is possible to mutate one half site without greatly affecting recombination efficiency as long as the other half site remains wild type. The compensatory effect of cooperativity has been used to impose asymmetry on Cre recombination (Albert *et al.*, 1995; Araki *et al.*, 1997). In this strategy, two mutant loxP sites, termed *lox66* and *lox71*, carry mutations in the right or left 13-bp binding sites, respectively (Fig. 1A). After recombination, one product RT will contain both wild-type binding half sites, and the other will contain both mutant binding half sites (Fig. 2A). The double-mutant product RT will have a greatly reduced ability to bind Cre; hence, the reverse recombination reaction will be disfavored. Second, the crossover region in the spacer can be altered. Because the sequence in the crossover region must be identical for productive recombination, a variety of "heterotypic" RTs have been generated, which permit different recombination events directed by one recombinase. Intensive work on heterotypic lox sites has revealed that the loxP crossover region cannot be freely mutated, and only certain mutations are possible (Langer *et al.*, 2002; Lee and Saito, 1998). Early work with heterotypic lox sites used singly mutated crossover regions; for example, lox511 (Fig. 1A; Lauth *et al.*, 2000).

However, a low but significant frequency of recombination between loxP and lox511 sites has been observed, such that doubly mutated lox sites, such as lox5171 or 2272, are now preferred (Fig. 1A; Kolb, 2001; Lauth *et al.*, 2002). Work on the FRT crossover region indicates that it is more freely mutatable than loxP and is mainly constrained by the GC content of the 8-bp crossover region (Umlauf and Cox, 1988). Increasing the GC content decreased recombination efficiency. The increased mutability of the FRT compared with loxP correlates with the looser synapse implicit in an 8-bp compared with a 6-bp crossover region, as revealed by the crystal structure (Chen and Rice, 2003; Chen *et al.*, 2000). The most commonly used heterotypic FRT is termed *F3* (Fig. 1A; Baer and Bode, 2001; Schlake and Bode, 1994).

When two RTs are placed in a DNA molecule so that their spacers are arranged as direct repeats, the DNA interval between the RTs is excised by the appropriate recombinase and released as a covalent circle (Fig. 1B). Because the reactions are inherently reversible, the covalent circle can

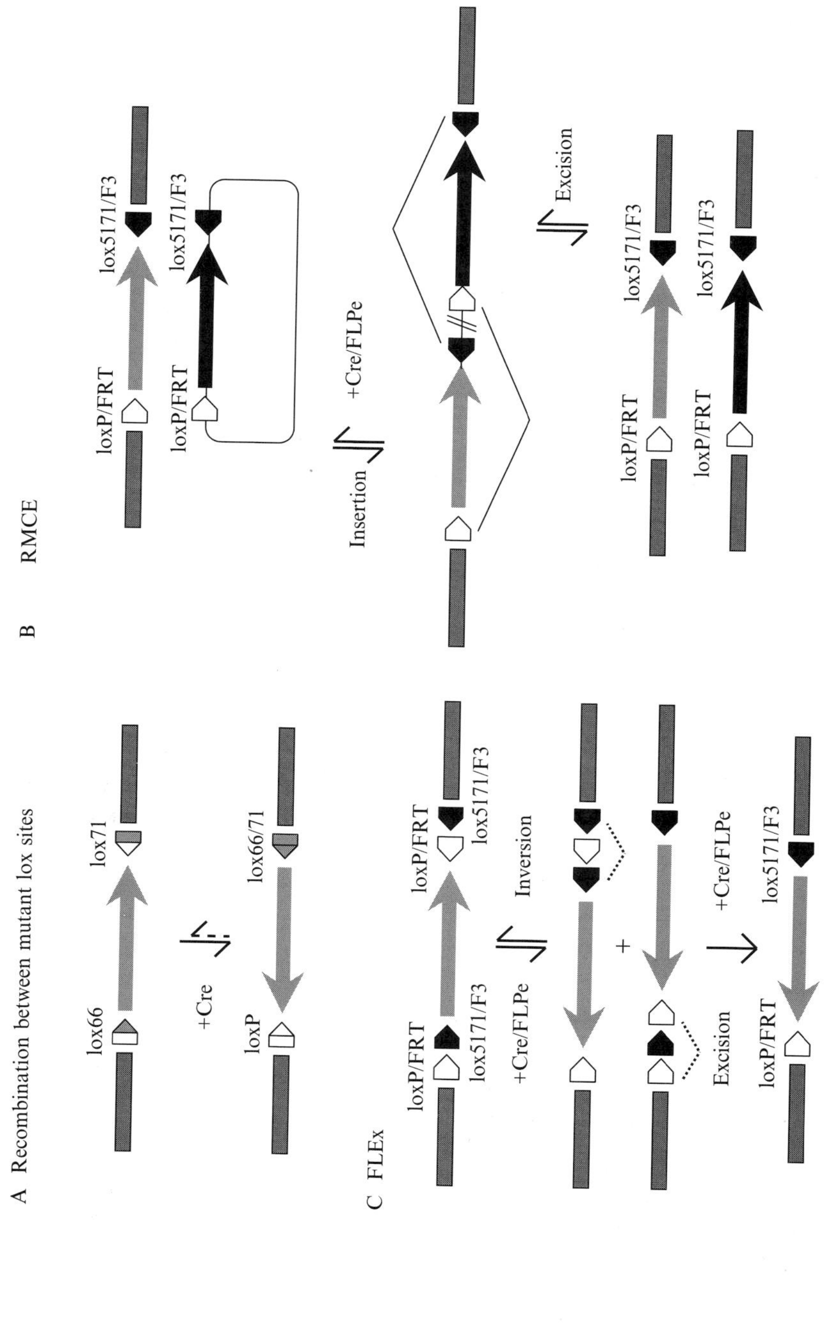

A Recombination between mutant lox sites
lox66
lox71
+Cre
loxP
lox66/71
B RMCE
loxP/FRT
lox5171/F3
loxP/FRT
lox5171/F3
Insertion
+Cre/FLPe
Excision
loxP/FRT
lox5171/F3
loxP/FRT
lox5171/F3
C FLEx
loxP/FRT
lox5171/F3
loxP/FRT
lox5171/F3
+Cre/FLPe
Inversion
+
Excision
+Cre/FLPe
loxP/FRT
lox5171/F3

reintegrate into the site from which it was excised. However, the intramolecular excision reaction is favored over the intermolecular integration reaction, because the two RTs can be separated by an infinite distance during intermolecular recombination but cannot separate by more than the distance between them when on the same DNA molecule.

Furthermore, in replicating cells, the excised circles are progressively diluted with each cell division, because they are not replicated, whereas the chromosomal excision product is (Logie and Stewart, 1995). When two RTs are placed in a DNA molecule so that their spacers are arranged as indirect repeats, recombination results in the inversion of the DNA interval between the two RTs. Because the reaction is reversible, the end product of recombination will be 50% in one orientation and 50% in the other, with an ongoing frequency of inversion if the recombinase continues to act (Fig. 1C). Finally, when RTs are placed in two different linear DNA molecules, a translocation occurs in which orientation is dictated by the direction of the spacers (Fig. 1D). Again, reversibility imposes an end product comprising a 50:50 mixture of the untranslocated and translocated molecules. The expected kinetics for these three reactions is depicted in Fig. 1E.

In addition to these three basic ways to deploy RTs, several more complicated designs have been described. Most notable is the use of pairs of RTs on two DNA molecules. Usually, this deployment involves a heterotypic RT pair and is the basis for recombinase mediated cassette exchange (RMCE) (Fig. 2B; Schlake and Bode, 1994). RMCE can also be based on two pairs of inverted homotypic RTs (Feng *et al.*, 1999). Also notable is the deployment of interwoven heterotypic RTs in the FlEx (flip excision) strategy (Fig. 2C; Schnütgen *et al.*, 2003). These applications are explored in more detail later.

FIG. 2. Directional recombination using Cre and FLP. (A) Inversion between mutant lox66 and lox71 generates a wild-type loxP site and a double mutant lox66/lox71 site that cannot recombine. (B) Recombinase-mediated cassette exchange (RMCE). Intermolecular recombination occurs between two different (heterotypic) RTs, here shown as wild-type (white pentagons) and mutant (black pentagons). Intramolecular recombination between heterotypic RTs is not possible. The RTs flank the exchange cassettes on a linear recipient molecule (in gray) and on a circular donor molecule (in black). The insertion of the donor cassette is followed by the excision of the recipient's cassette (gray) in 50% of cases. (C) Flip-excision (FLEx). Inversion of the RT flanked fragment occurs either at wild-type (white pentagons) or mutant (black pentagons) RTs. After either inversion, pairs of homotypic RTs in direct orientation flank a heterotypic RT. Excision between the directly repeated homotypic RTs excises the heterotypic RT, thus locking the recombination product. The final product is flanked by heterotypic RTs that cannot recombine.

Factors Affecting Cre and FLPe Recombination

After integration into a genome, the rate at which two RTs recombine in a population of cells is influenced by several factors, including:

1. The levels of active recombinase. Studies in ESCs using cell permeable Cre protein have shown that the recombination rate between two RTs inserted into the genome directly correlates with the amount of added enzyme. At high concentrations, recombination proceeds very quickly and is complete within a few hours (Peitz et al., 2002).

2. The physical distance between the two RTs. Site-specific recombination depends on random collision between two RTs. When the two RTs are positioned on the same naked DNA molecule, the rate of random collision is determined by the inherent flexibility of DNA, known as the *persistence length*, which is 50 nm (Ringrose et al., 1999). This is an inherent property of DNA as a polymer, which yields maximal random collision frequencies between two sites 400 bp apart. Hence, maximum recombination rates between two RTs are observed at a distance of 400 bp. Increased distance leads to a predictable and asymptotic decrease in recombination frequencies, whereas two RTs cannot randomly collide when the distance is too short (less than approximately 120 bp) because of the inherent stiffness of DNA (Fig. 1F; Ringrose et al., 1999).

3. The position of the RTs within chromosomes. DNA in cells is not naked but embedded in chromatin. Chromatin is not a uniform polymer but includes fundamental regional variations such as hetero-or euchromatin, as well as local, nucleosomal, specific variations and probably distinct local tertiary structures. These variations produce an influence of chromatin known as *position effect*, which has been reported to influence the recombination efficiency between two RTs (Vooijs et al., 2001). However, it is still unclear to what extent the chromatin environment affects recombination. The influence of variables such as gene expression levels, whether an RT is in a transcribed region, whether the two RTs are separated by a chromatin boundary, and many other considerations all remain unresolved. Nevertheless, the relationship between distance and recombination frequencies in active chromatin has been observed to conform to polymer predictions, albeit with an unexpected decrease of the persistence length to 25 nm (Ringrose et al., 1999).

Although the absence of understanding of position effects makes predictable design of recombination substrates impossible at this stage, the best guideline for design involves placing the RTs as close to each other as practically possible because increased distance will decrease the rate of collision between the RTs, which is the rate-limiting step (Ringrose et al., 1998).

Characteristics of ΦC31 Recombination

In principle, the preceding considerations for Cre and FLPe also apply to the large serine recombinases. However, the serine recombinases use a fundamentally different recombination mechanism (Oram *et al.*, 1995), which may impose a limitation on how they can be applied. ΦC31 mediates recombination between two different RTs, attP and attB, to produce attL and attR (Fig. 3). The minimal attP and attB sites, 39 and 34 bp, respectively, include imperfect inverted repeats and a three-nucleotide recombination site, which here again imposes directionality. Like Cre and FLPe, ΦC31 excises and inverts DNA intervals flanked by attP and attL in direct and indirect orientation, respectively. However, unlike with Cre and FLPe, ΦC31 reactions are irreversible, presumably because reversibility requires a cofactor that is not present in mammalian cells. Although directionality is an advantage in certain applications (see later), ΦC31's performance is presently no match for Cre and FLPe, despite early indications (Andreas *et al.*, 2002). ΦC31 has been successfully applied for insertional mutagenesis (Sclimenti *et al.*, 2001) and RMCE (Belteki *et al.*, 2003). Both of these applications involve intermolecular recombination. Interestingly, the Belteki *et al.* study revealed an unusual asymmetry in reaction products that seems to reflect inefficient intramolecular recombination. This could be because serine recombinases need to topologically wrap one of the substrates before recombination (Oram *et al.*, 1995).

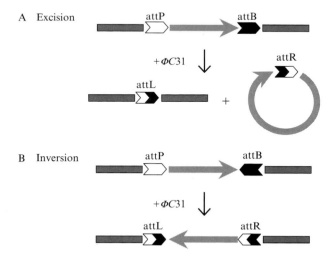

Fig. 3. Products of ΦC31 recombination. The ΦC31-specific RTs, attP and attB are shown in excision (A) or inversion (B) orientations. After recombination, the RTs are changed to attL and attR and cannot be recombined by ΦC31 in the reverse reaction.

Thus, ΦC31 inefficiency with intramolecular chromosomal recombination could be due to its inability to wrap a chromatin template, as opposed to an incoming transgenic template, before recombination.

Generation of Conditional Alleles

Two major gene-driven strategies have been used to induce mutations in ESCs, gene targeting and gene trapping. While gene targeting requires targeting vectors for each gene selected for inactivation, gene trapping induces mutations by inserting a generic gene disruption cassette throughout the genome (see Stanford *et al.*, Chapter 8, this issue). A combination of the two, called "targeted trapping" inserts a gene trap–style cassette into a gene of interest by homologous recombination (Friedel *et al.*, 2005).

Each of these strategies takes advantage of the ability of ESCs to pass mutations induced *in vitro* to the germ line of transgenic offspring *in vivo*, which provides a unique way to analyze gene function in living organisms. Consequently, more than 4000 mouse strains with functionally inactivated genes ("knockout" mice) have been generated using these technologies, and some have proven useful as models for human disease (Zambrowicz and Sands, 2003). However, for most of these mutant strains, the significance for human disease remains uncertain, because germline mutations can reveal only the earliest, nonredundant role of a gene. Moreover, approximately 30% of the genes targeted in ESCs are required for development and cause embryonic lethal phenotypes when passaged to the germline. These factors preclude accurate functional analysis in the adult.

Because most human disorders are the result of a late-onset gene dysfunction, strategies of conditional mutagenesis have been developed in ESCs that combine gene targeting or trapping with site-specific recombination. They fall into two main categories—strategies using excisions and strategies using inversions.

Strategies Using Excisions

The classic conditional allele is the so-called *floxed allele*. In a floxed allele, one or more exons of a target gene are flanked by loxP sites inserted into introns in a direct orientation. Introns are preferred insertion sites, because loxP sites in these positions are unlikely to have a mutagenic effect before recombination. As already mentioned, it is useful to place the loxP sites as close together as practically possible, so that Cre recombination deletes an essential section of the protein coding sequence. Alternatively, exons can be floxed whose deletion results in a shift of the protein translational reading frame (Shibata *et al.*, 1997).

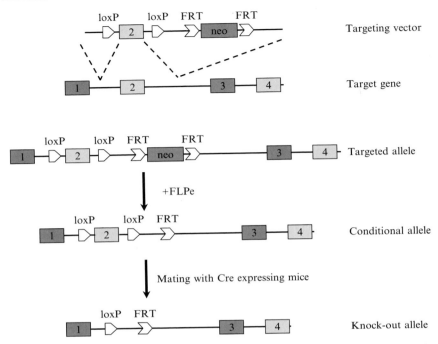

FIG. 4. A common strategy for creating conditional alleles in the mouse. In the targeting vector, an exon (here exon 2) of the target gene is flanked by loxP sites in direct (excision) orientation (white pentagons). The targeting vector contains a selection cassette (here neomycin; neo), which is flanked by FRT sites in direct orientation (white polygons). After introducing the vector into ESCs and selecting for homologous recombinants, the neomycin cassette is removed using FLPe, either in ESCs, mice, or oocytes. Homozygous mice for the conditional allele are crossed to mice expressing Cre in a spatially and/or temporally restricted manner. This deletes the loxP-flanked exon 2 from the target gene and causes a mutation.

Figure 4 illustrates a common strategy for generating conditional alleles. In the targeting vector, loxP sites flank the exon(s) of the target gene, and FRT sites flank the expression cassette of a selectable marker gene. After selecting for homologous recombinants in ESCs, the selectable marker is removed by FLPe (Rodriguez *et al.*, 2000; Schaft *et al.*, 2001).

By using FLPe for this task, the more potent Cre is reserved for conditional mutagenesis in the mouse. Although removal of the selectable marker gene is not essential, most investigators remove it because it can sometimes interfere with gene expression in the mouse (Kaul *et al.*, 2000). This can result in a hypomorphic mutation of the target gene, which can, however, have a merit of its own (Meyers *et al.*, 1998; Nagy *et al.*, 1998).

Strategies Using Inversions

Inversion strategies rely on insertional mutagenesis performed with cassettes designed to block gene expression when inserted into a gene. Originally developed for gene trapping, these cassettes consist of a reporter/selectable marker gene flanked by a splice acceptor sequence and a transcriptional termination signal (poly A). When inserted into an intron of an expressed gene, the cassette is transcribed from the endogenous promoter in the form of a fusion transcript in which the exon(s) upstream of the insertion site is spliced in frame to the reporter/selectable marker gene. Because transcription is terminated prematurely at the inserted polyadenylation site, the processed fusion transcript encodes a truncated and nonfunctional version of the cellular protein and the reporter/selectable marker. Thus, to cause a mutation the cassette needs to insert in the same transcriptional orientation relative to the target gene (also see Chapter 8). Cassette insertions in reverse orientations should not interfere with gene expression and therefore cause no mutation. Alternatively, conditional mutations can be induced by inserting an artificial intron into an exon of a target gene.

Although the intron splits the exon in two, its sense orientation is innocuous because it is removed by splicing, which reconstitutes the exon. However, in reverse orientation on the noncoding strand, the intron cannot be removed by splicing and causes a mutation (A. Economides and G. D. Yancopoulos, 2005, personal communication).

As discussed previously, both Cre and FLPe invert DNA fragments positioned between RTs with spacers arranged as indirect repeats. However, inversions induced by recombination between loxP or FRT sites are inherently reversible and equilibrate at an equal mixture of the two orientations. This is of limited usefulness in mutagenesis and has been superseeded by strategies that enable directional inversions.

The mutant loxP sites, lox66 and lox71, were the first to be used for this purpose (Fig. 2A; Oberdoerffer *et al.*, 2003). However, they recombine about three times less efficiently than the wild-type loxP sites (Oberdoerffer *et al.*, 2003). The lox66/71 strategy has been used in ESCs for inversions of immunoglobulin genes (Oberdoerffer *et al.*, 2003), of gene trap cassettes (Xin *et al.*, 2005), and of artificial introns inserted into exons (A. Economides and G. D. Yancopoulos, 2005, personal communication). However, directionality with the half site mutants is not absolute, because recombination can still occur between the loxP and loxP/lox66/71 sites at a low rate in both plants and ESCs (Albert *et al.*, 1995; Oberdoerffer *et al.*, 2003).

A second strategy, termed FlEx, uses pairs of inversely oriented heterotypic RTs to flank a cassette in inverse orientations. Recombination between either pair of homotypic RTs inverts the cassette and places the other homotypic RT pair near to each other in a direct orientation.

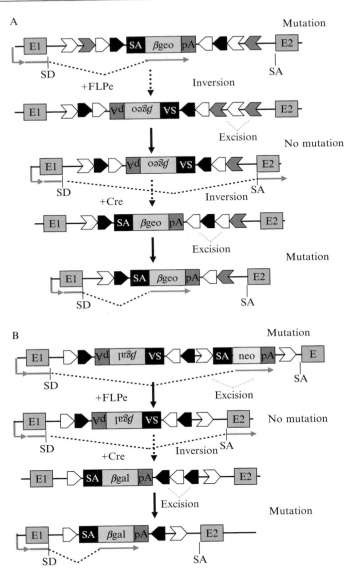

FIG. 5. Conditional gene inactivation by gene trap vectors. (A) Single cassette strategy. A flexed SAßgeopA gene trap cassette is illustrated after integration into an intron of an expressed gene. White polygons, FRT sites; gray polygons, F3 sites; white pentagons, loxP sites; black pentagons, lox5171 sites; ßgeo, ß-galactosidase/neomycin phosphotransferase fusion gene. Transcripts (shown as gray arrows) initiated at the endogenous promoter are spliced from the splice donor (SD) of an endogenous exon (here exon 1) to the splice acceptor (SA) of the SAßgeopA cassette. Thereby, the ßgeo reporter gene is expressed, and the

Recombination between this pair of directly repeated RTs excises one of the other heterotypic RTs, hence "locking" the recombination product against reinversion to the original orientation (Fig. 2B). The FlEx design was originally developed to monitor Cre recombination at cellular level in transgenic mice (Schnütgen et al., 2003). A targeting construct with an inversely oriented splice acceptor-ß–galactosidase-polyA (SAßgalpA) gene trap cassette was introduced into the retinoic acid receptor γ (RAR) gene by homologous recombination. In this construct, a RARγ exon and the SAßgalpA cassette were jointly flanked ("flexed") by pairs of heterotypic loxP/lox511 sites. When exposed to Cre, the gene trap cassette was inverted into a sense orientation on the coding strand, whereas the exon was placed into an antisense orientation on the noncoding strand. This caused a mutation and simultaneously activated the ß-gal reporter. Studies in mice carrying two flexed RARγ alleles showed that ß-gal accurately reported recombination at the cellular level and mirrored the expression pattern of the RARγ gene (Schnütgen et al., 2003).

FlEx arrays have been used recently in gene trap vectors developed for high-throughput conditional mutagenesis in ES cells (Schnütgen et al., 2005). These vectors rely on gene trap cassettes flexed by heterotypic FRT/F3 and loxP/lox5171 sites, which enable two-directional inversions if exposed to Cre and FLPe in succession. As exemplified in Fig. 5A, for a SAßgeopA cassette, FLPe inverts the gene trap cassette into an antisense orientation on the noncoding strand from where it is removed by endogenous splicing. This repairs the original mutation by restoring the normal gene expression. A second inversion induced by Cre places the cassette

---

endogenous transcript is captured and prematurely terminated at the cassette's polyadenylation sequence (pA), causing a mutation. FLPe inverts the SAßgeopA cassette onto the antisense, noncoding strand at either FRT (shown) or F3 (not shown) RTs and positions FRT and F3 sites between direct repeats of F3 and FRT RTs, respectively. By simultaneously excising the heterotypic RTs, the cassette is locked against reinversion, because the remaining FRT and F3 RTs cannot recombine. This reactivates normal splicing between the endogenous splice sites, thereby repairing the mutation. Cre-mediated inversion repositions the SAßgeopA cassette back onto the sense coding strand and reinduces the mutation (Schnütgen et al., 2005). (B) Double cassette strategy. Two gene trap cassettes in opposite orientation relative to each other are illustrated after integration into an intron of an expressed gene. Neo, neomycin phosphotransferase; ßgal, ß-galactosidase. The sense cassette (SAneopA) is flanked by wild-type FRT sites in direct orientation and is amenable to excision by FLPe. The antisense cassette (SAßgalpA) is flexed by heterotypic lox sites, hence invertable by Cre. Transcripts initiated at the endogenous promoter are spliced from the splice donor of the endogenous exon to the splice acceptor site of the SAneopA cassette, causing a mutation (see earlier). FLPe repairs the mutation by excising the SAneopA cassette and reactivating normal splicing between the endogenous splice sites. Cre-mediated inversion places the flexed SAßgalpA cassette onto the sense coding strand and reinduces the mutation.

back onto the coding strand, which reinduces the mutation. Thus, the gene trap vectors allow (1) high-throughput recovery of gene trap lines by selecting in G418, (2) inactivation of gene trap mutations before ESC conversion into mice by blastocyst injection, and (3) reactivation of the mutation at prespecified times in selected tissues of the resulting mice. Alternatively, the gene trap mutations can be directly passaged to the germ line and then repaired and reinduced by two successive breeding cycles to FLPe and Cre deleter mice.

Essentially similar results have been obtained with vectors containing two gene trap cassettes in opposite orientation relative to each other, one of which is flexed and the other floxed (Fig. 5B; J. Altschmied, F. S. Schnütgen, H.v. M, unpublished). In this strategy, the floxed cassette is used for trapped cell line selection and the flexed cassette for inducing the conditional mutation. Any of the gene trap cassettes described previously insert heterologous RTs into the genome, opening the possibility for a large variety of postinsertional modifications using RMCE. Examples include replacing the gene trap cassettes with Cre recombinase genes to expand the number of tissue-specific deleter strains or point-mutated minigenes to study point mutations. Further options are the induction of gain of function mutations or the ablation of specific cell lineages by inserting gain-of-function cassettes or toxin genes, respectively.

Recombinase Delivery to ES Cells

Recombinases are routinely delivered to cultured cells by transient transfection of recombinase expression plasmids. For ESCs, electroporation is the method of choice. Coexpression of a selectable marker gene can be useful, because it helps to enrich for recombinants. Promoter elements that are highly active in ESCs include the PGK and CMV/chicken ß-actin (CAGGS) promoters. Usually, between 10–40% of the electroporated cells express the transduced recombinase at levels high enough to cause recombination. This frequency increases if a short selection is applied. However, to avoid genome integration of expression plasmids, selection should not exceed 48 h.

For Cre, an alternative delivery method exists in the form of cell-permeable derivatives of the Cre enzyme (Jo *et al.*, 2001; Peitz *et al.*, 2002). Of the several cell-permeable Cre proteins described, the most widely used is HTN-Cre (HTNC). HTNC contains an N-terminal cell permeation domain derived from the HIV–TAT protein fused to a nuclear localization sequence (NLS) (Peitz *et al.*, 2002). Incubation of ESCs reporting Cre activity (see later) for 20 h with 2 μM of recombinant HTNC induced recombination in more than 95% of the cells without any noticeable toxicity

(Peitz *et al.*, 2002). This procedure is simple, efficient, and fast but does involve a period of cellular stress that may be deleterious for sensitive ESCs lines such as C57BL/6 lines. While large quantities of recombinant HTNC protein can be produced in *E. coli* and stored frozen without loss of activity (Peitz *et al.*, 2002), FLPe has thus far resisted conversion to a cell-permeable protein, and further efforts are in progress to achieve this goal.

Recombinase Delivery to Mice

To induce mutations in mice with conditional alleles, Cre is usually delivered by one of the following methods:

1. Spatial: crossing to a transgenic strain in which Cre is expressed from a tissue-specific promoter. Only tissues with Cre expression develop a target gene mutation in the double transgenic offspring and thus reveal its tissue-specific function.
2. Temporal: crossing to a transgenic strain containing a ubiquitously expressed, ligand-inducible Cre. Recombination occurs in all cells of double transgenic offspring after ligand induction, and thus the cell types requiring the target gene at the time of induction can be identified.
3. Spatiotemporal: crossing to a transgenic strain containing a tissue-specific, ligand-regulated Cre transgene. In double transgenic offspring, recombination occurs only in cell types expressing the transgene and after ligand induction. Depending on the inducible system, the ligand can be applied per os (tetracycline), topically, or by intraperitoneal injection (tamoxifen).
4. Local delivery of Cre, notably by adenoviruses, to specific cells and tissues. Unlike 1–3, this method does not require extensive breeding.

Major limitations encountered with conditional mutagenesis are presently (1) a relatively low number of tissue-specific promoters available for exclusive recombinase expression in somatic cells, (2) the leakiness of most inducible SSR systems, and (3) chromatin position effects affecting recombination efficiency between RTs, as well as the expression of the SSRs. Chromatin position effects can be weakened and tissue specificity improved by inserting the SSR genes into the mutant locus by gene targeting or RMCE (see later) to ensure an SSR expression pattern that is similar, if not identical, to that of the disrupted gene.

Recombinase-Mediated Cassette Exchange (RMCE)

RMCE is a gene knock-in strategy that provides a simple alternative to gene replacement by homologous recombination. RMCE was first described by Bode and colleagues using FLP recombinase but has found wider use with Cre (Baer and Bode, 2001; Schlake and Bode, 1994). RMCE in ESCs is performed in two steps.

First, a pair of inversely oriented heterotypic RTs is inserted into a genomic region of interest by homologous recombination. This step can be circumvented if a suitable conditional gene trap ESC line is available. As discussed previously, conditional gene trap vectors insert indirect repeats of heterotypic RTs across the genome. Hence, trapped ESC lines can be used directly for RMCE. More than 2000 ESC lines with conditional mutations in single genes have already been assembled by the International Gene Trap Consortium (IGTC; Nord *et al.*, 2006), and it is anticipated that a further 8000 lines will be available in the near future. All cell lines can be ordered from the IGTC (http://www.genetrap.org) and are freely available to the scientific community.

Second, a circularized DNA fragment containing a replacement cassette between the same pair of inversely oriented heterotypic RTs (incoming construct) is electroporated into ESCs with a recombinase expression plasmid. Recombination inserts the incoming construct into the locus in a two-step mechanism (Fig. 2B). Incoming cassettes almost always contain a positive selectable marker, so that selection for the replaced locus can be applied.

A potential limitation of RMCE relates to the length of the regions that can be exchanged. Placing the two genomic RTs more than a few kilobases apart has until now required two rounds of targeting in ESCs. Consequently, the relationship between the distance separating the genomic RTs and RMCE efficiencies has not been systematically explored. Similarly, the relationship between the distance separating RTs on the incoming construct and the efficiency of RMCE to insert or exchange long stretches of DNA has not been published.

Molecular Switches

Recombinase-mediated DNA excision can be applied as a molecular switch to achieve permanent gene activation after transient exposure to a recombinase activity (Angrand *et al.*, 1998; Russ, *et al.*, 1996; Thorey *et al.*, 1998). The core element of a SSR molecular switch is a DNA fragment flanked by directly orientated RTs. The fragment, commonly referred to as a "STOP" sequence, is used to block gene expression, hence it either disrupts the coding sequence of a gene or keeps the gene at a distance from an active promoter. STOP sequences used for spacing are frequently selectable marker or reporter genes, which are usually expressed before recombination. Recombination deletes the STOP sequence from the vector, which activates gene expression (Fig. 6A). The most widely used

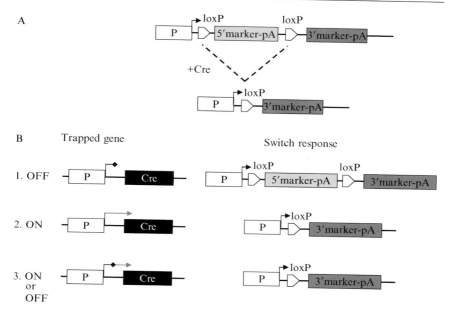

FIG. 6. Gene expression switch. (A) A selectable marker (5′marker-pA), flanked by loxP sites (white pentagons) in direct orientations, is expressed from a constitutively active promoter (P) and simultaneously blocks the expression of a downstream gene (3′marker-pA) by premature polyadenylation (pA). Cre deletes the upstream cassette, which activates the downstream gene. (B) Use of the gene expression switch in a genetic screen for inducible genes. A switch cassette is integrated into ESCs by selection for the upstream selection marker, which is flanked by loxP sites (white pentagons). The downstream marker is not expressed because of premature polyadenylation (pA). These cells are transduced with a Cre gene trap vector. Vector integrations into active genes express Cre so that these are eliminated by continued selection for the upstream marker. Hence, surviving cells do not express Cre, which must be integrated into silent genomic sites (1. OFF). Then, cells are treated with an inducer, which may be a cytokine, a hormone, or a differentiation protocol. If this change activates a gene trap insertion site to express Cre, recombination ensues, and selection applied for the activation of the downstream marker can be used to isolate these cells (2. ON). Regardless of whether Cre expression stays on or is subsequently turned off, the expression of the downstream marker continues (3. ON or OFF), hence facilitating the identification of transient sites of activation of Cre expression.

reporter gene encode is for ß-galactosidase, which is an easily detectable histochemical marker and is quantifiable in solution by spectrophotometry. Other popular reporter genes encode the firefly luciferase (LUC) or the enhanced green fluorescent protein (EGFP), which are both detectable in living cells and useful for *in vivo* imaging (Agah *et al.*, 1997; Constien *et al.*, 2001; Kolb *et al.*, 1999; Mao *et al.*, 2001; Pasqualetti *et al.*, 2002).

In their simplest application, switch vectors are used to monitor recombinase activity in cultured cells and mice. Because reporter activation is irreversible, switch vectors are well suited for tracing recombinase activity in transgenic mice and are applied routinely in pretesting the ability of Cre deleter strains to induce tissue-specific mutations.

The best reporter mouse lines have been obtained using vectors knocked into ubiquitously transcribed chromosomal regions such as ROSA26 or HPRT (Akagi *et al.*, 1997; Lallemand *et al.*, 1998; Soriano, 1999; Thorey *et al.*, 1998; Tsien *et al.*, 1996). From such locations, the expression of the reporter gene after recombination accurately reflects the expression of the Cre transgene. If the cells that express Cre are known, the expression pattern of the reporter gene charts the progenitor/progeny relationship (lineage tracing) and pattern of cell migration (fate mapping) during mouse development.

Switch vectors have also been used for conditional knock-downs in mice using short hairpin RNAs (shRNAs) for posttranscriptional gene silencing of gene expression. shRNAs are most efficiently expressed from polymerase III promoters. Unlike pol II promoters, inducible pol III promoters have not yet been described. Thus for conditional knock-downs in mice using shRNAs, a switch vector supporting pol III expression seems to be the best solution. The strategy has been successfully applied to inactivate the anti-apoptotic bcl2 family protein A1 in B cells (Oberdoerffer *et al.*, 2005) and the p53 tumor suppressor protein in mouse embryonic fibroblasts (Ventura *et al.*, 2004). Both strategies used a U6-lox-STOP-lox-shRNA switch inserted into the ESC genome. Cell type–specific knock-downs in U6-lox-STOP-lox-shA1 and U6-lox-STOP-lox-shp53 transgenic mice were achieved either by crossing to B cell–specific Cre deleter mice (Oberdoerffer *et al.*, 2005) or by infecting cultured fibroblasts with adenoviral Cre expression vectors (Ventura *et al.*, 2004).

Because activation of switch vectors requires only transient Cre expression, they have been used in combination with gene trapping to screen for genes induced during ESC differentiation (Chen *et al.*, 2004; Thorey *et al.*, 1998). The strategy uses an ESC line, which constitutively expresses a switch vector containing two selectable marker genes, of which the upstream one is flanked by loxP sites and blocks the expression of the downstream one (Fig. 6B). When this cell line is treated with gene trap vectors that insert a Cre gene randomly throughout the genome, insertions into active genes will express Cre, leading to deletion of the upstream gene by recombination. Selection for the deleted gene eliminates the ESCs with expressed gene trap integrations. The surviving ESCs are now enriched for insertions into "silent" genes and can be used to screen for genes that are activated by signals. Various signals can be used, such as signal transduction pathways activated by differentiation, cytokines, or hormones. If the signal activates the site of Cre insertion, Cre is expressed, and the upstream gene is deleted. Selection for the downstream gene, therefore, identifies the signal-responsive genes (Fig. 6B). Applied to retinoic acid–responsive genes, this strategy effectively selected for developmentally regulated genes (Chen *et al.*, 2004).

Protocols

General protocols for growing ES cells in tissue culture are described elsewhere in this issue. As a rule, if manipulated ESCs are to be converted into mice, they must be prevented from differentiating in the culture dish. In most cases, this is achieved by growing the cells in the presence of leukemia inhibitory factor (LIF) on mitotically inactivated feeder layers prepared with mouse embryonic fibroblasts (MEFs). If selection is required, MEFs need to be drug resistant. Feeder layers can be avoided by using ESCs adapted to feeder-free culture conditions.

Recombinase Delivery into ESCs (DNA Transfection)

This protocol is used for removing targeted DNA fragments flanked by FRT or loxP sites using site-specific FLPe-or Cre-recombinases, respectively. For higher efficiency of recombination (or reducing workload), the recombinases are bicistronically expressed with a puromycin resistance gene (pac) under the control of the CAGGs promoter. Thereby, transient selection for 48 h can be used to reduce background level (Taniguchi *et al.*, 1998). The expression vector, pCAGGs-Flpe-IRES-puro-pA has been described elsewhere (Schaft *et al.*, 2001). Similar vectors for Cre and ΦC31 integrase (pCAGGs-Cre-IRES-puro-pA and pCAGGs-ΦC31IRES-puro-pA) are available. Usually, the flanked fragments include selection cassettes, so that the efficiency of recombination can be checked afterwards by sensitivity assays to the selection pressure used previously.

1. Split confluent ESCs (usually 1×10^7 cells per 10-cm TC dish) and start with 2×10^6 cells per 10-cm TC dish so that after 24 h they are in the log phase of growth and have a density of 4–5×10^6 cells per dish.
2. After 24 h, wash cells with PBS and trypsinize with 1 ml 0.5% v/v trypsin solution for 5 min at 37°.
3. Inactivate trypsin with 9 ml ES medium and pipette the suspension using a 10-ml pipette (8–10 times) to get single cells.
4. Take an aliquot of 10 μl and count cells.
5. Centrifuge in 15-ml Falcon tube at 1000 rpm for 5 min at RT.
6. Resuspend the pellet in PBS at 1×10^7 cells in 900 μl PBS.
7. Mix the 900-μl suspension with the DNA (40 μg, circular), and transfer to an electroporation cuvette (4-mm gap).

8. Leave on ice for 5–10 min.
9. Electroporate using the following conditions: 250 Volt, 500 μF (Gene Pulser X-cell; BioRad).
10. After electroporation, immediately flick the cuvette to stabilize the pH.
11. Place the cuvette on ice.
12. Transfer the electroporated suspension using a 1-ml pipette into a 15-ml Falcon tube containing 9.5 ml ES medium. Total volume is approximately 10.4 ml.
13. Distribute the cells in 10-cm TC dishes (1 ml per dish in 10 dishes) that are already filled with 10 ml ES medium each.
14. After 24 h, replace the ES medium with one that contains 1 μg/ml puromycin (Sigma P-8833).
15. Keep the selection for 48 h, without changing the medium.
16. Remove the selection medium and replace with normal ES medium and change every day.
17. Ten–12 days after electroporation colonies become visible.

Other methods of recombinase delivery use transfection of *in vitro* transcribed RNA (Van den Plas *et al.*, 2003) or incubation with recombinase proteins fused to transduction domains (Peitz *et al.*, 2002). Detailed protocols can be found in the cited literature.

Low-Density Seeding of ESCs

If selection with puromycin is not possible or desired, the colonies will usually display a mosaic genotype for the recombination event. To purify the genotype, the cells have to be replated for growing clonal colonies.

1. Proceed as described previously until step 14. Instead of step 14, let the cells grow for 2 days.
2. Wash cells with PBS and trypsinize with 1 ml trypsin for 5 min at 37°.
3. Inactivate trypsin with 9 ml ES medium and pipette the suspension using a 10-ml pipette (8–10 times) to get single cells.
4. Take an aliquot of 10 μl and count cells.
5. Seed 500 cells onto gelatinized 6-cm dishes containing feeder layers.
6. Grow cells for 10–12 days with daily change of medium until colonies reach an appropriate size for picking.

Picking of Colonies

1. Seed feeder cells onto the appropriate number of freshly gelatinized 96-well plates 1 day before picking.

2. Aspirate culture medium and add prewarmed PBS. If colonies from more than one plate have to be picked, process them one by one. Break up the colonies using a Pipetman (P200) and sterile tips and collect the cells in 30 μl of PBS. Transfer the cell clumps to a 96-well plate and repeat until all colonies are picked.

3. Add 30 μl of 2× trypsin solution to each well and incubate until cells can be easily dispersed by tapping the plate. Add 100 μl of medium to each well and transfer cells onto 96-well plates containing feeder cells.

4. When cells approach confluence, trypsinize, and expand for freezing and further analysis.

In cases in which a selection cassette has been deleted, the colonies can be screened by applying selection pressure. For this reason, make duplicates or triplicates (depending on whether you want to see loss of selection markers in both alleles). One plate should contain normal medium, and the second should have medium-containing antibiotic corresponding to the deleted selection marker. Colonies that grow in normal medium but not in antibiotic-containing medium have been efficiently recombined.

Molecular Confirmation of Excisions

To confirm the deletion of an FRT-or loxP-flanked fragment, DNA should be prepared and analyzed by PCR or Southern blot. A detailed protocol for preparing genomic DNA from ESCs growing in 96-well plates has been described by Ramirez-Solis *et al.* (1993).

A schematic presentation of the Southern blot and PCR strategies is shown in Fig. 7. For the Southern blot, the DNA should be digested using an enzyme with recognition sequences upstream and downstream of the FRT-flanked selection cassette (enzyme x in Fig. 7B). It has become common practice to introduce the same restriction site in the targeting cassette.

For our purpose, a restriction site immediately downstream of the FRT-site is ideal. After Southern blot, the membranes can be hybridized using a probe situated between the sites (probe 1 in Fig. 7B). This probe can distinguish between wt-allele, targeted-allele (unrecombined), and recombined allele (Fig. 7B). If both unrecombined and recombined alleles are detectable, the recombination has been partial (colonies with a mixed population of cells). In addition, the DNA of the colonies should be analyzed for undesired integration of the recombinase expression plasmid (Southern blot using a puro-probe, probe 2 in Fig. 7A).

For the PCR analysis, one should design the primers so that all possible variations can be distinguished. Usually a set of three primers can be used.

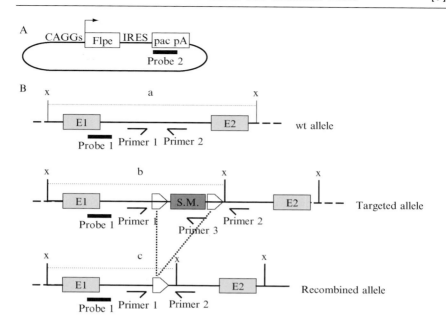

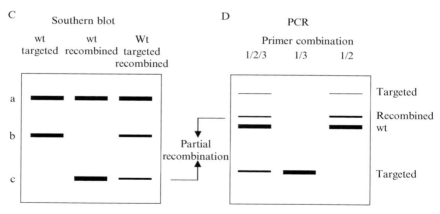

FIG. 7. Recombination in ESCs. (A) The expression vector pCAGGs-Flpe-IRES-puro-pA that is used for transfection in ESCs. (B) Schematic presentation of an imaginary gene in all three possible conformations: wt-allele, targeted allele, and recombined allele. Depicted are only exons 1 and 2 (gray boxes). The selection marker (S.M.) flanked by FRTsites (white pentagons) has been integrated in the first intron. Vertical arrows show positions of the hypothetical restriction site (x). Horizontal arrows represent the PCR primers used for testing recombination efficiency. Dashed horizontal lines that connect the restriction sites (x) represent the different fragments (a, b, c) that can be detected after hybridization with probe 1 (black bar). (C) Schematic presentation of Southern blot and the resulting fragments using probe 1. (D) Schematic presentation of PCR using different primer combinations.

Primers 1 and 2 amplify the wt- and the recombined- allele. Differences in size occur because of the recombinase target site left after recombination or additional sequences introduced with the targeted vector downstream of the cassette. One can also use the introduced restriction site for digesting the PCR product (only the recombined allele and not the wt will be digested). Primers 1 and 2 can also amplify the targeted allele (dashed line in Fig. 7D), but usually they lie far apart because of the introduced cassette, so they will rarely be amplified under standard PCR conditions. Therefore, primer 3, which anneals in the targeting cassette, can be used for detecting residual unrecombined alleles.

For relatively small deletions (less than 4 kb), the usual rate of recombination using pCAGGs FLPe–expression vector is approximately 5%. In the case where both alleles contain a cassette flanked by FRT sites, colonies carrying a deletion of one allele were observed about three times more often than colonies with the deletion of both alleles. The puromycin selection protocol includes the risk that the genomic integration of pCAGGs-FLPe-IRES-puro plasmid will be selected. In our experience, we observed integration in up to half of all transiently puromycin-selected colonies. It is quite likely that this frequency of undesired integration of the expression plasmid will be promoted by DNA breaks in the plasmid DNA preparation, so the use of supercoiled expression plasmid is recommended.

Tamoxifen Treatment of Primed ESCs

This approach is used in ES cells that contain a recombinase-LBD fusion integrated in the genome. The most widely used fusion is Cre-ERT2 (Feil et al., 1997). Integration of Cre-ERT2 in a locus that is ubiquitously expressed, such as the Rosa26, has been described (Seibler et al., 2003). In the inactive state, Cre-ERT2 is expressed in ES cells and is associated with the Hsp90 in the cytoplasm. Induction occurs on administration of a ligand such as 4-hydroxytamoxifen. Cre-ERT2 disassociates from Hsp90 and translocates to the nucleus. 4-Hydroxytamoxifen (4-OHT; Sigma H-6278) is dissolved at a concentration of 10^{-2} M in 100% ethanol and stored at $-20°$. An intermediate stock with a concentration of 10^{-4} M in 100% ethanol is also stored at $-20°$. The working concentration is 5×10^{-7} M in ES medium.

Recombination efficiencies of almost 100% (for deletion of fragments around 1 kb) have been observed within 1 day of tamoxifen induction. Factors affecting the efficiency of recombination are the levels of recombinase, the distance between the loxP sites, and their site of integration in the genome. Therefore, the efficiency of recombination for different loxP-flanked fragments should be experimentally tested. Ideally, one should set a time course and collect tamoxifen-treated cells at different time points. For each time point use two dishes so that you can analyze the efficiency of recombination at the DNA level and the effects at the RNA or protein level. Calculate the amount of plates you need (in duplicates) for your time course. A time course using uninduced, 6, 12, 24, 36, 48, 72, and 96 h induction will give you an idea of the kinetics of recombination. Do the inductions in reverse order, meaning induce the cells for the 6-h time point 6 h before collecting. This will facilitate your experiment, because you will have the same amount of cells for each different time point, and you can collect the cells at the same time.

1. Grow ESCs to confluence on 10-cm TC dishes in normal medium.
2. Split confluent ESCs (usually 1×10^7 cells per 10-cm TC dish) by trypsinization and start with 1×10^6 cells per 10-cm TC dish in medium containing 5×10^{-7} M 4-OHT.

Continue growing four plates of cells in normal medium (uninduced).

3. Change medium (4-OHT) after 24 h, and add 4-OHT in two of the uninduced plates (time point 72 h).
4. After 48 h, the ESCs usually reach confluence and should be split by trypsinization as described in step 2. Split the induced plates and continue culturing in 4-OHT–containing medium. Split the uninduced plate in at least 12 plates. Two of them already contain 4-OHT (time point 48 h). To the other eight plates add 4-OHT 36 h, 24 h, 12 h, and 6 h before collecting (two plates each time point). The last two plates remain uninduced.
5. After additional 48 h (96 h from the beginning of induction), collect cell pellets for DNA and protein extraction.
6. Wash twice with PBS.
7. Add 1 ml cold PBS per TC dish and scrape the cells using a rubber policeman. Transfer the scraped cells into 1.5-ml Eppendorf tubes, on ice.
8. Centrifuge at 4000 rpm for 4 min at 4°.
9. Aspirate supernatant and either freeze the cell pellet at −80° or proceed with DNA and protein extraction, using standard methods.

In Vitro *Verification of Conditional Constructs*

Because subsequent steps often represent a considerable investment of time and labor, it is desirable to verify at an early stage that introduced recombination target sites are competent for recombination. Therefore, we suggest pretesting conditional constructs before integration into ESCs.

Pretesting Conditional Constructs in Bacterial Strains

1. Generate competent 294-Cre or 294-Flp bacteria (Buchholz *et al.*, 1996) that contain stably integrated expression cassettes for Cre recombinase or FLPe recombinase, respectively.
2. Transform constructs to be tested into the appropriate bacterial strain and inoculate 5 ml of LB medium containing antibiotics

directly with the transformed bacteria without plating them onto LB agar plates. Grow overnight at 37°.

3. Isolate the plasmid DNA from these bacteria by standard procedures.
4. Transform appropriate lab strain (DH5a, XL1 blue) with 1 μl of Miniprep DNA and plate onto LB agar plates containing antibiotic and incubate overnight.
5. Pick colonies and check for recombination events by restriction digest or PCR screening.

Pretesting Conditional Constructs in Mammalian Cells

1. Seed 8×10^5 293T cells into a 6-cm TC dish and allow to adhere overnight.
2. Cotransfect the conditional construct (2 μg) with a fourfold excess of a recombinase expression plasmid (e.g., pCAGGs-Cre-IRES-puro-pA) using standard calcium phosphate precipitation.
3. Grow cells for 48 h with one medium change after 24 h.
4. Isolate DNA by standard procedures.
5. Transform *E. coli* (DH5a, XL1 blue) with 50 ng of DNA and inoculate 5 ml LB medium.
6. Incubate overnight at 37° in a bacterial shaker.
7. Miniprep plasmid DNA.
8. Analyze Miniprep DNA by PCR as described in Fig. 7.

Verification of Gene Trap Cassette Inversions

Conditional gene trap alleles contain gene disruption and selection cassettes that can be inverted twice by the successive application of FLPe and Cre recombinases. Although this sequence can be reversed for certain *in vitro* applications, it is advisable to use FLPe for the first inversion in ESCs and the more potent Cre for the second inversion in the mouse. For recombinase delivery *in vitro* follow the transfection protocol described previously. Recombinase delivery *in vivo* requires breeding of the gene trap line–derived transgenic mice to a FLPe or Cre deleter strain. Because the gene trap cassette is generic, the verification protocol applies to all ESC lines and mice produced with a particular gene trap vector. Here we describe the protocol for the FlipRosaβgeo vector and its derivatives (Schnütgen *et al.*, 2005), which have been used for the most of the ESC lines.

To monitor inversions, we use multiplex PCR with one forward primer complementary to the 3′ end of ßgeo (B048; 5′-CCT CCC CCG TGC CTT CCT TGA C-3′) and two reverse primers complementary to the 5′end of ßgeo and to viral sequences downstream of the 3′ RTs, respectively (B050; 5′-TTT GAG GGG ACG ACG ACA GTA T-3′ and (B045; 5′-CTC CGC

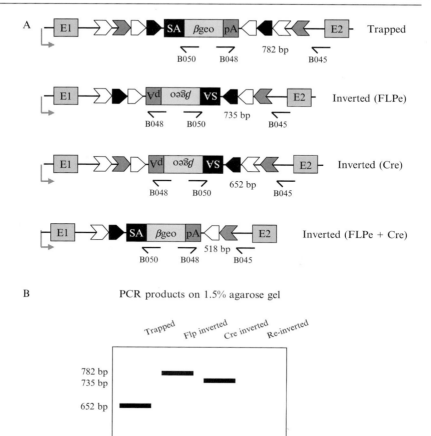

FIG. 8. Multiplex PCR strategy for the verification of gene trap cassette inversions in ESCs and mice. Positions of primers (A) and expected amplification products (B) from the three possible alleles inducible by recombination of the FlipRosaßgeo gene trap vector.

CTC CTC TTC CTC CAT C-3′) (Fig. 8). The size of the amplification product is diagnostic for the orientation of the gene trap cassette (Fig. 8).

1. Isolate DNA from ESCs or mouse tails by standard procedures (Laird *et al.*, 1991; Ramirez-Solis *et al.*, 1993).
2. For each reaction pipette 23 µl of a PCR-master mix containing 2.5 µl of 10× PCR buffer (Invitrogen), 0.75 µl of 2 m*M* MgCl$_2$, 0.5 µl

dNTPs (10 μM each), 1 μl of each B045, B048, and B050 primers (10 pmol/μl), 0.5 μl DMSO, and 0.2 μl Taq polymerase (Invitrogen) in H$_2$O into 0.2 ml PCR tubes.

3. Add approximately 500 ng of DNA in 2 μl to each tube and place the tubes into a appropriate thermocycler.

4. Allow amplification reactions to proceed for 30 cycles using 94° for 45 sec for denaturation, 61° for 45 sec for annealing, and 72° for 60 sec for elongation. Terminate the reaction with a final elongation cycle at 72° for 7 min.

5. Resolve amplification products on 1.5% agarose gels.

References

Agah, R., Frenkel, P. A., French, B. A., Michael, L. H., Overbeek, P. A., and Schneider, M. D. (1997). Gene recombination in postmitotic cells. Targeted expression of Cre recombinase provokes cardiac-restricted, site-specific rearrangement in adult ventricular muscle *in vivo*. *J. Clin. Invest.* **100**, 169–179.

Akagi, K., Sandig, V., Vooijs, M., Van der Valk, M., Giovannini, M., Strauss, M., and Berns, A. (1997). Cre-mediated somatic site-specific recombination in mice. *Nucleic Acids Res.* **25**, 1766–1773.

Albert, H., Dale, E. C., Lee, E., and Ow, D. W. (1995). Site-specific integration of DNA into wild-type and mutant lox sites placed in the plant genome. *Plant J.* **7**, 649–659.

Andreas, S., Schwenk, F., Kuter-Luks, B., Faust, N., and Kuhn, R. (2002). Enhanced efficiency through nuclear localization signal fusion on phage PhiC31-integrase: Activity comparison with Cre and FLPe recombinase in mammalian cells. *Nucleic Acids Res.* **30**, 2299–2306.

Angrand, P. O., Woodroofe, C. P., Buchholz, F., and Stewart, A. F. (1998). Inducible expression based on regulated recombination: A single vector strategy for stable expression in cultured cells. *Nucleic Acids Res.* **26**, 3263–3269.

Araki, H., Nakanishi, N., Evans, B. R., Matsuzaki, H., Jayaram, M., and Oshima, Y. (1992). Site-specific recombinase, R, encoded by yeast plasmid pSR1. *J. Mol. Biol.* **225**, 25–37.

Araki, K., Araki, M., and Yamamura, K. (1997). Targeted integration of DNA using mutant lox sites in embryonic stem cells. *Nucleic Acids Res.* **25**, 868–872.

Austin, C. P., Battey, J. F., Bradley, A., Bucan, M., Capecchi, M., Collins, F. S., Dove, W. F., Duyk, G., Dymecki, S., Eppig, J. T., Grieder, F. B., Heintz, N., Hicks, G., Insel, T. R., Joyner, A., Koller, B. H., Lloyd, K. C., Magnuson, T., Moore, M. W., Nagy, A., Pollock, J. D., Roses, A. D., Sands, A. T., Seed, B., Skarnes, W. C., Snoddy, J., Soriano, P., Stewart, D. J., Stewart, F., Stillman, B., Varmus, H., Varticovski, L., Verma, I. M., Vogt, T. F., von Melchner, H., Witkowski, J., Woychik, R. P., Wurst, W., Yancopoulos, G. D., Young, S. G., and Zambrowicz, B. (2004). The knockout mouse project. *Nat. Genet.* **36**, 921–924.

Auwerx, J., Avner, P., Baldock, R., Ballabio, A., Balling, R., Barbacid, M., Berns, A., Bradley, A., Brown, S., Carmeliet, P., Chambon, P., Cox, R., Davidson, D., Davies, K., Duboule, D., Forejt, J., Granucci, F., Hastie, N., de Angelis, M. H., Jackson, I., Kioussis, D., Kollias, G., Lathrop, M., Lendahl, U., Malumbres, M., von Melchner, H., Muller, W., Partanen, J., Ricciardi-Castagnoli, P., Rigby, P., Rosen, B., Rosenthal, N., Skarnes, B., Stewart, A. F., Thornton, J., Tocchini-Valentini, G., Wagner, E., Wahli, W., and Wurst, W. (2004). The European dimension for the mouse genome mutagenesis program. *Nat. Genet.* **36**, 925–927.

Baer, A., and Bode, J. (2001). Coping with kinetic and thermodynamic barriers: RMCE, an efficient strategy for the targeted integration of transgenes. *Curr. Opin. Biotechnol.* **12**, 473–480.

Belteki, G., Gertsenstein, M., Ow, D. W., and Nagy, A. (2003). Site-specific cassette exchange and germline transmission with mouse ES cells expressing phiC31 integrase. *Nat. Biotechnol.* **21,** 321–324.

Buchholz, F., Angrand, P. O., and Stewart, A. F. (1996). A simple assay to determine the functionality of Cre or FLP recombination targets in genomic manipulation constructs. *Nucleic Acids Res.* **24,** 3118–3119.

Buchholz, F., Angrand, P. O., and Stewart, A. F. (1998). Improved properties of FLP recombinase evolved by cycling mutagenesis. *Nat. Biotechnol.* **16,** 657–662.

Chen, Y., Narendra, U., Iype, L. E., Cox, M. M., and Rice, P. A. (2000). Crystal structure of a Flp recombinase-Holliday junction complex: Assembly of an active oligomer by helix swapping. *Mol. Cell* **6,** 885–897.

Chen, Y., and Rice, P. A. (2003). New insight into site-specific recombination from FLP recombinase-DNA structures. *Annu. Rev. Biophys. Biomol. Struct.* **32,** 135–139.

Chen, Y. T., Liu, P., and Bradley, A. (2004). Inducible gene trapping with drug-selectable markers and Cre/loxP to identify developmentally regulated genes. *Mol. Cell. Biol.* **24,** 9930–9941.

Constien, R., Forde, A., Liliensiek, B., Grone, H. J., Nawroth, P., Hammerling, G., and Arnold, B. (2001). Characterization of a novel EGFP reporter mouse to monitor Cre recombination as demonstrated by a Tie2 Cre mouse line. *Genesis* **30,** 36–44.

Cronin, C. A., Gluba, W., and Scrable, H. (2001). The lac operator-repressor system is functional in the mouse. *Genes Dev.* **15,** 1506–1517.

Danielian, P. S., Muccino, D., Rowitch, D. H., Michael, S. K., and McMahon, A. P. (1998). Modification of gene activity in mouse embryos in utero by a tamoxifen–inducible form of Cre recombinase. *Curr. Biol.* **8,** 1323–1326.

Ennifar, E., Meyer, J. E., Buchholz, F., Stewart, A. F., and Suck, D. (2003). Crystal structure of a wild-type Cre recombinase-loxP synapse reveals a novel spacer conformation suggesting an alternative mechanism for DNA cleavage activation. *Nucleic Acids Res.* **31,** 5449–5460.

Farley, F. W., Soriano, P., Steffen, L. S., and Dymecki, S. M. (2000). Widespread recombinase expression using FLPeR (flipper) mice. *Genesis* **28,** 106–110.

Feil, R., Brocard, J., Mascrez, B., LeMeur, M., Metzger, D., and Chambon, P. (1996). Ligand-activated site-specific recombination in mice. *Proc. Natl. Acad. Sci. USA* **93,** 10887–10890.

Feil, R., Wagner, J., Metzger, D., and Chambon, P. (1997). Regulation of Cre recombinase activity by mutated estrogen receptor ligand-binding domains. *Biochem. Biophys. Res. Commun.* **237,** 752–757.

Feng, Y. Q., Seibler, J., Alami, R., Eisen, A., Westerman, K. A., Leboulch, P., Fiering, S., and Bouhassira, E. E. (1999). Site-specific chromosomal integration in mammalian cells: Highly efficient CRE recombinase-mediated cassette exchange. *J. Mol. Biol.* **292,** 779–785.

Friedel, R. H., Plump, A., Lu, X., Spilker, K., Jolicoeur, C., Wong, K., Venkatesh, T. R., Yaron, A., Hynes, M., Chen, B., Okada, A., McConnell, S. K., Rayburn, H., and Tessier-Lavigne, M. (2005). Gene targeting using a promoterless gene trap vector ("targeted trapping") is an efficient method to mutate a large fraction of genes. *Proc. Natl. Acad. Sci. USA* **102,** 13188–13193.

Gu, H., Zou, Y. R., and Rajewsky, K. (1993). Independent control of immunoglobulin switch recombination at individual switch regions evidenced through Cre-loxP–mediated gene targeting. *Cell* **73,** 1155–1164.

Jo, D., Nashabi, A., Doxsee, C., Lin, Q., Unutmaz, D., Chen, J., and Ruley, H. E. (2001). Epigenetic regulation of gene structure and function with a cell-permeable Cre recombinase. *Nat. Biotechnol.* **19,** 929–933.

Kaul, A., Koster, M., Neuhaus, H., and Braun, T. (2000). Myf-5 revisited: Loss of early myotome formation does not lead to a rib phenotype in homozygous Myf-5 mutant mice. *Cell* **102,** 17–19.

Kolb, A. F. (2001). Selection-marker-free modification of the murine beta-casein gene using a lox2272 [correction of lox2722] site. *Anal. Biochem.* **290,** 260–271.

Kolb, A. F., Ansell, R., McWhir, J., and Siddell, S. G. (1999). Insertion of a foreign gene into the beta-casein locus by Cre-mediated site-specific recombination. *Gene* **227,** 21–31.

Laird, P. W., Zijderveld, A., Linders, K., Rudnicki, M. A., Jaenisch, R., and Berns, A. (1991). Simplified mammalian DNA isolation procedure. *Nucleic Acids Res* **19,** 4293.

Lallemand, Y., Luria, V., Haffner-Krausz, R., and Lonai, P. (1998). Maternally expressed PGK-Cre transgene as a tool for early and uniform activation of the Cre site-specific recombinase. *Transgenic Res.* **7,** 105–112.

Langer, S. J., Ghafoori, A. P., Byrd, M., and Leinwand, L. (2002). A genetic screen identifies novel non-compatible loxP sites. *Nucleic Acids Res.* **30,** 3067–3077.

Lauth, M., Moerl, K., Barski, J. J., and Meyer, M. (2000). Characterization of Cre-mediated cassette exchange after plasmid microinjection in fertilized mouse oocytes. *Genesis* **27,** 153–158.

Lauth, M., Spreafico, F., Dethleffsen, K., and Meyer, M. (2002). Stable and efficient cassette exchange under non-selectable conditions by combined use of two site-specific recombinases. *Nucleic Acids Res.* **30,** e115.

Le, Y., Gagneten, S., Tombaccini, D., Bethke, B., and Sauer, B. (1999). Nuclear targeting determinants of the phage P1 cre DNA recombinase. *Nucleic Acids Res.* **27,** 4703–4709.

Lee, G., and Saito, I. (1998). Role of nucleotide sequences of loxP spacer region in Cremediated recombination. *Gene* **216,** 55–65.

Lee, J. Y., Ristow, M., Lin, X., White, M. F., Magnuson, M. A., and Hennighausen, L. (2005). RIP-Cre revisited: Evidence for impairments of pancreatic beta-cell function. *J. Biol. Chem.* epub Dec 1.

Li, Z. W., Stark, G., Gotz, J., Rulicke, T., Gschwind, M., Huber, G., Muller, U., and Weissmann, C. (1996). Generation of mice with a 200-kb amyloid precursor protein gene deletion by Cre recombinase-mediated site-specific recombination in embryonic stem cells. *Proc. Natl. Acad. Sci. USA* **93,** 6158–6162.

Logie, C., and Stewart, A. F. (1995). Ligand-regulated site-specific recombination. *Proc. Natl. Acad. Sci. USA* **92,** 5940–5944.

Loonstra, A., Vooijs, M., Beverloo, H. B., Allak, B. A., van Drunen, E., Kanaar, R., Berns, A., and Jonkers, J. (2001). Growth inhibition and DNA damage induced by Cre recombinase in mammalian cells. *Proc. Natl. Acad. Sci. USA* **98,** 9209–9214.

Madsen, L., Labrecque, N., Engberg, J., Dierich, A., Svejgaard, A., Benoist, C., Mathis, D., and Fugger, L. (1999). Mice lacking all conventional MHC class II genes. *Proc. Natl. Acad. Sci. USA* **96,** 10338–10343.

Mao, J., Barrow, J., McMahon, J., Vaughan, J., and McMahon, A. P. (2005). An ES cell system for rapid, spatial and temporal analysis of gene function *in vitro* and *in vivo*. *Nucleic Acids Res.* **33,** e155.

Mao, X., Fujiwara, Y., Chapdelaine, A., Yang, H., and Orkin, S. H. (2001). Activation of EGFP expression by Cre-mediated excision in a new ROSA26 reporter mouse strain. *Blood* **97,** 324–326.

Meyers, E. N., Lewandoski, M., and Martin, G. R. (1998). An Fgf8 mutant allelic series generated by Cre-and Flp-mediated recombination. *Nat. Genet.* **18,** 136–141.

Nagy, A., Moens, C., Ivanyi, E., Pawling, J., Gertsenstein, M., Hadjantonakis, A. K., Pirity, M., and Rossant, J. (1998). Dissecting the role of N-myc in development using a single targeting vector to generate a series of alleles. *Curr. Biol.* **8,** 661–664.

Nord, A. S., Chang, P. J., Conklin, B. R., Cox, A. V., Harper, C. A., Hicks, G. G., Huang, C. C., Johns, S. J., Kawamoto, M., Liu, S., Meng, E. C., Morris, J. H., Rossant, J., Ruiz, P., Skarnes, W. C., Soriano, P., Stanford, W. L., Stryke, D., von Melchner, H., Wurst, W., Yamamura, K., Young, S. G., Babbitt, P. C., and Ferrin, T. E. (2006). The International

Gene Trap Consortium Website: A portal to all publicly available gene trap cell lines in mouse. *Nucleic Acids Res.* **34,** D642–D648.

O'Gorman, S., Dagenais, N. A., Qian, M., and Marchuk, Y. (1997). Protamine-Cre recombinase transgenes efficiently recombine target sequences in the male germ line of mice, but not in embryonic stem cells. *Proc. Natl. Acad. Sci. USA* **94,** 14602–14607.

Oberdoerffer, P., Kanellopoulou, C., Heissmeyer, V., Paeper, C., Borowski, C., Aifantis, I., Rao, A., and Rajewsky, K. (2005). Efficiency of RNA interference in the mouse hematopoietic system varies between cell types and developmental stages. *Mol. Cell. Biol.* **25,** 3896–3905.

Oberdoerffer, P., Otipoby, K. L., Maruyama, M., and Rajewsky, K. (2003). Unidirectional Cre-mediated genetic inversion in mice using the mutant loxP pair lox66/lox71. *Nucleic Acids Res.* **31,** e140.

Okabe, M., Ikawa, M., Kominami, K., Nakanishi, T., and Nishimune, Y. (1997). 'Green mice' as a source of ubiquitous green cells. *FEBS Lett.* **407,** 313–319.

Olivares, E. C., Hollis, R. P., Chalberg, T. W., Meuse, L., Kay, M. A., and Calos, M. P. (2002). Site-specific genomic integration produces therapeutic Factor IX levels in mice. *Nat. Biotechnol.* **20,** 1124–1128.

Oram, M., Szczelkun, M. D., and Halford, S. E. (1995). Recombination. Pieces of the site-specific recombination puzzle. *Curr. Biol.* **5,** 1106–1109.

Pasqualetti, M., Ren, S. Y., Poulet, M., LeMeur, M., Dierich, A., and Rijli, F. M. (2002). A Hoxa2 knockin allele that expresses EGFP upon conditional Cre-mediated recombination. *Genesis* **32,** 109–111.

Peitz, M., Pfannkuche, K., Rajewsky, K., and Edenhofer, F. (2002). Ability of the hydrophobic FGF and basic TAT peptides to promote cellular uptake of recombinant Cre recombinase: A tool for efficient genetic engineering of mammalian genomes. *Proc. Natl. Acad. Sci. USA* **99,** 4489–4494.

Ramirez-Solis, R., Davis, A. C., and Bradley, A. (1993). Gene targeting in embryonic stem cells. *Methods Enzymol.* **225,** 855–878.

Ramirez-Solis, R., Liu, P., and Bradley, A. (1995). Chromosome engineering in mice. *Nature* **378,** 720–724.

Ringrose, L., Angrand, P. O., and Stewart, A. F. (1997). The Kw recombinase, an integrase from *Kluyveromyces waltii*. *Eur. J. Biochem.* **248,** 903–912.

Ringrose, L., Chabanis, S., Angrand, P. O., Woodroofe, C., and Stewart, A. F. (1999). Quantitative comparison of DNA looping *in vitro* and *in vivo*: Chromatin increases effective DNA flexibility at short distances. *EMBO J.* **18,** 6630–6641.

Ringrose, L., Lounnas, V., Ehrlich, L., Buchholz, F., Wade, R., and Stewart, A. F. (1998). Comparative kinetic analysis of FLP and cre recombinases: Mathematical models for DNA binding and recombination. *J. Mol. Biol.* **284,** 363–384.

Rodriguez, C. I., Buchholz, F., Galloway, J., Sequerra, R., Kasper, J., Ayala, R., Stewart, A. F., and Dymecki, S. M. (2000). High-efficiency deleter mice show that FLPe is an alternative to Cre-loxP. *Nat. Genet.* **25,** 139–140.

Russ, A. P., Friedel, C., Ballas, K., Kalina, U., Zahn, D., Strebhardt, K., and von Melchner, H. (1996). Identification of genes induced by factor deprivation in hematopoietic cells undergoing apoptosis using gene-trap mutagenesis and site-specific recombination. *Proc. Natl. Acad. Sci. USA* **93,** 15279–15284.

Saam, J. R., and Gordon, J. I. (1999). Inducible gene knockouts in the small intestinal and colonic epithelium. *J. Biol. Chem.* **274,** 38071–38082.

Sauer, B., and McDermott, J. (2004). DNA recombination with a heterospecific Cre homolog identified from comparison of the pac-c1 regions of P1-related phages. *Nucleic Acids Res.* **32,** 6086–6095.

Schaft, J., Ashery-Padan, R., van der Hoeven, F., Gruss, P., and Stewart, A. F. (2001). Efficient FLP recombination in mouse ES cells and oocytes. *Genesis* **31,** 6–10.

Schlake, T., and Bode, J. (1994). Use of mutated FLP recognition target (FRT) sites for the exchange of expression cassettes at defined chromosomal loci. *Biochemistry* **33**, 12746–12751.

Schlake, T., Schupp, I., Kutsche, K., Mincheva, A., Lichter, P., and Boehm, T. (1999). Predetermined chromosomal deletion encompassing the Nf-1 gene. *Oncogene* **18**, 6078–6082.

Schmidt, E. E., Taylor, D. S., Prigge, J. R., Barnett, S., and Capecchi, M. R. (2000). Illegitimate Cre-dependent chromosome rearrangements in transgenic mouse spermatids. *Proc. Natl. Acad. Sci. USA* **97**, 13702–13707.

Schnütgen, F., De-Zolt, S., Van Sloun, P., Hollatz, M., Floss, T., Hansen, J., Altschmied, J., Seisenberger, C., Ghyselinck, N. B., Ruiz, P., Chambon, P., Wurst, W., and von Melchner, H. (2005). Genomewide production of multipurpose alleles for the functional analysis of the mouse genome. *Proc. Natl. Acad. Sci. USA* **102**, 7221–7226.

Schnütgen, F., Doerflinger, N., Calleja, C., Wendling, O., Chambon, P., and Ghyselinck, N. B. (2003). A directional strategy for monitoring Cre-mediated recombination at the cellular level in the mouse. *Nat. Biotechnol.* **21**, 562–565.

Schwenk, F., Kuhn, R., Angrand, P. O., Rajewsky, K., and Stewart, A. F. (1998). Temporally and spatially regulated somatic mutagenesis in mice. *Nucleic Acids Res.* **26**, 1427–1432.

Sclimenti, C. R., Thyagarajan, B., and Calos, M. P. (2001). Directed evolution of a recombinase for improved genomic integration at a native human sequence. *Nucleic Acids Res.* **29**, 5044–5051.

Seibler, J., Zevnik, B., Kuter-Luks, B., Andreas, S., Kern, H., Hennek, T., Rode, A., Heimann, C., Faust, N., Kauselmann, G., Schoor, M., Jaenisch, R., Rajewsky, K., Kuhn, R., and Schwenk, F. (2003). Rapid generation of inducible mouse mutants. *Nucleic Acids Res.* **31**, e12.

Shibata, H., Toyama, K., Shioya, H., Ito, M., Hirota, M., Hasegawa, S., Matsumoto, H., Takano, H., Akiyama, T., Toyoshima, K., Kanamaru, R., Kanegae, Y., Saito, I., Nakamura, Y., Shiba, K., and Noda, T. (1997). Rapid colorectal adenoma formation initiated by conditional targeting of the Apc gene. *Science* **278**, 120–123.

Shimshek, D. R., Kim, J., Hubner, M. R., Spergel, D. J., Buchholz, F., Casanova, E., Stewart, A. F., Seeburg, P. H., and Sprengel, R. (2002). Codon-improved Cre recombinase (iCre) expression in the mouse. *Genesis* **32**, 19–26.

Smith, M. C., and Thorpe, H. M. (2002). Diversity in the serine recombinases. *Mol. Microbiol.* **44**, 299–307.

Soriano, P. (1999). Generalized lacZ expression with the ROSA26 Cre reporter strain. *Nat. Genet.* **21**, 70–71.

Sternberg, N., Sauer, B., Hoess, R., and Abremski, K. (1986). Bacteriophage P1 cre gene and its regulatory region. Evidence for multiple promoters and for regulation by DNA methylation. *J. Mol. Biol.* **187**, 197–212.

Taniguchi, M., Sanbo, M., Watanabe, S., Naruse, I., Mishina, M., and Yagi, T. (1998). Efficient production of Cre-mediated site-directed recombinants through the utilization of the puromycin resistance gene, pac: A transient gene-integration marker for ES cells. *Nucleic Acids Res* **26**, 679–680.

Thorey, I. S., Muth, K., Russ, A. P., Otte, J., Reffelmann, A., and von Melchner, H. (1998). Selective disruption of genes transiently induced in differentiating mouse embryonic stem cells by using gene trap mutagenesis and site-specific recombination. *Mol. Cell. Biol.* **18**, 3081–3088.

Thorpe, H. M., and Smith, M. C. (1998). *In vitro* site-specific integration of bacteriophage DNA catalyzed by a recombinase of the resolvase/invertase family. *Proc. Natl. Acad. Sci. USA* **95**, 5505–5510.

Tsien, J. Z., Chen, D. F., Gerber, D., Tom, C., Mercer, E. H., Anderson, D. J., Mayford, M., Kandel, E. R., and Tonegawa, S. (1996). Subregion-and cell type-restricted gene knockout in mouse brain. *Cell* **87**, 1317–1326.

Umlauf, S. W., and Cox, M. M. (1988). The functional significance of DNA sequence structure in a site-specific genetic recombination reaction. *EMBO J.* **7**, 1845–1852.

Van den Plas, D., Ponsaerts, P., Van Tendeloo, V., Van Bockstaele, D. R., Berneman, Z. N., and Merregaert, J. (2003). Efficient removal of LoxP-flanked genes by electroporation of Cre-recombinase mRNA. *Biochem. Biophys. Res. Commun.* **305**, 10–15.

Van Duyne, G. D. (2001). A structural view of cre-loxp site-specific recombination. *Annu. Rev. Biophys. Biomol. Struct.* **30**, 87–104.

Ventura, A., Meissner, A., Dillon, C. P., McManus, M., Sharp, P. A., Van Parijs, L., Jaenisch, R., and Jacks, T. (2004). Cre-lox-regulated conditional RNA interference from transgenes. *Proc. Natl. Acad. Sci. USA* **101**, 10380–10385.

Vooijs, M., Jonkers, J., and Berns, A. (2001). A highly efficient ligand-regulated Cre recombinase mouse line shows that LoxP recombination is position dependent. *EMBO Rep.* **2**, 292–297.

Wunderlich, F. T., Wildner, H., Rajewsky, K., and Edenhofer, F. (2001). New variants of inducible Cre recombinase: A novel mutant of Cre-PR fusion protein exhibits enhanced sensitivity and an expanded range of inducibility. *Nucleic Acids Res.* **29**, E47.

Xin, H. B., Deng, K. Y., Shui, B., Qu, S., Sun, Q., Lee, J., Greene, K. S., Wilson, J., Yu, Y., Feldman, M., and Kotlikoff, M. I. (2005). Gene trap and gene inversion methods for conditional gene inactivation in the mouse. *Nucleic Acids Res.* **33**, e14.

Zambrowicz, B. P., and Sands, A. T. (2003). Knockouts model the 100 best-selling drugs will they model the next 100? *Nat. Rev. Drug Discov.* **2**, 38–51.

Zheng, B., Sage, M., Sheppeard, E. A., Jurecic, V., and Bradley, A. (2000). Engineering mouse chromosomes with Cre-loxP: Range, efficiency, and somatic applications. *Mol. Cell. Biol.* **20**, 648–655.

[8] Gene Trapping in Embryonic Stem Cells

By WILLIAM L. STANFORD, TREVOR EPP,
TAMMY REID, and JANET ROSSANT

Abstract

Gene trapping in embryonic stem cells (ESCs) generates random, sequence-tagged insertional mutations, which can often report the gene expression pattern of the mutated gene. This mutagenesis strategy has often been coupled to expression or function-based assays in gene discovery screens. The availability of the mouse genome sequence has shifted gene trapping from a gene discovery platform to a high-throughput mutagenesis platform. At present, a concerted worldwide effort is underway to develop a library of loss-of-function mutations in all mouse genes. The International Gene Trap Consortium (IGTC) is leading the way by making a first pass of the genome by random mutagenesis before a high-throughput gene targeting program takes over. In this chapter, we provide a methods guidebook to exploring and using the IGTC resource, explain the different kinds of vectors and insertions that reside in the different libraries, and provide advice and methods for investigators to design novel expression-based "cottage industry" screens.

METHODS IN ENZYMOLOGY, VOL. 420   0076-6879/06 $35.00

Introduction

With the completion of the human and mouse genome sequence, there has been renewed interest in developing tools for genome-wide mutagenesis in the mouse, with the goal of analyzing function of all genes in the genome in the context of the intact organism. Gene trap insertional mutagenesis in mouse embryonic stem (ES) cells is an important component of a comprehensive approach to functional annotation of the mouse genome, providing the possibility of efficiently generating a resource of insertional mutations across a large proportion of the genome (Stanford et al., 2001). Insertional mutagenesis has been widely used in genetic screens in many different model organisms, including mice, because of the ease of identifying the genes mutated using the insertion vector as a tag. Early studies in mice used exogenous transgene or retroviral vectors to generate novel insertional mutations in a number of different genes, whereas recent studies have suggested that transposase-activated hopping transposons, such as Sleeping Beauty (Keng et al., 2005) and piggyBac (Ding et al., 2005), can also be mutagenic in the mouse germline. Gene trap technology can be grafted onto any of these different means of introducing DNA into the genome, and it adds considerable functionality to the insertion event. A variety of different gene trap vectors have been developed, but all essentially work by insertion of a promoterless reporter gene into an endogenous gene, such that the insertion simultaneously reports on expression of the endogenous gene, mutates that gene, and allows cloning of the disrupted gene from the inserted DNA tag. Application of this technique in a genome-wide manner has the potential to identify most, if not all, of the active transcripts in the genome, including alternatively spliced forms and low-abundance transcripts and is thus an important tool in genome annotation. Importantly, the use of this mutagenesis approach in ESCs allows generation of libraries of sequence-tagged mutations across the genome. Such ESC libraries are easily archived and distributed, providing a community resource for production of mutant mice and exploration of mammalian biology.

Lexicon Genetics, a mouse genetics-based biotechnology company, was the first to move gene trapping from a "cottage industry" to a robust, high-throughput technology with rapid isolation and annotation of large numbers of gene trap insertions in ESCs, and they have reported generation of a library of more than 270,000 mouse ESC clones, representing insertions in up to 60% of the genes in the genome (Zambrowicz et al., 2003). However, although the sequence tags associated with these insertions are deposited in the public databases, it is not currently cost-effective for most investigators to access this resource. Several academic-based centers have also been funded over the past few years to generate a public domain resource of gene trap insertions. These centers together formed the International Gene Trap Consortium with the goal of generating a well-annotated and publicly available resource of gene trap insertions in ESCs. This public effort now has a database of nearly 45,000 ESC clones, representing 29% of the genes in the genome (personal communication, Deanna Church, NCBI). The availability of these clones is already having a major impact on the mouse genetics community, obviating in many cases the need to generate expensive targeted mutations to explore gene function.

Common Types of Gene Trap Vectors in IGTC

Several essential features are common to any gene trap vector, including the ability to:

- Allow rapid identification of the trapped gene
- Disrupt function of the trapped gene
- Provide a reporter to easily detect endogenous gene expression

The most common types of gene trap vectors used to date all share these common features (Fig. 1). The most widely used vectors are variations on the splice-acceptor–β-geo vectors first developed in the Soriano laboratory (Friedrich and Soriano, 1991). In these vectors, insertions into the intron of a gene expressed in ESCs results in a fusion transcript between the upstream exon and the β-galactosidase–neo fusion construct, resulting in neomycin resistance and β-galactosidase expression dependent on the host gene regulatory elements (Fig. 1A). Because the only clones that grow in G418 are by definition gene trap insertions, this is a simple and effective way of isolating gene trap clones. Other type of vectors used include the U3neo gene entrapment vectors (Hicks *et al.*, 1997; Fig. 1B), which contain no splice acceptor sequence and are designed to trap insertions within exons of genes (although cryptic splice acceptor sequences in these vectors means that half of the insertions are actually in introns [Osipovich *et al.*, 2004]) and the original splice acceptor–β-galactosidase vectors, with a separate drug resistance cassette (Gossler *et al.*, 1989; Skarnes *et al.*, 1992; Fig. 1C). The efficiency of isolating gene trap clones from either of these vectors is much lower than with β-geo vectors, but both are effective mutagens. The U3neo vectors have the advantage of being able to trap single exon genes and potentially noncoding transcripts.

With the combined use of these different vectors in the international consortium, it has been demonstrated that the accrual rate of new gene insertions seems to be higher than that in the Lexicon data set, in which only a single vector type was used (Skarnes *et al.*, 2004). This suggests that different vectors may have different biases for insertions and that multiple

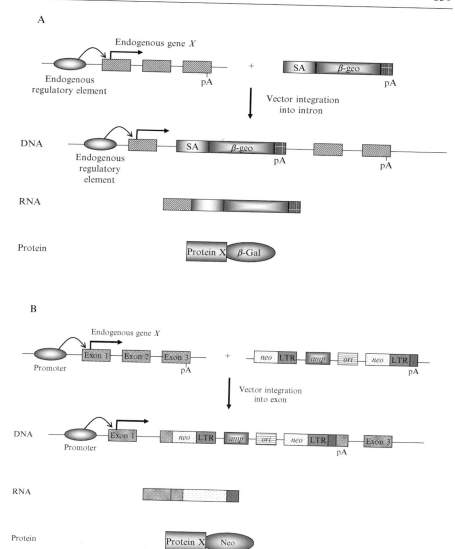

FIG. 1. (*continued*)

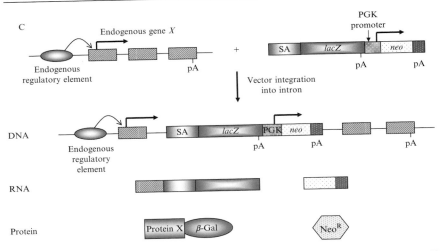

Fig. 1. Three common gene trap vectors. Each vector is depicted inserting into gene X. (A) The β-geo vector contains a splice acceptor (SA) immediately upstream of a promoterless β-galactosidase–neomycin resistance gene fusion. The insertion of the β-geo vector into an intron generates a fusion transcript and protein from the β-geo reporter and the upstream exon of gene X, providing that gene X is transcriptionally active in undifferentiated ESCs. (B) The U3neo promoter trap provirus contains the ampicillin resistance gene (*amp*) and a plasmid origin of replication flanked by the *neo* gene in each LTR. Selecting for neo-resistant clones identifies those cells in which an endogenous gene has been disrupted as a result of the proviral insertion into an exon (shown) or into an intron such that the upstream splice donor of gene X splices to a cryptic splice acceptor site within the *neo* gene (not shown). (C) The β-gal vector depicted contains a splice acceptor immediately upstream of the *lacZ* reporter followed by a *neo* selectable marker driven by an autologous promoter. All insertions, regardless of whether the insertion occurs within an intron (as shown) or in intergenic regions, lead to neomycin resistance and selection. If the insertion occurs in an intron, a fusion transcript is generated between the *lacZ* reporter and the upstream exon of gene X on transcriptional activation of the locus.

vector use ensures broader genome coverage. However, the largest number of insertions still comes from β-geo gene traps, which require that the trapped gene is expressed in ESCs for identification of the clones. Clearly β-geo is a very sensitive marker, and insertions in many genes expressed at low levels in ESCs can be detected. It has been estimated that approximately 60–70% of the genome could potentially be trapped by β-geo vectors (Austin *et al.*, 2004). However, there will always be a subset of genes not expressed in ESCs that cannot be trapped by β-geo vectors.

To overcome this, there has been considerable interest in developing vectors that trap genes irrespective of expression levels in ESCs. PolyA trap vectors, first developed in Yamamura's laboratory (Niwa *et al.*, 1993) and later used in initial studies at Lexicon Genetics (Zambrowicz *et al.*, 1998), have the potential to achieve this goal. In these vectors, a splice-acceptor–reporter construct remains to trap upstream exons and report gene expression, but the polyA sequence of the promoter–neo construct is replaced by a splice donor sequence. Neo-resistant clones can only arise when the vector lands in an intron and the neo gene can find a polyA sequence by splicing to downstream exons. Because neo has its own promoter, this expression does not depend on the active transcription of the trapped gene. Although this kind of vector has been shown to effectively trap genes not trapped by other methods, there have been problems in implementing polyA trapping on a large scale, because of concerns about a 3' bias in polyA trap insertions. This bias tends to limit the mutagenicity of the insertions because large pieces of intact protein can be made from the upstream, nondisrupted exons. An elegant study by Ishida has recently shown that this 3' bias is a result of loss of insertions that occur in more upstream exons because of nonsense-mediated decay (NMD) (Shigeoka et al., 2005). Nonsense-mediated decay targets transcripts with premature termination codons for destruction by the cellular machinery and is presumably a cellular defense mechanism. Because the polyA trap insertions will generate fusion transcripts of host gene exons downstream of the neo gene, the stop codon in neo will lead to NMD of transcripts other than those close to the 3' end. After demonstrating that this mechanism was in play, Ishida also showed that NMD could be overcome in polyA trap vectors by placing an IRES sequence downstream of neo and upstream of the splice donor (Fig. 2).

We have recently developed novel polyA trap vectors that co-opt NMD as a mutagenesis agent by engineering an internal exon containing a premature stop codon downstream of a fluorescent reporter. For this strategy, 3' terminal integrations are desired, because Cre-mediated recombination will often rescue the allele, replacing it with a C-terminal fluorescently tagged allele, which can be used for real-time subcellular localization studies (Fig. 3). Implementation of these vectors on a large scale will now be needed to validate that polyA trap insertional mutagenesis can, indeed, extend the application of gene trapping to a large segment of the non-ESC–expressed genome.

In addition to the basic features of trapping and disrupting host gene transcripts and reporting host gene expression, new generations of gene trap vectors have been developed that have other functionalities. Inclusion of a membrane-targeting sequence has allowed the specific selection of membrane-associated and secreted factors, in the so-called *secretory trap* vector (Skarnes et al., 1995). Several groups are developing vectors that allow postinsertion modification of the gene trap insertion, using a variety of recombinase-mediated exchange mechanisms. And, finally, there is considerable interest in generating gene trap vectors that are "conditional ready," which can be used to generate null mutations or tissue-specific or inducible

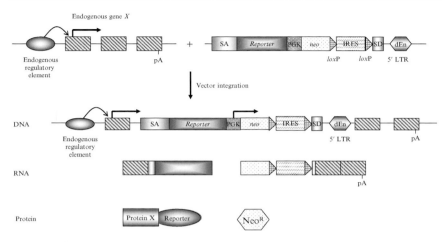

FIG. 2. Overcoming nonsense-mediated decay using the UPATrap vector. The polyA trap vector is a modification of the β-gal vector (Fig. 1C), such that the *neo* gene polyA site is replaced by a splice donor (SD). This requires insertion of the vector upstream of a splice acceptor site and polyA sequence to produce neo protein. Nonsense-mediated decay (NMD) is activated by the *neo* fusion transcript if the neo termination codon is more than 55 bp upstream of the final splice junction site. NMD is suppressed by introducing a floxed internal ribosome entry site (IRES) sequence upstream of initiation codons in all three reading frames inserted between the *neo* gene and the splice donor sequence of UPATrap polyA trap vector (Shigeoka *et al.*, 2005). The resulting bicistronic message escapes NMD and is translated. To increase mutagenicity, Cre recombination is performed after selection and cloning *in vitro* or *in vivo* to prevent expression of the 3′ portion of the trapped gene. The IRES sequence inserted downstream of the termination codon of the *neo* gene prevented activation of NMD, allowing trapping of transcriptionally silent genes without a bias in the vector-integration site.

mutations. One published approach is the FlEx strategy that is being implemented in the German Gene Trap initiative (Schnütgen *et al.*, 2005). In this strategy, the SA-β–geo vector is surrounded by paired recombination sites for several different recombinases so that the mutagenic insertion can first be rescued by promoting an inversion of the β-geo in the intron. The inverted sequence should not be mutagenic because there is no longer a fusion protein made with the host gene. In this configuration, the vector is ready for conditional mutagenesis; when crossed with appropriate Cre lines, the β-geo can be inverted again, and the mutation generated in a tissue-specific or inducible manner. Although this is an attractive strategy, there still remain some questions about whether the silent inverted insertion will be neutral always or whether it may have some deleterious effects on its own. More data are needed and will be available soon to assess the success of these vectors.

Whatever strategy is used, all gene trapping has one common feature: the generation of a sequence tag for the trapped gene. This is the common

A Vector design

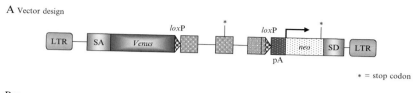

* = stop codon

B Transcript-trapped allele (– Cre)

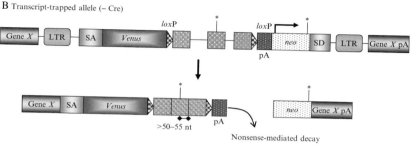

>50–55 nt

Nonsense-mediated decay

C Protein-tagged allele (+Cre)

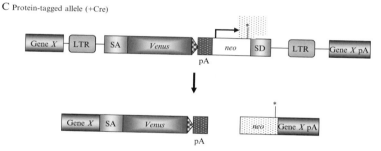

FIG. 3. Co-opting nonsense–mediated decay as a mutagenesis agent. Because NMD is exceptionally proficient at degrading transcripts, we reasoned that co-opting NMD as a mutagenesis agent could be at least, if not more, mutagenic than conventional gene trap vectors. Although insertions within the final intron of genes are disadvantageous from a mutagenesis standpoint, it does offer improved functionality as an expression marker. The 3′ insertions of gene trap vectors containing a fluorescent reporter allows high-throughput random protein tagging that can be used to resolve expression profiles at the subcellular level—an important and useful tool for the characterization of new genes. We wanted to maintain this functionality in our gene trap vector design while still allowing mutagenesis of the trapped gene. Our NMDi polyA trap vector was engineered by inserting three floxed internal exons containing premature stop codons downstream of a fluorescent reporter, targeting the trapped gene for NMD. For this strategy, 3′ terminal integrations are desired, because Cre-mediated recombination will often rescue the allele, replacing it with a C-terminal fluorescently tagged allele, which can be used for real-time subcellular localization studies.

currency of all active gene trap programs, and it is the feature that connects the gene trap resource with the broader genomic databases. As the gene trap effort grows, the International Consortium is dedicated to ensure that the resource has maximal value for the community and to encourage researchers to visit the existing web sites and access the reagents therein.

A User's Guide to the International Gene Trap Consortium Resource

As discussed previously, a number of international laboratories (Table I) supported by numerous funding agencies are currently generating a resource of sequence-tagged gene trap ESC clones. This resource for the generation of mutagenized mice is freely available on a noncollaborative basis. The IGTC sequence–tagged resource obviates the need for independent investigators to generate mutations by homologous recombination for a substantial proportion of the mouse genome and the need to describe protocols to enable independent investigators to perform their own sequence-based gene trap screens. Instead, in this section of the chapter we will overview how investigators can use the IGTC resource, including requesting clones, verifying their identify, generating mice, and developing genotyping strategies for the resulting mutant mice.

A Repository of Sequence-tagged ESC Lines

The member laboratories of the IGTC work in parallel, using different gene trap vectors, transfection parameters (viral or plasmid), and parental ESC lines. This ensures the greatest coverage of the genome with as many different types of alleles that can be generated by gene trapping. Each center generates its own sequence tags, performs sequence analysis, and posts the sequences in its own databases maintained on its own web sites (Table I). Most of the IGTC member websites have similar user modalities to those on the CMHD website (To *et al.*, 2004).

1. Sequence-based querying of the database by means of a BLAST interface
2. Keyword-based querying of the database (e.g., gene name, GO annotations...).

Each website has specific information about requesting clones, as well as protocols associated with the resource, including critical protocols concerning the generation of mutant mice using that center's ESCs or developing geno-typing strategies specific for a particular vector. All member IGTC labora-tories also upload sequences into the NCBI dbGSS (genome survey sequence) database. Beacuse dbGSS sequence submissions are immediately publicly

TABLE I
IGTC MEMBER LABORATORIES AND THEIR WEB SITES

IGTC member	Web site
Baygenomics (USA)	www.baygenomics.ucsf.edu/
Centre for Modelling Human Disease (Toronto, Canada)	http://www.cmhd.ca/genetrap/
Embryonic Stem Cell Database (University of Manitoba, Canada)	www.escells.ca/
Exchangeable Gene Trap Clones (Kumamoto University, Japan)	http://egtc.jp/show/index
German Gene Trap Consortium (Germany)	http://tikus.gsf.de/
Sanger Institute Gene Trap Resource (Cambridge, UK)	www.sanger.ac.uk/PostGenomics/genetrap
Soriano Lab Gene Trap Database (FHCRC, Seattle, USA)	www.fhcrc.org/labs/soriano/trap.html
International Gene Trap Consortium	www.genetrap.org

accessible, this repository remains the most up-to-date and comprehensive source for gene trap sequence data.

All gene trap insertions matching any given query sequence can be retrieved from NCBI using BLASTN or MegaBLAST (http://www.ncbi.nlm.nih.gov/BLAST). From the BLAST GUI (graphical user interface) enter your sequence, select dbGSS under "sequence database," and enter "gene trap" under "limit by entrez query." It is often beneficial to include the full genomic sequence rather than just the cDNA sequence, to also identify gene trap tags isolated by genome-based approaches (e.g., inverse polymerase chain reaction [PCR], plasmid rescue) or those isolated by cDNA approaches (especially 3′-RACE), where the context of the integration site has led to use of cryptic splicing signals. In either case, it is important to mask any repetitive elements in your query sequence to avoid nonspecific hits. Online resources for masking repeats can be found at http://www.repeatmasker.org or http://www.girinst.org/censor/. From the dbGSS sequence reports, links to the individual gene trap project sites allow the user to access further information such as vector features, methods used, and associated protocols.

Gene trap sequence tags can be visualized by means of the NCBI Map Viewer (http://www.ncbi.nih.gov/mapview). A keyword or BLAST query will display the genomic interval of interest. From there, gene trap insertions (IGTC and Lexicon Genetics) can be graphically displayed by making the appropriate selection under the "Maps & Options" toggle button. Currently, a subset of gene trap insertions can be displayed on the UCSC Genome Browser using a custom annotation track provided by Bay Genomics (http://genome.cse.ucsc.edu/goldenPath/customTracks). Alternately, the entire IGTC data set can be displayed on the Ensembl genome browser (http://www.ensembl.org). First, use the BLAST sequence query or a text-based search for the gene of interest to obtain the genomic interval to be displayed ("ContigView"). The "Detailed View" window of the Contig-View page contains a dropdown menu labeled "DAS" for distributed annotation system wherein a check-box will allow the user to display the mapped gene trap sequence tags to the interval of interest. Note that, because annotation of gene trap sequence data occurs intermittently, recent dbGSS submissions will often not be accessible by means of these genome browsers.

Most groups, including ours, use parallel BLAST alignments of sequence tags with cDNA and entire genome databases, with congruous results interpreted as correctly identifying the locus. Sometimes these annotations do not distinguish sense from antisense alignments, so the user is advised to manually confirm the annotation results with the original dbGSS sequence report or trace file. Highly conserved paralogous genes or pseudogenes may also lead to misannotations or annotation conflicts that we have found can often be resolved by calculation of inferred splice site scores. Thus, as a user, it is advisable to try different approaches to obtain gene trap data. If several gene trap clones exist for your gene of interest, it is then possible to further discriminate according to the different sites of insertion and various features of the specific vectors, such as type of reporter, presence and orientation of any recombination signals presence of protein affinity tags.

In an effort to simplify this data acquisition process, the IGTC has recently launched its own website (www.genetrap.org), enabling users to begin their search for gene trap clones at a single source (Nord *et al.*, 2006). The IGTC website allows users to browse and search the database for trapped genes based on sequence identity, gene name, or accession numbers. In addition, searches can be performed for gene trap clones that fall within a particular biological pathway, expression pattern, chromosomal location, or Gene Ontology (GO) classifications. Also, the IGTC web site hosts a gene trap tutorial and links to all of the member sites for clone requests and additional IGTC member-specific information including protocols associated with each center.

As computational biology and genome annotation analysis continues to grow in new directions, the IGTC resource will also develop or link to new resources to better annotate clones and place trapped genes within specific pathways. For example, building on support vector machines, Bayesian analysis, and other computation strategies, we are currently developing gene functional prediction software that will be first tested on our own web site (CMHD) and then maintained on the IGTC web site.

Requesting Clones

Once an investigator has identified a clone with an insertion within a "gene of interest," they must determine whether it is mutagenic. Gene traps should not be considered as necessarily equivalent to knockouts. These random insertions are usually mutagenic, even leading to null mutations. However, the insertion site in a clone is a critical determinant of the type of mutation generated. Insertions occurring in the 5' coding region will likely generate a null mutation, whereas other types of insertions lead to hypomorphic or neomorphic mutations, or even to dominant negative mutations. This is dependent on the gene structure and function, as well as the type of gene trap vector used. On a clone request, we assess and inform the requisitioning scientist of the likelihood of the insertion being mutagenic and will offer advice on genotyping strategies. If more than one ESC line is available for a gene of interest, especially if the insertions are made with different vectors integrating in different introns, it is possible that the investigator could investigate an allelic series. Although a high percentage of IGTC ESC lines yield germline-transmitting chimeras, not all do. Thus, requesting multiple lines also will increase the chances of successful mutant mouse generation. We and other IGTC members will verify that the requested clones grow well after thawing and demonstrate morphologically undifferentiated characteristics. Furthermore, investigators should request the IGTC member laboratory to confirm gene insertion identity on the thawed clone before shipment, because the original PCR-generated sequence was generated using high-throughput 96-well or 384-well protocols, with inevitable possibilities for mistakes. Ideally, gene identity should be validated by a different assay from the original strategy (i.e., inverse PCR to identify genomic insertion versus cDNA identification by RACE-PCR). Protocols for both approaches are vector specific; thus, each IGTC member's website has the appropriate downloadable protocols.

Many IGTC members, including ourselves, require a nominal payment to help defray the ongoing cost of cryopreservation and maintenance of stocks and shipping of clones as well as a signed nonrestrictive Materials Transfer Agreement (MTA). There has been a concerted effort to standardize the MTA by the various host institutions within the IGTC. For example, our MTA is designed primarily to require the investigators using our gene trap clones to notify us of publications in which our clones were used, as well as to ensure that our resource is acknowledged (without authorship) within manuscripts. Acknowledgment is critical for sustained support of the resource by granting agencies.

Clone and Mutant Analysis

On receipt of a gene trap clone, it is advisable to further characterize the site of integration. Knowledge of the precise genomic site of integration will allow design of a PCR genotyping strategy. Often only a 5′ or 3′-RACE sequence is known, with the inference that the vector has inserted somewhere in the adjoining intron, which can sometimes encompass hundreds of kilobases in length. There are many approaches to identifying unknown flanking DNA sequence, including inverse PCR, splinkerette PCR, anchored PCR, or plasmid rescue (reviewed in Hui *et al.* [1998]) as well as more recent strategies such as universal fast walking (Myrick and Gelbart, 2002). However, in practice, it is usually most convenient to perform straight genomic PCR designed using sequence information from the original dbGSS sequence. A protocol describing long and accurate (LA) PCR can be found in an earlier volume in this series (Chen and Soriano, 2003). Finally, mapping the integration locus by genomic Southern blotting will uncover any undesirable occurrence of local deletions and rearrangements. Although uncommon, these mutations have been described previously (Niwa *et al.*, 1993) and, if present, could lead to incorrect conclusions being made from the phenotypic analysis of the gene trap line.

Investigator-Initiated Screens

Because reporter genes lie within most gene trap vectors, gene trapping lends itself to screening for particular gene expression characteristics, given an appropriate expression assay. Thus, although the IGTC is saturating the trappable mouse genome with sequence tags, there is still a role for investigator-initiated screens, so-called *cottage industry gene trapping*. Although large-scale *in vivo* gene trap expression screens have been successfully performed (Leighton *et al.*, 2001; Wurst *et al.*, 1995), a more efficient strategy is to use the *in vitro* differentiation capacity of ESCs or the ability of ESCs to respond to physiological stimuli (Bautch *et al.*, 1996; Doetschman *et al.*, 1985; Nakano *et al.*, 1994) as a surrogate assay for *in vivo* expression or gene function. We, and other groups, have used this strategy to identify gene trap insertions within genes differentially regulated in specific developmental pathways such as hematopoiesis and angiogenesis or regulated by retinoic acid or ionizing radiation (for example, Forrester *et al.* [1996]; Kuhnert and Stuhlmann [2004]; Mainguy *et al.* [2000]; Stanford *et al.* [1998]; Tarrant *et al.* [2002]; Vallis *et al.* [2002]). Although potentially labor-intensive, this strategy can be very fruitful, providing the *in vitro* differentiation or response assay is efficient.

Using *in vitro* ESC–based assays requires that the pathway of interest is accessible in either undifferentiated or differentiated ESCs. Computational analysis of large-scale gene expression data can be used to identify potential ESC clones harboring gene trap insertions within genes responsive to specific stimuli or differentially expressed in various cell types, which can then be analyzed for phenotype *in vivo*. The Soriano and Ishida groups have used an alternative strategy in which transcriptional profiling is performed on custom cDNA microarrays generated from high throughput 3'RACE sequence tagging of gene trap insertions (Chen *et al.*, 2004; Matsuda *et al.*, 2004). An advantage of arraying 3'RACE products is that all potential genes available to gene trap mutagenesis are analyzed, preserving one of the tenets of gene trapping—gene discovery. Using a 2000 ROSAFARY gene trap array, the Soriano laboratory identified 23 genes that were differentially expressed by PDGF-BB, whereas the Ishida group used the NAISTrap gene trap array to identify differentially expressed genes among various tissues. However, many investigators may not have array facilities accessible to them for such experiments. Furthermore, depending on the specificity of the microarray experiment, this strategy may require tens or possibly hundreds of thousands of RACE products to be arrayed to identify specific targets of the pathway of interest.

Design of Screens

The future of boutique ESC gene trap screens is limited principally by the imagination of the investigator. An advantage of *in vitro* expression screens over computational expression strategies is that expression can be analyzed in individual cells and structures rather than as a signal average. Thus, screens built around the coexpression of genes of interest and trapped genes are particularly attractive. This strategy has not been exploited extensively despite the fact that highly sensitive fluorescent reporters are now available. We have found that the modified yellow fluorescent reporter Venus (Nagai *et al.*, 2002) is roughly as sensitive as β-galactosidase in gene trap vectors (Tanaka *et al.*, in preparation), enabling us to proceed with coexpression screens. Extending this strategy, fluorescent gene trap screens could also be used with fluorescence resonance energy transfer (FRET) to identify protein–protein interactions. Furthermore, we anticipate that gene trapping in human ESCs offers enormous potential to investigate early human development. In addition, a library of sequence-tagged gene trap insertions combined with *in vitro* differentiation screens would generate reporter cell lines for the optimization of ESC–derived cell lineages using tissue engineering strategies.

For investigators contemplating boutique screens, we believe the following questions should be kept in mind in your screen design:

- *Are the target genes expressed in ESCs or cells undergoing* in vitro *differentiation?* This will certainly dictate the choice of vector. If the assay is performed in undifferentiated cells, β-geo or similar vectors should be used; otherwise, polyA trap vectors should be used.
- *Is the assay robust?* As with all screens, the quality of the results hinges entirely on having specific, robust, high-throughput screens. Do you have secondary or validation screens? We have begun to use high-content screening with a Cellomics Incorporated ArrayScan automated fluorescent microscope to enable real-time screening and quantification.
- *What percentage of the genome would deliver a hit in your screen?* As discussed previously, collectively the IGTC has generated 45,000 gene trap ESC clones, representing approximately 29% of the genome. How many clones must be screened to identify critical hits? The more clones required to screen, the more we encourage the investigator to use viral-based vectors, which are much more efficient.

Below are protocols that we have used for our screens, including procedures for freezing clones in 96-well tubes and various *in vitro* differentiation assays, as well as molecular analysis. All the culture-related protocols were optimized using the R1 parental ES cell line (Nagy and Rossant, 1993). These protocols may need to be modified for other cell lines.

More detailed protocols can be found online at: http://www.cmhd.ca/genetrap/protocols.html.

ESC Culture Media

ESCs are cultured in Dulbecco's modified Eagle medium (Gibco #11960-044) containing 15% of ESC-qualified fetal bovine serum (FBS; should still be screened to ensure suitability), 100 units/ml leukemia inhibitory factor (ESGRO, Chemicon), 2 mM L-glutamine (Invitrogen 35050-061), 100 μM 2-mercptoethanol (Sigma, M7522), 0.1 mM nonessential amino acids (Invitrogen, 11140-050), 1 mM sodium pyruvate (Gibco, 11360-070), and penicillin/streptomycin (Invitrogen #15140-148, final concentration 50 μg/ml each).

General Culturing of ESCs

All procedures are performed under sterile conditions in a laminar flow hood using sterile instruments and detergent-free glassware. All reagents used for culturing ESCs should be "tissue culture tested" or "tissue culture grade." For ESCs to remain in an undifferentiated state, they must be cultured in the presence of LIF (Esgro, Chemicon), and the tissue culture plates must be specifically treated before seeding the ESCs. This is performed either by coating the plates with 0.1% gelatin (Sigma #G-1890) or preparing a layer of mitotically inactivated embryonic fibroblasts (MEFs) (Specialty Media). We do not recommend growing ESCs for long periods of time in LIF alone (i.e., on gelatin-coated plates) without a feeder layer unless using commercially purchased LIF with known activity units (Esgro, Chemicon). Also, if the ESCs grow to overconfluency, it can result in their differentiation and loss of germline competence. ESCs should be fed every day and split every second day (approximately 70–80% confluency, colonies almost touching each other). To passage cells, the media is aspirated, and the cells are rinsed with PBS without calcium or magnesium. The cells are dissociated for 5 min with a 0.05% solution of trypsin–ethylenediaminetetraacidic acid (EDTA; Invitrogen). The trypsin reaction is stopped by the addition of at least twice the volume of ESC culture medium, and the cells are resuspended and passaged onto a previously prepared plate using a 1:5 ratio (this may need to be adjusted depending on the cell line).

Freezing of Clones in 96-Well Plates

Clones are frozen in individual 0.6-ml tubes, which are racked in 96-well boxes (CLP #mini2600, Continental Lab Products). Freezing plates are prepared ahead of time by placing 150 μl of a 2× freezing media (20% DMSO, 40% FBS, and 50% media) into each well. Plates containing ESC clones that are ready to be frozen (60–80% confluent) are then washed with 50 μl/well of PBS (minus Mg_2, Ca^+); 50 μl/well of trypsin (0.05%) is added, and the plates are incubated for 5 min at 37°. After incubation, 100 μl of media is added to each well, and the clones are resuspended well. It is important to create a single cell suspension, because clumps of cells will not be protected by the dimethyl sulfoxide (DMSO) during the freezing process, resulting in cell death. Once the well is resuspended, the cells are transferred to the prepared freezing plate and mixed with the freezing media, resulting in a total of 300 μl/vial. Pliable caps (Falcon, capbands #352117) in strips of eight are used to seal the individual tubes, allowing retrieval of a single clone. It is important to use soft plastic caps because hard plastic ones will pop off during storage in cryotanks. Plates are frozen overnight at −86° and transferred to vapor phase liquid nitrogen tanks (ESBE, CBS model) within 48 h.

Thawing ESC Clones

For most efficient recovery, ESC clones should be thawed onto feeders. The easiest way to thaw an entire 96-well plate is to remove the bottom of the plate and immerse the tubes, still in the rack, into a 37° water bath to rapidly thaw cells. Quickly add 200 μl of ESC media to each well and then centrifuge the plate at 1000 rpm for at least 5 min. Aspirate the freezing media, resuspend the cells in 150 μl of ESC media, and transfer to a 96-well plate containing a MEF layer and 100 μl of ESC media. Incubate at 37° overnight and change the media the next day. To thaw individual tubes, remove the vial from the plate and quickly thaw in a 37° water bath. The contents of the tube can either be directly added to one well of a 24-well plate (with feeders and 2 ml of ESC media) or by washing the cells by centrifugation with 2 ml of media. We routinely thaw directly into a well, and the cells recover well.

Introduction of Vectors into ESCs—Retroviral Infection of ESCs

We have used both the pGen$^-$ and pGep$^-$ vector backbones for the generation of retroviral vectors for gene trapping (Chen *et al.*, 2004; Soriano *et al.*, 1991). Viral stocks were prepared using a Phoenix packaging cell line, and the multiplicity of infection (MOI) was determined before use to ensure an MOI of 0.1–0.5. Viral stocks are stored in −86° and aliquoted for single-use retrieval, because the freeze–thaw cycle results in a decreased infection rate. One day before infection, ESCs are plated at a density of 3×10^6 cells in a 10-cm dish with ESC medium and incubated overnight. The next day the supernatant containing the packaged retrovirus is thawed and diluted with ESC medium containing 4 μg/ml of polybrene (hexadimethrine bromide; Sigma H9268-5G) to produce an MOI of 0.1–0.5. This dilution enhances the probability of a single virus infection per cell. The ESC medium is removed from the ESCs, and 3–4ml of the virus polybrene mixture is added per 10-cm plate. Cells and virus are incubated on a rocker platform at 37°, 5% CO_2 for 3–5 h, after which time another 6–7 ml of ESC medium containing 4 μg/ml polybrene is added per plate. The rocking motion during the initial incubation is important for the virus to tumble across the cells and adhere to their surface. The cells are then incubated for another 20 h without rocking. After 24 h of virus incubation, the medium is removed, and the drug selection is initiated (Geneticin, Gibco #10131-035; 167 μg/ml in ESC medium with LIF).

Electroporation of Gene Trap Vectors into ESCs

Linearized gene trap vectors are introduced into ESCs by electroporation using 1 μg of DNA per 1.5 million cells with a minimum of 10 million cells and maximum of 20 million cells per cuvette. From a 10-cm plate that is 80% confluent, cells are rinsed with PBS and dissociated using 1.5 ml of a 0.05% solution of trypsin–EDTA (Invitrogen, #25300-054) for 5 min at

37°. Once the cells have detached from the plate, 4 ml of media is added, and the cells are resuspended to create a single cell suspension. This is essential for an efficient electroporation because the current will not travel through each cell in a cell clump, resulting in an inefficient uptake of DNA. Also, if the cells are too dense within the cuvette, the current will take too long to traverse the cuvette, resulting in a high time constant value and damage to the cells. The cells are then centrifuged for 5 min at 1000 rpm. After centrifugation, cells are washed in ESC electroporation buffer (Specialty Media) to remove salts and media components. If the ion concentration is too high within the cuvette, the current will traverse through the cuvette too quickly and not make the cells competent for DNA uptake. High ion concentration can also cause a surge of current, killing essentially all of the cells. Cells are then resuspended at the correct concentration in ESC electroporation buffer for a final volume of 0.8 ml per cuvette. Linearized vector DNA is added to the cells, and the cuvette is placed on ice for 5 min. The electroporation is performed using 250V and 500 μF capacity (BioRad). Time constants should be noted and should not be more than 9 or less than 6. Immediately place the cuvette back on ice for 5–10 min to allow the cells to recover. Then, using a 1-ml pipette, gently transfer the contents of the cuvette to 5 ml of media in a 15-ml tube and leave for another 5–10 min at room temperature. The cells are very fragile at this stage and easily damaged if vigorously resuspended. White clumps or strings of debris indicate that the cells were damaged during the electroporation, and the efficiency may be lower than expected. However, viable colonies will still be produced so the experiment should be continued. The content of each tube is then plated onto two gelatin-coated 10-cm plates in a total volume of 10 ml and placed at 37° with 5% CO_2. Selection with ESC media containing the appropriate antibiotic (160 μg/ml Geneticin [G418]; 3.5 μg/ml Blasticidin; 1–2 μg/ml Puromycin, Invitrogen, for R1 cells) is started 24 h after electroporation, and the medium is changed every day.

Colony Picking

Resistant colonies will be ready for picking within 7–10 days (for electroporated cells) or 10–12 days (for infected cells). The surviving ESC colonies should have smooth margins and a raised three-dimensional appearance, with individual cells not readily apparent. Avoid picking colonies with obvious necrosis (dark center) or those containing flat differentiated cells. The surviving ES clones are picked using a dissecting microscope within a laminar flow hood and placed into individual wells of a V-bottom 96-well dish (CoStar #3894) containing 50 μl/well of trypsin (0.05%). The plate can be stored on ice, which will prevent over-trypsinization of the cells during the picking process. After picking 96 clones, the entire 96-well plate is incubated for 3 min at 37° and then 200 μl of ES media is added to each well. The cells are resuspended and transferred to a new 96-well plate prepared with a MEF feeder layer. Generally, after 3–4 days, most of the wells should be at least 80% confluent. The clones can then be expanded using a 1:4 split onto three plates containing MEFs to produce replicas for freezing and differentiation assays and one plate treated with gelatin for RNA and DNA isolation. Once these are confluent, two replicates of each plate are frozen for future retrieval, and the other two plates can be further expanded for genetic screening and/or used for the creation of differentiation assays.

High-Throughput Differentiation Assays

Certain assays will work better if the ESCs are grown on feeders, whereas others require growing on gelatin. Single cell suspensions of ESC clones grown in 96-well plates are prepared by aspirating the medium and washing the clones with 50 μl/well of PBS (minus Mg_2, Ca^+). Then, 50 μl/well of trypsin (0.05%) is added, and the plates are incubated for 5 min at 37°. After incubation, 150 μl of media is added to each well, and the clones are resuspended well. From one 96-well plate, the single cell suspension can be used to produce a variety of differentiation assays or screens.

OP9 Assay

Coculture of ESCs in the absence of LIF with the OP9 stromal cell line, which was derived from the M-CSF–deficient mouse strain *op/op*, promotes mesodermal lineage differentiation and hematopoietic cell propagation (Nakano *et al.*, 1994). One of the most important factors in achieving good differentiation on OP9 is the media used for the assay. We have discovered that the OP9 cells grow better when the alpha-MEM medium is made fresh from powder as opposed to commercially prepared medium and also results in better differentiation of the ESCs on the OP9 layer. Minimum essential medium-alpha (α-MEM) powdered media is used (Gibco #12000-022), and the powder is prepared according to the package directions in 900 ml of sterile distilled water with stirring. Once the powder has dissolved, we add 2.2 g of sodium bicarbonate (tissue culture tested), 6 ml of L-glutamine (200 m*M* stock, GIBCO), 6 ml of diluted ß-mercaptoethanol (made by adding 70 μl of 2-mercaptoethanol [Sigma, M7522] to 100 ml of water), and 5 ml of penicillin \streptomycin solution (Gibco #15140-148, 50 μg/ml final concentration).

The total volume is then brought up to 1 L and filter-sterilized (0.22-μm). Different serum lots also influence the differentiation of cells cocultured on OP9, and serum should be screened for optimal performance. For standard culturing, one confluent 10-cm plate of OP9 is trypsinized as usual, and a 1:3 split is performed every 2 days. Overconfluent plates or improper media will result in the OP9 differentiating into adipocytes.

For each set of clones picked, two 96-well plates of OP9 cells are required to set up the assay. One 10-cm plate of a 2-day culture can make a maximum of eight 96-well plates, and the 96-well plates can be prepared 1 or 2 days in advance. The media is aspirated from a 2-day-old 10-cm plate of OP9 cells, rinsed with 4 ml of PBS and 2 ml of trypsin is added. After incubation at 37° for 5 min, the cells are resuspended well in 6 ml of OP9 media. For preparation of the OP9 layers 1 day in advance, use a 1:4 dilution of a 2-day-old OP9 culture (10-cm dish). For each 96-well plate required, dilute 2 ml of resuspended OP9 cells into 8.2 ml of media and dispense 100 μl/well into the plate. If preparing the layers 2 days in advance, use a 1:8 dilution of the 2-day-old OP9 culture (10-cm dish). For each 96-well plate required, dilute 1 ml of resuspended OP9 cells into 9.2 ml of media and dispense 100 μl/well into the plate. Cells are grown for 24–48 h until the OP9 layer is approximately 80% confluent. On the day of use, the plates are subjected to gamma-irradiation (5 Gy). This will limit their proliferative capacity and prevent the layers detaching from the plate bottom during the assay. Add fresh media to each well before use in the OP9 assay.

In our hands, single cell suspensions of ESCs made from plates containing feeders produce more consistent results then ones originating from gelatin. The OP9 plates are irradiated, and then the media is replaced with 100 μl of fresh medium. An aliquot of 0.5 μl/well of the single cell suspension, prepared from the 96-well plate containing ESC clones and feeders, is added to each plate. Duplicate plates are required for assaying both mesodermal (day 5) and hematopoietic (day 8–10) differentiation. An additional 150 μl of media is then added to each well to distribute the cells and bring the final volume to 250 μl. ESCs differentiate into primitive mesoderm within 3–5 days as judged by Brachyury expression, followed by endothelial and hematopoietic cell emergence on days 4–5 (Hidaka et al., 1999). Cultures are fed by replacing half the media on day 3. On day 5 of culture, a single cell suspension is made, in a total volume of 200 μl, using one of the replica plates (50 μl trypsin [0.05%], 150 μl OP9 medium), and 5 μl from each well is transferred to a freshly prepared γ-irradiated OP9 plate to expand the hematopoietic progenitors. Plates are fed on day 7 and then left to develop hematopoietic colonies between days 8–10. The untouched duplicate plate containing the mesodermal colonies is fixed and/or assayed for gene expression.

Collagen IV Assay

Culture of ESCs in the absence of LIF on the extracellular matrix protein collagen type IV promotes mesoderm development along the vascular endothelial and smooth muscle lineages (Hirashima *et al.*, 1999 and unpublished data). Media for the collagen IV assay is prepared as described previously for the OP9 assay with the exception that only 10% FBS is added. Before the addition of ESC cell single cell suspensions, duplicate 96–well plates are coated with 40 μl/well of collagen type IV (250 μg/ml) (Sigma C5533), and incubated for 15 min at 37°, and then the collagen is aspirated and the plates are allowed to dry. After the addition of 100 μl of collagen IV medium to each well of the prepared plates, an aliquot of 3 μl/well of the single cell suspension is added. This is followed by an additional 150 μl of media to distribute the cells. Clones are fed every second day, and the cells are assayed for reporter gene activity on days 4 and 7.

Embryoid Body (EB) Assay

ESC clones from the original single cell suspension are transferred at a 1:5 ratio to a freshly prepared 0.1% gelatin-coated plate and grown to approximately 70% confluency. ESC colonies are washed with PBS and then subjected to Dispase treatment (Roche) using 40 μl/well of a 1:4 dilution (in PBS). After incubation in diluted Dispase for 30 sec–1 min, EB media (same as ESC medium with the exclusion of LIF) is added to each well, and the colonies are gently resuspended between 5–10 times. One half to one third of the well is then transferred to an "ultra low cluster" 96-well plate (Costar 3474) that has been previously prepared by adding 100 μl of EB media and incubated at 37° for at least 15–20 min before use. After the addition of the ESC colonies, an additional 100 μl of media is added to distribute the colonies. After 2 days, the EBs must be fed by very carefully removing half of the media and replacing it with fresh EB media, because the EBs are growing in suspension and are not attached to the plate. On day 4, the EBs are split from one "ultra low cluster" plate using a 1:6 or 1:8 split ratio onto gelatin coated 96-well tissue culture plates containing EB media, and the EBs are allowed to attach to the plate. These plates can then be used for a variety of different induction assays or immunohistochemistry-based analysis. EB plates can be grown for an additional 4–8 days, with feeding every 2 days, and subjected to different media conditions or environmental changes and analyzed for reporter gene activity or immunohistochemistry.

Induction Assays

Hypoxia and γ-Irradiation

Clones can also be analyzed for reporter gene regulation by specific physiological parameters such as hypoxia and γ-irradiation. Undifferentiated

ESCs (50–60% confluent) and EBs are subjected to hypoxic conditions of 1–2% O_2 for 24 h of culture. The plates are then removed and immediately analyzed for a change in reporter gene activity in comparison with a control plate grown in normoxic conditions. For γ-irradiation, undifferentiated ESCs and EBs are subjected to γ-irradiation at an appropriate dosage (such as 5 Gy). Clones are then incubated for 24 h at 37° in CO_2 and then compared with an unexposed control plate for a change in reporter gene activity.

Retinoic Acid

Growth or morphogenetic factor screens, such as retinoic acid, can also be performed. The media used in the retinoic acid assay is the same as the EB media with the exception that only 5% FBS is added and retinoic acid is added at a concentration of 1 μM. To condition the cells to the change in FBS concentration, media containing only 10% FBS is used for the media change 2 days before the retinoic acid is added. Clones treated with retinoic acid are incubated for 48 h during the developmental stage of interest and then assayed for changes in reporter gene activity compared with an untreated control plate grown in 5% FBS.

Gene Trap Insertion Identification—cDNA-Based Strategies

Gene trap insertions result in fusion transcripts between the reporter gene and the gene into which it is inserted. Consequently, flanking sequences can be amplified by 5'RACE PCR using RNA isolated from the gene trap line. Successful isolation of the 5' sequence is dependant on adequate expression levels in ESCs. Sometimes, *in vitro* differentiation of the gene trap line will activate the trapped locus, thereby permitting amplification by 5'RACE. PolyA trap vectors can also be characterized using 3'RACE, and because expression of the selectable marker fusion transcripts is driven by a constitutive reporter, the success rate in isolating PCR products is greater. Many commercial kits are available for conducting RACE experiments; we use the SMART RACE kit (Clontech Laboratories, Inc. Mountain View, CA). Note that RACE requires use of a gene-specific primer (GSP), which will be specific for the gene trap vector used. If designing a GSP for 3'RACE, you should attempt to use sequence 3' of the selectable marker; otherwise transgenes present in the feeder cells can interfere with amplification.

Gene Trap Insertion Identification—Genomic-Based Strategy

Inverse PCR is used to clone sequences flanking a known sequence. Flanking sequences are digested and ligated to make a circular DNA. PCR primers pointing away from the known sequences are then used to amplify the flanking sequences. Usually 4-base cutters are used for digestion because the shorter fragments are more efficiently circularized and PCR amplified. This is true for retroviral insertions, where the boundary between the known and unknown sequences is defined precisely because the long terminal repeats (LTRs) are conserved in the integrated provirus. However, problems are soon encountered when applying inverse PCR to plasmid-based constructs because unpredictable and often quite extensive amounts of endonucleolytic digestion occur. Losses of up to 1.8 kb from the

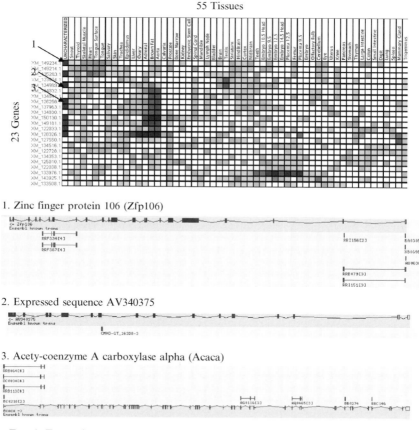

FIG. 4. Expression patterns of 23 genes known or predicted to be involved in insulin receptor signaling (GO:0008286). Predictions were made at a precision of 25% or greater as described (Zhang, 2004). Of the nine predicted genes (indicated by colored boxes in the left column), three have been trapped by members of the IGTC (arrows). The genomic structure of these three genes, together with the position of gene trap sequence tags, are illustrated in the bottom panel. (See color insert.)

5'-end and 3 kb from the 3'-end have been reported (Voss *et al.*, 1998). Therefore, to generate inverse PCR products where there has been moderate end digestion that would have otherwise destroyed primer sites used in conjunction with the frequent 4-base cutters, we use a series of 6-base cutters. The approach is similar to standard inverse PCR protocols with the exception of longer extension times during PCR cycling and the inclusion of a polymerase with proofreading activity. Without the greater processivity of these enzyme mixes, internal deletions are usually observed in the PCR products.

Bioinformatic-Driven Screens

Although the mandate of public gene trap resources is to enable a more rapid and cost-efficient characterization of gene function, currently there is still a fear to commit time and resources to novel genes, because they may lead the investigator away from their specific areas of expertise. *In silico* predictions, such as those based on transcriptional coexpression (Zhang *et al.*, 2004), can provide testable hypotheses regarding the functions of thousands of unannotated genes in the mouse genome.

Quantitative genome-wide expression profiles over multiple tissues are analyzed for clusters of coexpression, because coregulated genes are predicted to more likely share biological function. Indeed, functional annotations using gene ontology (GO) terms are often clustered. Moreover cross-validation studies using machine-learning algorithms indicate that patterns of gene coexpression within many functional categories are "learnable" and distinguishable from other categories. Machine-learning algorithm-based functional predictions with an associated level of statistical precision can be queried using a user-friendly graphical interface provided by the Tim Hughes laboratory at the University of Toronto (http://mgpd.med.utoronto.ca). An example of this strategy to identify IGTC gene traps within genes predicted to be involved in insulin receptor signaling is shown in Fig. 4.

References

Austin, C. P., Battey, J. F., Bradley, A., Bucan, M., Capecchi, M., Collins, F. S., Dove, W. F., Duyk, G., Dymecki, S., Eppig, J. T., Grieder, F. B., Heintz, N., Hicks, G., Insel, T. R., Joyner, A., Koller, B. H., Lloyd, K. C., Magnuson, T., Moore, M. W., Nagy, A., Pollock, J. D., Roses, A. D., Sands, A. T., Seed, B., Skarnes, W. C., Snoddy, J., Soriano, P., Stewart, D. J., Stewart, F., Stillman, B., Varmus, H., Varticovski, L., Verma, I. M., Vogt, T. F., von Melchner, H., Witkowski, J., Woychik, R. P., Wurst, W., Yancopoulos, G. D., Young, S. G., and Zambrowicz, B. (2004). The knockout mouse project. *Nat. Genet.* **36,** 921–924.
Bautch, V. L., Stanford, W. L., Rapoport, R., Russell, S., Byrum, R. S., and Futch, T. A. (1996). Blood island formation in attached cultures of murine embryonic stem cells. *Dev. Dyn.* **205,** 1–12.

Chen, W. V., Delrow, J., Corrin, P. D., Frazier, J. P., and Soriano, P. (2004). Identification and validation of PDGF transcriptional targets by microarray-coupled gene-trap mutagenesis. *Nat. Genet.* **36,** 304–312.

Chen, W. V., and Soriano, P. (2003). Gene trap mutagenesis in embryonic stem cells. *Methods Enzymol.* **365,** 367–386.

Ding, S., Wu, X., Li, G., Han, M., Zhuang, Y., and Xu, T. (2005). Efficient transposition of the piggyBac (PB) transposon in mammalian cells and mice. *Cell* **122,** 473–483.

Doetschman, T. C., Eistetter, H., Katz, M., Schmidt, W., and Kemler, R. (1985). The *in vitro* development of blastocyst-derived embryonic stem cell lines: Formation of visceral yolk sac, blood islands and myocardium. *J. Embryol. Exp. Morph.* **87,** 27–45.

Forrester, L., Nagy, A., Sam, M., Watt, A., Stevenson, L., Bernstein, A., Joyner, A. L., and Wurst, W. (1996). Induction gene trapping in ES cells: Identification of developmentally regulated genes that respond to retinoic acid. *Proc. Natl. Acad. Sci. USA* **93,** 1677–1682.

Friedrich, G., and Soriano, P. (1991). Promoter traps in embryonic stem cells: A genetic screen to identify and mutate developmental genes in mice. *Genes Dev.* **5,** 1513–1523.

Gossler, A., Joyner, A. L., Rossant, J., and Skarnes, W. C. (1989). Mouse embryonic stem cells and reporter constructs to detect developmentally regulated genes. *Science* **244,** 463–465.

Hicks, G. G., Shi, E. G., Li, X. M., Li, C. H., Pawlak, M., and Ruley, H. E. (1997). Functional genomics in mice by tagged sequence mutagenesis. *Nat. Genet.* **16,** 338–344.

Hidaka, M., Stanford, W. L., and Bernstein, A. (1999). Conditional requirement for the Flk-1 receptor in the *in vitro* generation of early hematopoietic cells. *Proc. Natl. Acad. Sci. USA* **96,** 7370–7375.

Hirashima, M., Kataoka, H., Nishikawa, S., Matsuyoshi, N., and Nishikawa, S. (1999). Maturation of embryonic stem cells into endothelial cells in an *in vitro* model of vasculogenesis. *Blood* **93,** 1253–1263.

Hui, E. K., Wang, P. C., and Lo, S. J. (1998). Strategies for cloning unknown cellular flanking DNA sequences from foreign integrants. *Cell Mol. Life Sci.* **54,** 1403–1411.

Keng, V. W., Yae, K., Hayakawa, T., Mizuno, S., Uno, Y., Yusa, K., Kokubu, C., Kinoshita, T., Akagi, K., Jenkins, N. A., Copeland, N. G., Horie, K., and Takeda, J. (2005). Region-specific saturation germline mutagenesis in mice using the Sleeping Beauty transposon system. *Nat. Methods* **2,** 763–769.

Kuhnert, F., and Stuhlmann, H. (2004). Identifying early vascular genes through gene trapping in mouse embryonic stem cells. *Curr. Top. Dev. Biol.* **62,** 261–281.

Leighton, P. A., Mitchell, K. J., Goodrich, L. V., Lu, X., Pinson, K., Scherz, P., Skarnes, W. C., and Tessier-Lavigne, M. (2001). Defining brain wiring patterns and mechanisms through gene trapping in mice. *Nature* **410,** 174–179.

Mainguy, G., Montesinos, M. L., Lesaffre, B., Zevnik, B., Karasawa, M., Kothary, R., Wurst, W., Prochiantz, A., and Volovitch, M. (2000). An induction gene trap for identifying a homeoprotein-regulated locus. *Nat. Biotechnol.* **18,** 746–749.

Matsuda, E., Shigeoka, T., Iida, R., Yamanaka, S., Kawaichi, M., and Ishida, Y. (2004). Expression profiling with arrays of randomly disrupted genes in mouse embryonic stem cells leads to *in vivo* functional analysis. *Proc. Natl. Acad. Sci. USA* **101,** 4170–4174.

Myrick, K. V., and Gelbart, W. M. (2002). Universal Fast Walking for direct and versatile determination of flanking sequence. *Gene* **284,** 125–131.

Nagai, T., Ibata, K., Park, E. S., Kubota, M., Mikoshiba, K., and Miyawaki, A. (2002). A variant of yellow fluorescent protein with fast and efficient maturation for cell-biological applications. *Nat. Biotechnol.* **20,** 87–90.

Nagy, A., and Rossant, J. (1993). Production of completely ES cell derived fetuses. *In* "Gene Targeting: A Practical Approach" (A. Joyner, ed.), pp. 147–179. IRL Press, New York.

Nakano, T., Kodama, H., and Honjo, T. (1994). Generation of lymphohematopoietic cells from embryonic stem cells in culture. *Science* **265**, 1098–1101.

Niwa, H., Araki, K., Kimura, S., Taniguchi, S., Wakasugi, S., and Yamamura, K. (1993). An efficient gene-trap method using poly A trap vectors and characterization of gene-trap events. *J. Biochem.* **113**, 343–349.

Nord, A. S., Chang, P. J., Conklin, B. R., Cox, A. V., Harper, C. A., Hicks, G. G., Huang, C. C., Johns, S. J., Kawamoto, M., Liu, S., Meng, E. C., Morris, J. H., Rossant, J., Ruiz, P., Skarnes, W. C., Soriano, P., Stanford, W. L., Stryke, D., von Melchner, H., Wurst, W., Yamamura, K., Young, S. G., Babbitt, P. C., and Ferrin, T. E. (2006). The International Gene Trap Consortium Website: a portal to all publicly available gene trap cell lines in mouse. *Nucleic Acids Res.* **34**, D642–648.

Osipovich, A. B., White-Grindley, E. K., Hicks, G. G., Roshon, M. J., Shaffer, C., Moore, J. H., and Ruley, H. E. (2004). Activation of cryptic 3′ splice sites within introns of cellular genes following gene entrapment. *Nucleic Acids Res.* **32**, 2912–2924.

Schnutgen, F., De-Zolt, S., Van Sloun, P., Hollatz, M., Floss, T., Hansen, J., Altschmied, J., Seisenberger, C., Ghyselinck, N. B., Ruiz, P., Chambon, P., Wurst, W., and von Melchner, H. (2005). Genomewide production of multipurpose alleles for the functional analysis of the mouse genome. *Proc. Natl. Acad. Sci. USA* **102**, 7221–7226.

Shigeoka, T., Kawaichi, M., and Ishida, Y. (2005). Suppression of nonsense-mediated mRNA decay permits unbiased gene trapping in mouse embryonic stem cells. *Nucleic Acids Res.* **33**, e20.

Skarnes, W. C., Auerbach, B. A., and Joyner, A. L. (1992). A gene trap approach in mouse embryonic stem cells: the lacZ reporter is activated by splicing, reflects endogenous gene expression, and is mutagenic in mice. *Genes Dev.* **6**, 903–918.

Skarnes, W. C., Moss, J. E., Hurtley, S. M., and Beddington, R. S. P. (1995). Capturing genes encoding membrane and secreted proteins important for mouse development. *Proc. Natl. Acad. Sci. USA* **92**, 6592–6596.

Skarnes, W. C., von Melchner, H., Wurst, W., Hicks, G., Nord, A. S., Cox, T., Young, S. G., Ruiz, P., Soriano, P., Tessier-Lavigne, M., Conklin, B. R., Stanford, W. L., and Rossant, J. (2004). A public gene trap resource for mouse functional genomics. *Nat. Genet.* **36**, 543–544.

Soriano, P., Friedrich, G., and Lawinger, P. (1991). Promoter interactions in retrovirus vectors introduced into fibroblasts and embryonic stem cells. *J. Virol.* **65**, 2314–2319.

Stanford, W. L., Caruana, G., Vallis, K. A., Inamdar, M., Hidaka, M., Bautch, V. L., and Bernstein, A. (1998). Expression trapping: Identification of novel genes expressed in hematopoietic and endothelial lineages by gene trapping in ES cells. *Blood* **92**, 4622–4631.

Stanford, W. L., Cohn, J. B., and Cordes, S. P. (2001). Gene trap mutagenesis: past, present and beyond. *Nat. Rev. Genet.* **2**, 756–768.

Tarrant, J. M., Groom, J., Metcalf, D., Li, R., Borobokas, B., Wright, M. D., Tarlinton, D., and Robb, L. (2002). The absence of Tssc6, a member of the tetraspanin superfamily, does not affect lymphoid development but enhances *in vitro* T-cell proliferative responses. *Mol. Cell. Biol.* **22**, 5006–5018.

To, C., Epp, T., Reid, T., Lan, Q., Yu, M., Li, C. Y., Ohishi, M., Hant, P., Tsao, N., Casallo, G., Rossant, J., Osborne, L. R., and Stanford, W. L. (2004). The Centre for Modeling Human Disease Gene Trap resource. *Nucleic Acids Res.* **32**, Database issue, D557–559.

Vallis, K. A., Chen, Z., Stanford, W. L., Hill, R. P., and Bernstein, A. (2002). Identification of radiation-responsive genes in vitro using a gene trap strategy predicts for modulation of expression by radiation *in vivo*. *Radiat. Res.* **157**, 8–18.

Voss, A. K., Thomas, T., and Gruss, P. (1998). Compensation for a gene trap mutation in the murine microtubule-associated protein 4 locus by alternative polyadenylation and alternative splicing. *Dev. Dyn.* **212**, 258–266.

Wurst, W., Rossant, J., Prideaux, V., Kownacka, M., Joyner, A. L., Hill, D. P., Guillemot, F., Gasca, S., Cado, D., Auerbach, A., and Ang, S.-L. (1995). A large-scale gene-trap screen for insertional mutations in developmentally regulated genes in mice. *Genetics* **139**, 889–899.

Zambrowicz, B. P., Abuin, A., Ramirez-Solis, R., Richter, L. J., Piggott, J., Beltran del Rio, H., Buxton, E. C., Edwards, J., Finch, R. A., Friddle, C. J., Gupta, A., Hansen, G., Hu, Y., Huang, W., Jaing, C., Key, B. W., Jr., Kipp, P., Kohlhauff, B., Ma, Z. Q., Markesich, D., Payne, R., Potter, D. G., Qian, N., Shaw, J., Schrick, J., Shi, Z. Z., Sparks, M. J., Van Sligtenhorst, I., Vogel, P., Walke, W., Xu, N., Zhu, Q., Person, C., and Sands, A. T. (2003). Wnk1 kinase deficiency lowers blood pressure in mice: a gene-trap screen to identify potential targets for therapeutic intervention. *Proc. Natl. Acad. Sci. USA* **100**, 14109–14114.

Zambrowicz, B. P., Freidrich, G. A., Buxton, E. C., Lilleberg, S. L., Person, C., and Sands, A. T. (1998). Disruption and sequence identification of 2,000 genes in mouse embryonic stem cells. *Nature* **392**, 608–611.

Zhang, W., Morris, Q. D., Chang, R., Shai, O., Bakowski, M. A., Mitsakakis, N., Mohammad, N., Robinson, M. D., Zirngibl, R., Somogyi, E., Laurin, N., Eftekharpour, E., Sat, E., Grigull, J., Pan, Q., Peng, W. T., Krogan, N., Greenblatt, J., Fehlings, M., van der Kooy, D., Aubin, J., Bruneau, B. G., Rossant, J., Blencowe, B. J., Frey, B. J., and Hughes, T. R. (2004). The functional landscape of mouse gene expression. *J. Biol.* **3**, 21.

[9]   GeneChips in Stem Cell Research

By JASON HIPP and ANTHONY ATALA

Abstract

An understanding of the genes and signaling networks responsible for stem cell growth and differentiation will be essential for their ultimate therapeutic application. GeneChips are miniature platforms of nucleotides capable of monitoring the expression levels of almost every known and unknown gene. Performing a GeneChip experiment is like snapping a picture of a cell's mRNA (transcripts), thus giving a static view and measurement of gene expression inside the cell. Taking multiple "pictures" of stem cells as they grow and differentiate will provide insight into the genetic mechanisms of "stemness" or can be used to create "transcriptional signatures" to assess differentiation and variability between stem cell lines. The first half of this chapter covers the many components involved in a GeneChip experiment, illustrating the many variables at each step and describing a protocol for analysis that is inexpensive and requires minimal computer skills. The chapter then describes how researchers are currently applying GeneChips to stem cell biology. We conclude that the true potential of GeneChip technology lies in the *in silico* analysis—their integration and comparison of diverse data sets, where the biological questions are the driving force in the analysis.

METHODS IN ENZYMOLOGY, VOL. 420
0076-6879/06 $35.00
DOI: 10.1016/S0076-6879(06)20009-0

Introduction

Embryonic stem cells (ESCs) have the ability to grow indefinitely and ultimately differentiate into any cell type. With these capabilities, they could potentially *cure* a disease rather than simply delay its progression. In addition, they will serve as models for studying the genetic mechanisms of regeneration and provide novel insights into diseases such as cancer, diabetes, Alzheimer's disease, and Parkinson's disease. Despite great excitement over the potential of ESCs, little is known about how they grow and differentiate. The genes that are unique to ESCs and responsible for their self-renewal (ability to grow indefinitely) and pluripotentiality (ability to differentiate into any cell type) are referred to as "stemness" genes.

Of the estimated 20,000–25,000 genes in the human genome (Stein, 2004), there are only a handful of genes that are known to be ESC-specific "stemness" genes (Brivanlou *et al.*, 2003). This chapter will use the Mendelian definition of gene as a unit of inheritance, referring frequently to its transcriptional form (noncoding/coding RNA) and will further define it when necessary. An understanding of "stemness" genes and the signaling networks responsible for their differentiation will be essential for their ultimate therapeutic application. Currently, millions of patients are suffering from degenerative diseases that could potentially be cured by stem cells, and new technologies must be applied to quickly and efficiently solve the riddle of stem cells and provide for this medical need.

With the ability to monitor the expression levels of almost every known and unknown gene, GeneChip technology could provide the answers (Lipshutz *et al.*, 1999; Lockhart *et al.*, 1996). GeneChips are miniature platforms with approximately 1 million 25-base nucleotide sequences that measure the transcriptional expression levels of 47,000 transcripts and variants, including 38,500 well-characterized human genes (HG-U133 Plus 2.0, www.affymetrix.com). These platforms include almost every known gene in the human *transcriptome*—the mRNA equivalent of the human genome.

Performing a GeneChip experiment is like snapping a picture of a cell's mRNA (transcripts), thus giving a static view and measurement of gene expression inside the cell. By taking multiple "pictures" and comparing them to one another, the researcher can gain insight into the mechanisms and kinetics of a cellular process such as differentiation or can create a "transcriptional signature" to be used to compare and contrast different ESC and their differentiated progeny. What would take years to analyze by quantifying the expression of 660,000 genes with RT-PCR now takes but a few days (30 GeneChips × ~22,000 genes/GeneChip were used in the experiments described later). Such an understanding will provide insight into controlling ESC growth and lineage directed differentiation for clinical application, including

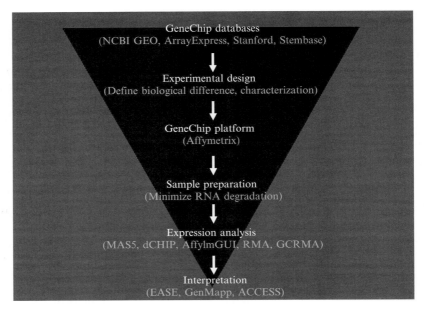

FIG. 1. Outline of the chapter illustrating the multiple components of a GeneChip experiment.

regeneration methods that could allow one to stimulate regeneration *in vivo* through either genetic manipulation, new chemical entities (NCE), or with biomaterials. The first half of this chapter covers the many components involved in a GeneChip experiment (Fig. 1), illustrating the many variables at each step and describing a protocol for analysis. The chapter then describes how researchers are currently applying GeneChips to ESC biology.

Protocol

GeneChip Databases

The first step of a GeneChip experiment begins with a thorough search of the publicly available databases for GeneChip data. Among the most commonly searched databases are: NCBI GEO (Barrett *et al.*, 2005), ArrayExpress (Parkinson *et al.*, 2005; Sarkans *et al.*, 2005), Stanford (Ball *et al.*, 2005), Stembase (Ball *et al.*, 2005; Perez-Iratxeta *et al.*, 2005), and Public Expression Profiling Resource (Chen *et al.*, 2004). These databases contain hundreds of GeneChips and other downloadable microarray data files both raw and analyzed, including Affymetrix GeneChips and other microarray platforms. Reviewing these databases may eliminate the need to perform specific experiments and also provides tremendous insight into how others are designing and implementing GeneChip technology.

Archived microarray databases serve as a permanent archive that can be constantly reanalyzed and reinterpreted in the context of new software or biological advances. Such capabilities serve as an efficient and inexpensive way to cross-validate data, a method called *in silico post hoc*. Because *in silico* comparisons are not limited by biological, time, or financial constraints, they offer the possibility of an almost limitless number of comparisons, the extent and novelty of such being limited only by one's creativity. This ability to perform numerous comparisons *in silico* and integrate data sets derived from diverse cells and conditions is a tremendous power of this technology.

Experimental Design: Defining the Biological Phenotype

If the cornerstone of a good GeneChip experiment is the experimental design, and the experimental design is only as good as the biological question, then the first and most important step in a GeneChip experiment is to clearly define the biological and phenotypical differences. Such differences might often include changes in cell function, signal transduction, or protein expression. Because the power of GeneChips lies in their ability to *provide a global genetic explanation for a biological difference,* often consisting of hundreds to thousands of genes differentially expressed, valuable answers can be hidden within the mass of data. Clearly defining this biological difference will improve the likelihood that the gene expression data relates to the important biological questions.

The question of required number of replicates to perform is often dependent on the difficulty of generating enough sample RNA and by one's budget. The more replicates performed (per condition) in the analysis, the more statistical power there will be in identifying differentially expressed genes. Typically, three replicates are sufficient to overcome the variance in data and enable good statistical power. A recommended approach is to be prepared to perform GeneChip experiments by harvesting copious amounts of RNA from multiple replicate cell or tissue samples.

GeneChip Platform

Many factors influence which platform to use for GeneChip analysis. Depending on the expertise of a laboratory, one can print custom microarray platforms or use commercially available GeneChip platforms. The benefit of printing custom microarrays is the reduced cost if one performs many microarrays. One form of custom arrays involves generating a platform-specific cDNA library using RNA from the cell type of interest (Saha *et al.*, 2002; Velculescu *et al.*, 1995). However, these techniques tend to lack reproducibility. Minor errors can be introduced in generating the probes, their printing, hybridization, labeling of RNA, and validation. Thus, many samples must be run to identify potential errors. With the commercially available platforms, these problems have already been addressed.

The advantage of using commercially available platforms is their user-friendly nature. Typically, one needs only to generate the sample (tissue/cells). Although most groups isolate their own RNA, there are some commercial enterprises (e.g., Genome Explorations, www.GenomeExplorations.com) that will do this and perform the GeneChip analysis. The choice of GeneChip platform is influenced by the level of depth needed in the genetic explanation and by the budget. The next question is whether to screen the entire transcriptome or specific pathways. If one is focused on a particular pathway, Superarrays can be ideal, because they are pathway specific (www.superarray.com). If one is interested in covering as many genes as possible, then Affymetrix, Agilent, or GE Healthcare platforms are more appropriate (www.agilent.com, www.GEHealthcare.com). Platforms capable of scanning the entire transcriptome come as single (Affymetrix) versus dual channel chips (Agilent, GE Healthcare). *Dual channel* means that the two samples are labeled with different color dyes and simultaneously hybridized to the chip. Affymetrix uses *single channel*, meaning that the sample is labeled with only one dye, and the difference in intensity of this dye is measured. The Affymetrix GeneChip platform design allows for the absolute detection of whether a gene is present or absent (described later), as well as absolute quantification enabling sample comparison among other chip sets. Numerous software analysis programs have been developed specifically for the Affymetrix GeneChip design. For the field of ESC biology, the authors prefer the Affymetrix platform for additional reasons described later in this chapter.

Sample Preparation

It is important to have a pure cellular or tissue population for GeneChip analysis to limit contaminating RNA from other cell types. Accordingly, cell lines are easier to use than biopsy specimens. Laser microdissection can be used to minimize contaminating cell types.

The quantity and quality of RNA isolated will directly influence the quality of GeneChip data generated. Because RNA has a free 2′-OH that can serve as a nucleophile, one must be careful to prevent RNA degradation during isolation. Numerous protocols exist, including commercially available kits, for purification of RNA. Most of the protocols are appropriate for GeneChip studies if care is taken to avoid RNAse contamination. The quality of RNA should be confirmed by spectrophotometric analysis (A260/280 should be 1.8–2.1 in TE buffer or 1.6–1.9 in water) and by running an RNA gel for the identification of two tight bands (18s and 28s peaks with a ratio of 1:2).

The investigator must be extremely careful when dealing with small amounts of RNA and using RNA amplification techniques. In these circumstances, the effects of a small amount of RNA degradation will be amplified. In many experiments, the amount of RNA is the limiting factor.

The advantage of using Affymetrix is that its labeling and hybridization protocol has been standardized and thoroughly tested. Labeling and hybridization are usually done by a core facility. Many prefer to use core facilities because of the experience and consistency provided by the core. The core facility reverse transcribes the provided RNA (1–15 μg) into double-stranded cDNA with a T7 olig(dT) promoter primer (Affymetrix, 4 A.D.). The double-stranded cDNA is then transcribed with biotin-labeled nucleotides to make cRNA. The cRNA is then fragmented and hybridized to the GeneChip. Because the RNA is reverse transcribed, 11 probes (25-mer nucleotide sequences) are chosen to match (Perfect Match, PM) the gene transcript, a unique feature of the Affymetrix GeneChip. Each of these PM probes has a corresponding MisMatch (MM) probe which differs in that the 13th nucleotide is mutated. The core facility performs a quality control check on the final data output by examining the number of present genes, 5′ and 3′ ratio, and signal to background ratio, and then provide a set of data files. The .DAT file is the scanned array image file. The .CEL file is the cell-intensity data file derived from the .DAT and contains the PM–MM values. The .CHP is the analyzed and saved .CEL file. The .RPT is the summary report file (Affymetrix, 4 A.D.).

Expression Analysis

Overview of Programs

Data analysis by the biologist with minimal computer training can become overwhelming with the many different ways GeneChip data can be analyzed, coupled with the inherent complexity of some analytical programs (sometimes requiring code writing, in addition to converting and transferring files between different programs). Analysis often becomes a self-limiting task. Although commercial packages are available, these tend to be expensive, and the different methods of analysis remain difficult to understand. This chapter provides an overview of some of the more commonly used data analysis programs and discusses how to apply them in a relatively inexpensive manner, catering to biologists with limited computer expertise.

The main difference among the programs is in the way they adjust for nonbiological variability that occurs during the labeling and hybridization procedure, referred to as data normalization. Although there are numerous programs for analyzing GeneChip data, each offering a particular advantage/disadvantage, the most commonly used programs are MAS5, dCHIP, and RMA (a comparison of different GeneChip analysis methods can be found at http://affycomp.biostat.jhsph.edu [Cope *et al.*, 2004; Irizarry *et al.*, 2005]). Of the files generated by the core facility, the .CEL files (which are approximately 5 MB and contain the signal intensities of all the probes on the GeneChip) are the ones most often analyzed by these programs.

MAS5. MAS5 is the program created by Affymetrix, and because of its size, usually it runs on its own workstation (Affymetrix, 2001, 2005). Using a Turkey–Biweight formula, it determines whether the PM intensities are greater than MM and then assigns a p value to determine whether a gene is either present ($p < 0.04$), marginal ($0.04 < p < 0.06$), or absent ($p > 0.06$) (Affymetrix, 2001, 2005). Before data from separate GeneChips can be compared with one another, they first need to be normalized to minimize discrepancies among multiple GeneChips because of sample preparation and hybridization. MAS5 normalizes the average intensities of one GeneChip to a baseline GeneChip using either a specific value, all probe sets, or a selected group of probe sets (Affymetrix, 2001). This software is limited by a 1-by-1 comparison. Often, the MAS5 analysis is provided by a core facility.

DCHIP. Li and Wong (2001) noticed that some probes had an outlying expression value consistent across GeneChips and, therefore, developed dCHIP, which can be downloaded at www.dchip.org. dCHIP uses a nonlinear normalization method to remove outlying probe effects (noise) by first normalizing all GeneChip intensities to the median GeneChip intensity and then computing a model-based expression index (MBEI) to estimate gene expression levels. The program is easy to use with a graphical user interface (GUI), is free to the public, and can be run on a laptop computer.

RMA. Irizarry *et al.* (2003a) compared Robust Multichip Analysis (RMA) to dCHIP and MAS5 and demonstrated that RMA has better precision, particularly for genes with low expression levels. RMA provides a greater than fivefold reduction of the within-replicate variance compared with dCHIP and MAS5, provides more consistent estimates of fold change, and provides higher specificity and sensitivity when using fold change analysis to detect differential expression. The group judges MAS5 to be more accurate than RMA but believes this modest loss of accuracy with RMA is offset by a gain in precision (Irizarry *et al.*, 2003a).

RMA is unique in that it adjusts for background noise, performs a quantile normalization, log transforms the data, and then summarizes the multiple probes into one intensity (Bolstad *et al.*, 2003, 2004; Cope *et al.*, 2004; Irizarry *et al.*, 2003a,b). It uses only the PM probes and ignores the MM probes, which can cause exaggerated variance (Cope *et al.*, 2004). Quantile normalization was chosen because it has been shown to have the best performance and works by making the distribution of intensities at the probe level, rather than by choosing a baseline GeneChip or standard intensity (Bolstad *et al.*, 2003).

GCRMA. GCRMA is an adaptation of RMA but differs in that it uses a model-based background correction determined by G–C content and Partial Match–MisMatch values (Wu and Irizarry, 2005). GCRMA was shown to be even more accurate than MAS5 without losing precision in identifying differential gene expression. However, in terms of both accuracy and precision, RMA is best at higher RNA concentrations, whereas GCRMA is better at lower concentrations (Wu and Irizarry, 2005).

AffyPLM. AffyPLM is another program similar to RMA, but the summarization method differs in that it uses a probe linear model instead of a median polish (Affymetrix, 2005; Bolstad, 5 A.D.; Bolstad, 2005). A detailed comparison of different GeneChip analysis methods can be found at http://affycomp.biostat.jhsph.edu (Cope *et al.*, 2004; Irizarry *et al.*, 2005; Rosenberg *et al.*, 2004b). AffyPLM, GCRMA, and RMA are all free of charge to the public and all run in the open source programming language R (www.r-project.org); all can be downloaded from www.bioconductor.org.

Data Analysis

Depending on the biological question, two fundamentally distinct types of analysis can be performed. One is based on call detection (whether a gene is present or absent) using the program MAS5. The other type of analysis is to quantify the relative levels of gene expression. To do this, the authors use the all-in-one package affylmGUI, which contains affyPLM/RMA/GCRMA and LIMMA in a GUI environment (http://bioinf.wehi.edu.au/affylmGUI).

ABSENT/PRESENT CALL DETECTION. The authors believe the strength of MAS5 is in its Present/Absent call detection. This program is recommended to identify a "transcriptional signature" or "transcriptome" of genes that are flagged as Present. A comparison of signatures can identify genes that are Present/Absent between cell types.

Core facilities usually provide free of charge or a minimal fee for data analysis using the Affymetrix Software. Some laboratories have their own workstations. However, if one is only using the Present/Absent/Marginal detection calls, the core facility can provide the MAS5 output, and the laboratory can make "transcriptome" comparisons using Excel and MS Access.

RELATIVE EXPRESSION LEVELS. To quantify the relative differences in gene expression, affylmGUI, the sister program of LimmaGUI (Wettenhall, 2004; Wettenhall and Smyth, 2004), is recommended. AffylmGUI is an all-in-one package that reads the raw Affymetrix .CEL files directly, summarizes gene expression values with either RMA, affyPLM, or GCRMA, and uses the program Linear Modeling of Microarray data (Smyth, 2004) to identify statistically significant differentially expressed genes, all in a GUI. AffylmGUI can be downloaded at http://bioinf.wehi.edu.au/affylmGUI free of charge. Within affylmGUI, LIMMA fits a linear model for every gene (like an ANOVA or multiple regression), then hypothesis tests and adjusts *p* values for multiple testings (Smyth, 2004, 2005). A moderated *t* statistic is calculated for each gene, in which the standard errors are shrunk to a common value using a Bayesian model (Smyth, 2005). Although multiple methods of moderation can be chosen, the most common is Benjamini and Hochberg's (1995) method to control false discovery rate. In addition, it computes a B statistic that is similar to that of Lonch and Speed (Lockhart *et al.*, 1996); however, this is reformulated using a moderated *t* statistic in which posterior residual standard deviations are used in place of ordinary standard deviations (Smyth, 2005).

Running affylmGUI is relatively simple and time efficient. One begins by creating a text file that identifies the .CEL files and a design matrix (associating the .CEL files with contrast groups). Once the .CEL files are incorporated, the investigator has the choice of summarizing the gene expression values with RMA, GCRMA, or affyPLM. A linear model is then computed, and the desired contrasts are made. The results can then be opened in Excel. The output file consists of columns representing the Affymetrix probe set (gene identification), M value (fold change in log based 2), A value (average signal intensity), *t* statistic, *p* value, and B statistic (Fig. 2). A FDR adjusted *p* value of <0.001 means that those genes that are selected are expected to have a proportion of false discovery that is controlled to be less than 0.1%. A B statistic of 2 is an odds of differential expression of 4, which means that there is an 80% chance of differential expression.

Interpretation of GeneChip Data

Once lists of differentially expressed genes are identified, one faces the most difficult task: deriving biological meaning. This immense challenge is analogous to putting together the pieces of a puzzle in which there is no picture as a guide.

A

	GCRMA	RMA	affyPLM
GCRMA	844	760	793
RMA	760	1114	1063
affyPLM	793	1063	1231

C

GCRMA	844
GCRMA not RMA	84
GCRMA not affyPLM	51
GCRMA not RMA-affyPLM	39
RMA	1114
RMA not GCRMA	354
RMA not affyPLM	51
RMA not GCCRMA-affyPLM	39
affyPLM	1231
affyPLM not RMA	168
affyPLM not GCRMA	438
affyPLM not RMA-GCRMA	123
Identified by all 3	**748**

B

	GCRMA	RMA	affyPLM
GCRMA	1	0.9	0.939
RMA	0.682	1	0.954
affyPLM	0.644	0.863	1

FIG. 2. The data set provided by D'Amour *et al.* (2003) was analyzed with RMA, GCRMA, affyPLM. (A) The matrix here represents the number of genes in common between both methods. (B) The values from Fig. 2A were converted to ratios. GCCRMA has 90% of its genes in common with RMA and 94% in common with affyPLM. RMA has 68% of its genes in common with GCRMA and 95% in common with affyPLM. affyPLM has 64% of its genes in common with GCRMA and 86% in common with RMA. (C) The number of genes identified with each method.

EASE

An initial analysis should begin with those genes that have the greatest B statistic or FC. These genes can be annotated with EASE (Dennis *et al.*, 2003; Hosack *et al.*, 2003), which is a GUI program downloaded onto a desktop computer (http://david.niaid.nih.gov/david/). Affymetrix probe set (gene ids) can be pasted directly into the window, and then the different databases for annotation can be chosen. Lists can be annotated with gene name, gene symbol, alias symbol, chromosomal location, geneRIF, and OMIM. An HTML file is generated that consists of a table of genes with all the desired annotations. The advantage of this program is that it can be used to annotate thousands of genes in less than 30 sec, a process that would take years to do by hand.

Those genes that are identified as differentially expressed, using a B statistic > 0, can be used to identify biological themes with the "find overrepresented gene categories" function. The lists of genes are loaded into EASE as before and a categorical system such as gene ontology, chromosomal location, or protein domains is chosen. Gene ontology is a collaborative effort to develop a controlled vocabulary (ontologies) that describes gene products in terms of their biological processes, cellular components, or molecular functions in a species-independent manner (Ashburner *et al.*, 2000). A reference file is then chosen, which contains all the possible categories for every gene on the GeneChip. EASE then compares the researcher's list this reference file and depending on which statistical method is chosen (Bonferroni or EASE score—a conservative variant of the Fisher Exact probability), it will generate a *p* value for the most overrepresented themes in less than 30 sec.

GenMapp

When comparing multiple data sets, one can use GenMapp. GenMapp is a program consisting of hundreds of premade pathway maps (Dahlquist *et al.*, 2002; Doniger *et al.*, 2003) and can be downloaded at http://www. genmapp.org. Lists of genes (in the Affymetrix probe set format) are loaded directly into GenMapp and assigned a color on the basis of expression. Hundreds of pathways can then be viewed in which each gene is color-coded on the basis of its cell type and direction of change (up-regulated or down-regulated). This allows one to efficiently identify pathways with significant genetic changes (Fig. 3). Information on each gene is integrated from multiple databases and is easily accessed by right-or-left clicking the name.

Effects of Normalization

To understand how the three normalization programs offered in affylm-GUI (RMA, GCRMA, AffyPLM) affect the numbers and types of genes, fold change, and biological significance, the authors created sets of genes that were down-regulated on mouse ESC differentiation using the data set provided by D'Amour and Gage (2003). Of the 12,422 genes present on the MG-U74aV2 GeneChip, there were 748 genes identified by all three methods. Figure 2 further describes the number of genes identified by each method and provides a comparison of genes identified by one method and not another.

These data demonstrate that GCRMA is the most conservative of the three, identifying the fewest number of genes—many of which were also identified by RMA (90%) and affyPLM (94%). affyPLM and RMA identified a similar number of genes, and 95% of the genes identified by RMA were also identified by affyPLM, and 86% of the genes identified by affyPLM were also identified by RMA. There were only a small number of genes that were exclusively identified by one method—39 for GCRMA, 39 for RMA, and 123 for affyPLM (Fig. 2).

The authors then were interested in the types of genes that were identified with the greatest Fold Change in each of the three methods. The top 15 ranked genes identified by FC that had a B statistic > 0 were then compared (Fig. 3), if a gene was ranked in the top 15 with one method and not another, its corresponding rank was then included). All methods identified the classic ESC markers Nanog, POU domain, class 5, transcription

A

AffyPLM	RMA	GCRMA
Amyotrophic lateral sclerosis 2 (juvenile) homolog (human)	Amyotrophic lateral sclerosis 2 (juvenile) homolog (human)	Amyotrophic lateral sclerosis 2 (juvenile) homolog (human)
Developmental pluripotency associated 2	Developmental pluripotency associated 2	Developmental pluripotency associated 2
Developmental pluripotency associated 5	Developmental pluripotency associated 5	Developmental pluripotency associated 5
F-box only protein 15	F-box only protein 15	F-box only protein 15
Kruppel-like factor5	Kruppel-like factor 5	Kruppel-like factor 5
Nanog homeobox	Nanog homeobox	Nanog homeobox
POU domain, class 5, transcription factor 1	POU domain, class 5, transcription factor 1	POU domain, class 5, transcription factor 1
Secreted phosphoprotein1	Secreted phosphoprotein 1	Secreted phosphoprotein 1
Tumor rejection antigen P1A	Tumor rejection antigen P1A	Tumor rejection antigen P1A
Uridine phosphorylase 1	Uridine phosphorylase 1	Uridine phosphorylase 1
Zinc finger protein 42	Zinc finger protein 42	16
Expressed sequence AI467481	Expressed sequence AI467481	22
Kruppel-like factor 4 (gut)	Kruppel-like factor 4 (gut)	21
Phosphofructokinase, platelet	Phosphofructokinase, platelet	23
Serum/glucocorticoid regulated kinase	Serum/glucocorticoid regulated kinase	20
25	31	Undifferentiated embryonic cell transcription factor 1
21	20	Apolipoprotein E
31	26	Fibroblast growth factor 4
73	69	Growth differentiation factor 3
20	17	RNA binding protein gene with multiple splicing

FIG. 3. (*continued*)

B

GCRMA	AffyPLM	RMA
Alcohol catabolism	Alcohol catabolism	Alcohol catabolism
Alcohol metabolism	Alcohol metabolism	Alcohol metabolism
X	X	Amine biosynthesis
X	X	Amino acid biosynthesis
Aromatic compound metabolism		Aromatic compound metabolism
Biosynthesis	Biosynthesis	Biosynthesis
Carbohydrate catabolism	Carbohydrate catabolism	Carbohydrate catabolism
Carbohydrate metabolism	Carbohydrate metabolism	Carbohydrate metabolism
Cell proliferation	Cell proliferation	Cell proliferation
Cytoplasm organization and biogenesis	X	X
Energy derivation by oxidation of organic compounds	Energy derivation by oxidation of organic compounds	Energy derivation by oxidation of organic compounds
Energy pathways	Energy pathways	Energy pathways
Glucose catabolism	Glucose catabolism	Glucose catabolism
Glucose metabolism	Glucose metabolism	Glucose metabolism
Glycolysis	Glycolysis	Glycolysis
X	Heterocycle metabolism	Heterocycle metabolism
Hexose catabolism	Hexose catabolism	Hexose catabolism
Hexose metabolism	Hexose metabolism	Hexose metabolism
Macromolecule biosynthesis	Macromolecule biosynthesis	X
Main pathways of carbohydrate metabolism	Main pathways of carbohydrate metabolism	Main pathways of carbohydrate metabolism
Metabolism	Metabolism	Metabolism
Monosaccharide catabolism	Monosaccharide catabolism	Monosaccharide catabolism
Monosaccharide metabolism	Monosaccharide metabolism	Monosaccharide metabolism
Protein biosynthesis	Protein biosynthesis	X
X	Protein metabolism	X
Ribosome biogenesis	Ribosome biogenesis	Ribosome biogenesis
Ribosome biogenesis and assembly	Ribosome biogenesis and assembly	Ribosome biogenesis and assembly

factor 1 (OCT4), etc. These also show that the top 15 genes identified by one method were also included in the top 75 in the other (Fig. 3A).

These data sets were then clustered on the basis of their GO Biological Process using EASE, and processes that had a $p < 0.01$ were selected and compared (Fig. 3B). These data demonstrate very little difference in the biological themes identified by each of the three normalization methods, RMA, GCRMA, and affyPLM. Therefore, because of the ease, efficiency, and inexpensiveness of affylmGUI and to ensure a broad coverage, the authors recommend analyzing data with either RMA or affyPLM and GCRMA.

ESC Differentiation

The most widely used application of GeneChips for ESC biology is to identify stemness genes. An understanding of stemness—the ability to self-renew and differentiate into almost any cell type—will uncover the secrets of human development and regeneration and provide insights into degenerative and chronic diseases. Knowledge of stemness genes could potentially allow one to genetically manipulate and reprogram somatic cells (Cowan *et al.*, 2005), design novel cell culture conditions for the *ex vivo* expansion of progenitor cells for tissue engineering, and improve the quality and efficiency of lineage-directed differentiation. With the proper experimental design, GeneChips can begin to explain how stem cells are capable of regenerating themselves, or how they differentiate into any tissue in the body, or possibly explain the pathogenesis of cancer. By comparing stem cell data sets of diverse origins, one can begin to identify novel stem cell functions. GeneChips, because of their ability to screen almost every known and unknown gene, represent an important tool in understanding stemness and bringing us closer to the clinical application of ESC.

FIG. 3. (A) How do the genes with the greatest FC differ among RMA, GCRMA, and affyPLM? Using the data provided by D'Amour *et al.* (2003), the top 15 ranked genes with the greatest decrease in FC on differentiation (with a corresponding B statistic >0) were identified by RMA, GCRMA, and affyPLM. When a gene was ranked by one method and not another, its corresponding rank was then included. The identification of many known ESC markers such as Nanog and POU domain, class 5, transcription factor 1 (OCT4), not only validates the quality of the data but their slight differences might also demonstrate some advantages of using one program over another. (B) Genes identified with GCRMA, affyPLM, and RMA as being up-regulated on differentiation were clustered with EASE using their GO Biological Process. Genetic themes with an EASE score $p < 0.01$ were selected. Many of the genetic themes are conserved when either program is used to summarize gene expression values.

GeneChip Experiments

The initial stem cell GeneChip studies presented in a series of *Science* articles describing the elusiveness of stemness genes were met with controversy. Ramalho-Santos *et al.* (2002) and Ivanova *et al.* (2002) used Gene-Chips to identify stemness genes by comparing the transcriptome profiles among ESC, HSC, and NSC. Using ESC, NPC, and RPC, Fortunel *et al.* (2003) identified sets of stemness genes, and when all three data sets were intersected, there was only one gene in common. However, when stemness genes were identified in a cell-specific manner were identified 332 ESC–specific and 236 NPC–specific. Rao and Stice (2004) ascribe this discrepancy to differences in method, stem cell populations, and stringency in data analysis. Suarez-Farinas *et al.* (2005) believe that the different results are due to the various protocols used for analysis and that raw data should be analyzed with exactly the same statistical methods, cutoffs, and only on the common genes. Larkin *et al.* (2005) believe that the data disagreement is a failure not of the platform or biological system but rather a reflection of the metrics used. However, this controversy involves not only the stem cell field but also the microarray field in general.

Stemness genes can be identified with GeneChips by comparison of ESC gene expression to that exhibited by their differentiated progeny or other somatic cells. Integration and comparison of ESC GeneChip data derived with different experimental designs will allow one to identify novel ESC-specific genes and provide insights into the genetics of ESC self-renewal and differentiation.

A true understanding of data from ESC gene expression studies requires a familiarity with the data analysis protocols used, including the appropriateness of a given analytic approach, the strengths and limitations of each approach, and the analytic steps executed that result in the final statistical conclusions. Unfortunately, many of GeneChip analytical software programs are neither intuitive nor user-friendly. In the following, we have provided an example of a step-by-step analysis of GeneChip data with corresponding screen-shots (Appendix 1) The data files examined were made publicly available by Sato *et al.* (2003), who compared the undifferentiated HESC H1 line with their differentiated progeny (differentiated for 26 days on matrigel [BD, NJ] with nonconditioned medium) using the Affymetrix U133a GeneChip.

Step-by-Step Analysis of GeneChip Data

The programs used in the representative analysis are RGui, affylmGUI, and EASE. This is accomplished by consolidating the .CEL files into a single folder and then creating a Hybridization file that allows affylmGUI to identify and group the .CEL files accordingly (Fig. A). This is a text file

(.txt) that can be made in Notepad, consisting of three tab-delimitated columns: Name (a unique name), Filename (name of the .CEL file), and Target (the name of the group) (Fig. A). It is important that the columns are separated by a tab space and each line is followed by a return with no spaces after each line of text.

RGui

The next step is to open the program RGui (Fig. B). Because the amount of memory on your computer determines the speed and number of files that can be analyzed, it is important to increase the amount of memory available to RGui to the maximum. If there is 4000 MB of memory available in the computer, this can be accomplished by entering the following command (Fig. C):

> memory.limit(size = 4000)

When this is finished, "Null" should appear below (Fig. D). The next thing to do is to open affylmGUI. This is done by entering the following case-sensitive command (Fig. E):

> library(affylmGUI)

A window will then appear asking to begin affylmGUI (Fig. F).

AffylmGUI

The affylmGUI main menu will appear (Fig. G). Import the .CEL files by clicking on *File* and then *Open* in the upper left corner of the menu bar in affylmGUI and navigate to the folder where the .CEL files are located. The program will then ask one to locate the .txt file made earlier and then enter a name for this data set. The files have now been incorporated into affylmGUI.

The next step is to normalize the data by clicking *Normalization* on the menu bar, then selecting *Normalize* from the dropdown menu and choosing the normalization method (RMA, GCRMA, affyPLM). The authors recommend creating two sets of data: one analyzed with RMA or affyPLM and the other by GCRMA but will use RMA only for this example. The next step is to compute a linear model by clicking on *Linear Model* on the menu bar and then *Compute Linear Model*. Next click on *Linear Model* and then *Compute Contrasts*, then select the desired group comparisons. A window with a series of pull-down menus appears, allowing you to choose the comparisons to be made (Fig. H). In this data set, the differentiated versus undifferentiated HESC are compared. To do this, click on the pull-down menu at the left and select *differentiated* group. The pull-down menu to the right of this should have "minus" selected, and to the right of this, select *undifferentiated* group

(Fig. I). This orientation of the data sets will determine the direction of fold change. Thus, the differentiated minus undifferentiated comparison indicates a change from undifferentiated to differentiated. In other words, if a gene has a positive fold change, it has a higher expression level in the differentiated group relative to the undifferentiated group.

After entering a name, a pop-up window will indicate that the calculation of the contrasts fit is complete. To calculate the comparison between groups, click on *TopTable* on the menu bar and then *Table of Genes Ranked in Order of Differential Expression*. It will then ask what contrasts parameterization this is for, and then select the group and click *OK*. A top table Options menu will pop up (Fig. J), allowing you to select the number of genes to output into the table (select *All genes*); how you would like to rank the list of genes (the authors select *B statistic*); and the Adjust method for the *p* value (the authors select *FDR*). A window will pop up containing the data analysis; save it to the computer (Fig. K).

Excel

Open the saved file from above with EXCEL (Fig. L) and paste those genes with a B > 0 into a new Excel sheet. Because the fold change (M value) is in Log2, add a column next to the B statistic for Fold Change, then enter the following command into the first cell of the Fold Change column (Fig. M1):

$$= 2^{\wedge}(\text{then click on the corresponding M value})$$

Copy this formula into every cell of the fold change column.

Next, sort the column data by fold change by clicking *Data* then *Sort*. A window will pop up, and in the pull-down menu select the fold change column. (Optional: we prefer to create separate files for the up-regulated and down-regulated and paste them into a new document, which makes later interpretation easier).

To summarize, the raw .CEL files were incorporated into affylmGUI, normalized with RMA, p values were adjusted using FDR, and those genes ranked with a B statistic of >0. This process identified 704 genes as being down-regulated and 1175 genes as being up-regulated. As expected, those genes that were most significantly down-regulated were known ESC genes such as Oct-4, TDGF1, SOX2, Nanog, and Telomerase (Fig. 2). However, there were many other genes that had similar expression profiles such as LeftyB, Thy1, FGF13, Galanin, and DNMT3B.

EASE

EASE can be used to provide a detailed annotation of those genes that were identified as differentially expressed. Open the EXCEL file containing the genes identified as down-regulated on HESC differentiation. Select the probe sets under the column "ID" and paste them into "Input Genes" located at the left of the main EASE menu (Fig. N). Click on *Select Annotation Fields* at the bottom right corner of the EASE menu under the Annotation option. A window will appear. Click *Add fields.* Here is the option of choosing a number of different annotation parameters. Select as many annotation parameters as desired, such as Gene Name, GeneRIF, and then click on *Open.* Click on *Add fields* again, but this time in the upper right, click on the folder *Class.* This will allow the choice of even more parameters, such as the PFAM domain, biochemical function, after which click *Open* and then *Done.* This will take you back to the main menu. Then, in the bottom right, click on *Annotate Genes.* This will create an HTML file with all the probesets (genes) with their corresponding annotations (Fig. O). The example identifies numerous growth factors that HESC seem to secrete in an auto/paracrine manner such as FGF2, FGF13, EGAF, TDGF1, GDF3, and nucleostemin.

To identify common themes present in the data set, genes may be grouped on the basis of their gene ontology. Begin by opening EASE. At the top of the main menu is a heading "1. Select Output," where there should be a check in the box that says "Display output in web browser." In the EXCEL file containing those genes down-regulated on differentiation of HESC, copy all the probesets (these are the Affymetrix gene identifiers that correspond with a gene) in the ID column, and click *Paste* above the "Input Genes" window located to the left of the EASE main menu.

Once the probesets (genes) are loaded into EASE, click on select *Categorical System* under Analysis options located at the bottom right of the EASE main menu, and then chose the ontology for examining the genes. For this example, click on *GO Biological process, Open,* and then *Done.* This navigates back to the main screen of EASE. Click on *Find Overrepresented Gene Categories.* Another window will pop up asking to input "list Identifiers for ALL genes assayed" (Fig. P). In the pull-down menu, select *Affymetrix probeset,* then click on the button *from a population file* and chose the file that corresponds to the type of GeneChip used (*HU133A*) and click *Open* (Fig. Q). Click on "*Run basic analysis.*" An HTML file will pop up containing all the GO Biological Processes in the data set with the processes with the greatest statistical significance ranked at the top (Fig. R). This file can be saved to a folder and then opened and edited in EXCEL. The entire process can be repeated for each of the different ontologies.

In the representative analysis, the most overrepresented theme using GO Biological Process is mitotic cell cycle. When SwissProt Keyword is the selected Ontology, transit peptides and mitochondrion are most overrepresented. GO Cellular Component identifies mitochondrion, and GO Molecular Function identifies catalytic activity as most overrepresented. Clustering a data set in this manner serves to validate/confirm a data set in its biological context. For example, one would expect to identify numerous genes involved in mitosis to be down-regulated on differentiation, which was the case here. However, other processes might be revealed that might not have been as obvious, such as genes involved in mitochondria and ATP metabolism that provide insight into energy demands of cell division, chromatin assembly, and remodeling.

The next step is to identify and annotate those genes that were associated with a particular ontological process. For example, cluster the list of down-regulated HESC genes using GO Biological Process (as earlier) and SwissProt. In the GO Biological Process data set, scroll down to the Gene Category "Growth" (Fig. R) and for the SwissProt data set "Growth Factor." At the far right of these rows is a column containing all "Affymetrix probesets" for these categories. Select and paste the corresponding probesets for these ontological processes into Input Genes at the left of the main EASE menu and annotate as described earlier (Fig. R). This will create an HTML file with all the probesets (genes) that were clustered under "Growth" and "Growth Factor." This analysis identifies numerous genes that HESC seem to secrete in an auto/paracrine manner such as FGF2, FGF13, EGAF, TDGF1, and GDF3.

ACCESS

With this and every analysis performed, those genes that are identified as differentially expressed and the "transcriptomes" that were identified by Present calls are imported into an ACCESS database. In ACCESS, every possible comparison can be made between data sets such as identifying genes that are present in one data set and not another or those common to multiple data sets. These data sets are then interpreted with EASE.

Parthenogenetic Embryonic Stem Cells

A similar approach to understanding nonhuman primate parthenogenetic embryonic–like stem cell (PGESC) differentiation (Cibelli *et al.*, 2002; Vrana *et al.*, 2003) was applied. Parthenogenesis entails the *in vitro* activation of oocytes, which stimulates their growth and development as though fertilized by sperm. These parthenotes cannot develop past the blastocyst stage, even if transferred *in vivo*. Embryonic-like stem cells can be isolated from the inner cell mass. These cells express hESC markers and are capable of differentiating into all three germ layers (Cibelli *et al.*, 2002; Vrana *et al.*, 2003), into neuronal progenitors, and then on to neurons that express functional voltage-dependent sodium channels. The Human U133A GeneChip was used to profile undifferentiated PGESC, and PGESC differentiated into neuronal progenitors. The .CEL files were analyzed as described previously; 658 genes were identified as down-regulated and 647 as up-regulated. As an inherent biological control, the ES markers Oct-4, TDGF1, and telomerase were identified as well (SOX2 was not identified in this data set because it also serves as a neural progenitor marker). Clustering this data set reveals many of the same ontological processes identified in the hESC data set. The intersection of this data set with those that were down-regulated in hESC from above identified 126 genes in common. This analysis demonstrates that there were a number of genes down-regulated on differentiation in PGESC and not hESC and vice versa. Does this mean that there are many distinct genes or combinations responsible for pluripotency and self-renewal? Or are there different shades of pluripotency as suggested by Rao *et al.* (2004)?

Because this GeneChip data set was differentiated along the neuronal lineage, those genes that were up-regulated to assess differentiation or identify new genetic markers can be analyzed. For example, some of the most significantly up-regulated genes are Neurofilament 68KD, Neurofilament 3, and neural cell adhesion molecule. When this data set is clustered using GO Biological Function, the most overrepresented processes are antigen processing (MHC I) and neurogenesis. However, when analyzing the large list of genes that are up-regulated on differentiation, it is difficult to distinguish those genes responsible for "differentiation" and those differentiation genes that are neuronal lineage specific.

Genomic imprinting is an epigenetic mechanism that is species-specific, temporally-specific, and tissue-specific, and controls allelic gene expression on the basis of its parent of origin. Although there are approximately 70 imprinted genes, it is estimated that there are 100–500 imprinted genes in humans (Jirtle, 2004; Murphy and Jirtle, 2003). The authors believe GeneChip analysis of PGESC will provide an understanding of imprinting's role in stem cell growth and differentiation. To understand imprinted gene expression, a "transcriptome" signature of genes that were identified as Present by MAS5 was created for PGESC (purely maternal origin) and hESC (biparental) (Hipp *et al.*, 2004). Lists of known imprinted genes were compiled from the human imprinted gene databases: Imprinted Gene Catalogue (IGC) (Morison *et al.*, 2001), http://www.otago.ac.nz/igc), Harwell (Beechey *et al.*, 2005) (http://www.mgu.har.mrc.ac.uk/research/imprinting/), and Gene Imprint (www. geneimprint.com). Figure 4 demonstrates the presence of known PEG (paternally expressed genes) in HESC but not PGESC. Although the imprinting status and expression pattern of some of the genes in the table are unknown in humans (Gabrb3, Kip2, Igf2r), our data demonstrate that genes such as Gabrb3 and Kip2 are not paternally expressed genes; Par5, Peg10, and Znf264 are paternally expressed; but Igf2r could be purely maternally expressed (Hipp *et al.*, 2004).

PGESC	HESC	Imprinted status
-	Ipw	PEG- human
-	Mest	PEG- human
-	Ndn	PEG- human
-	Peg3	PEG- human
-	Sdhd	PEG- human
-	Sgce	PEG- human
-	Snrpn	PEG- human
-	Snurf	PEG- human
-	Impact	PEG- mouse
-	Slc38a4	PEG- mouse
M6pr	M6pr	MEG- ?
-	Igf2r	MEG- ?
-	-	MEG- ?
Gnas	Gnas	MEG- human
grb10	grb10	MEG- human
tssc3	tssc3	MEG- human
Ube3a	Ube3a	MEG- human
CD81	CD81	MEG- mouse
Dcn	Dcn	MEG- mouse
Gatm	Gatm	MEG- mouse
-	Napll4	MEG- mouse
Cdkn1c	Cdkn1c	?-human
-	Par5	?-human
-	Peg10	?-human
-	Ppp1r9a	?-mouse
-	Znf264	?-mouse
Gabrb3	Gabrb3	?-?
Kip2	Kip2	?-?

FIG. 4. Table of imprinted genes present in PGESC and HESC: (–) = the gene was not detected as present; (?) = unknown expression pattern). This table demonstrates that PGESC express maternally expressed genes (MEG) but not paternally expressed genes (PEG).

Mouse ESCs

Using a novel experimental design, D'Amour and Gage (2003) used GeneChips to define the genetic signature of pluripotency and multipotency. mESCs were transfected with EGFP-labeled SOX2, a gene expressed by ESCs and NSC. These cells were then injected into a blastocyst that was transferred *in utero* and developed to day 14. NSC from the fetal telencephalon were isolated and sorted. Some of these were cultured for 5 days *in vitro*. Thus, pure populations of ESC and those that had undergone *in vivo* differentiation into NSC were generated by selecting for SOX2 expression and then analyzed with the Affymetrix U74Av2.

This study is unique in that it selected for homogenous cellular populations of ESCs and NSCs, ensuring full differentiation and the removal of contaminating cell types such as glia or astrocytes. Because ESCs are pluripotential and NSCs are multipotential, this biological model allows for the identification of pluripotential versus multipotential stemness genes (Fig. 5B, F). Furthermore, it provides insight into the effect of *in vitro* culturing on gene expression (Fig. 5C, D).

The authors reanalyzed the .CEL files of D'Amour and Gage (2003) with the protocol described previously and identified numerous genes that were up-regulated (A, 1393) and down-regulated (B, 1114) when ESCs differentiated into freshly isolated NSC (fNSC). These genes were then clustered (B) on the basis of their ontology and the most overrepresented themes were catabolic pathways involved in energy production. The themes predominant in (A) are involved in neurogenesis. Cultured NSC (cNSC) were then compared with fNSC, and a similar number of genes that were identified as up-regulated (D, 727) and down-regulated (E, 1062) on 5 days of *in vitro* culturing. Metabolism was the predominant theme involved in (D), and DNA modification and neurogenesis were the predominant themes in (E).

To compare these results with other studies that typically compare cultured ESC to their progeny differentiated *in vitro*, the authors then compared ES with cNSC and identified 1253 (F) genes that were up-regulated and 1430 (G) genes that were down-regulated. Among the genes in (G) are those involved in cell growth and cell cycle and those in (F) are involved in neurogenesis. Those genes that were up-regulated and down-regulated in ESC versus fNSC were compared with those that were up-regulated and down-regulated between ESCs versus cNSCs. This comparison identified 610 genes

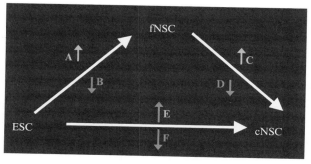

FIG. 5. Experimental design. ESCs were compared with freshly isolated NSCs (fNSCs) and with cultured NSCs(cNSCs), and fNSCs were compared with cNSCs. The red arrows represent those genes that were up-regulated, and the blue arrows were those that were down-regulated.

(A not E) that were up-regulated and 281 genes (B not F) down-regulated on *in vivo* differentiation (ESCs vs fNSCs) and not "*in vitro*" differentiation (ESCs vs cNSCs). Of the genes that were up-regulated, only the GO Biological ontology identified statistically significant themes, which were involved in neurogenesis and behavior. Of the down-regulated genes, catabolism was identified. Of the genes that were up-regulated (E not A, 470) on *in vitro* differentiation (ESCs vs cNSCs) and not on *in vivo* differentiation (ESCs vs fNSCs) were genes involved in lipid metabolism and cell cycle arrest. Of the genes that were down-regulated (F not B, 597) on *in vitro* differentiation (ESCs vs cNSCs) and not down-regulated on *in vivo* differentiation, (ESCs vs fNSCs) were genes involved in cell cycle.

To understand the genes that are up-regulated and down-regulated on 5 days of *in vitro* culturing, the authors compared these data sets to the differentially regulated *in vivo* differentiation. Of those genes that were up-regulated on *in vitro* culturing, 62 genes were also up-regulated on *in vivo* differentiation (C and A). The significant processes identified were neurogenesis and behavior; 87 genes were both down-regulated on *in vitro* culturing and down-regulated on *in vivo* differentiation (D not B). The ontological processes identified in this data set were those involved in "response to stimulus/DNA damage." There were 517 genes that were identified as both down-regulated on *in vitro* culturing and up-regulated on *in vivo* differentiation (D and A). The predominant process identified in this data set was neurogenesis; 150 genes were both up-regulated on *in vitro* culturing and down-regulated on *in vivo* differentiation (C and B). The predominant theme in this data set was catabolism.

The authors then loaded these data sets into GenMapp that allows one to compare and contrast the multiple data sets in the context of premade pathways (Fig. 6). The predominance of "red" in the Wnt GenMapp illustrates that the Wnt pathway is up-regulated on ESC differentiation into NSCs (Fig. 6A). Figure 6B notes the number of genes down-regulated on differentiation (blue) involved in "translation factors." Figure 6C demonstrates the differential expression of multiple data sets of genes involved in "Growth."

ESC Genes and *In Vivo* Regeneration

As a way to understand and categorize the ESC genes identified previously in an *in vivo* context, the data sets were compared with GeneChip data from an injury induced *in vivo* regeneration model (Zhao *et al.*, 2002). This group sought to use mouse Affymetrix GeneChips to identify the downstream targets of MyoD in myogenic regeneration. To induce regeneration, tissue damage was induced by cardiotoxin injection into the gastrocnemii muscle. GeneChips were performed on gastrocnemii muscle at 0, 12 h, 1 day, 2 days,

4 days, and 10 days after injury. Hematoxylin-eosin staining demonstrated progressive inflammation from 12 h–2 days, regenerating muscle fibers at day 4. At day 10, approximately 50% of the muscle fibers demonstrated regeneration. Zhao *et al.* identified Slug and calpain 6 as targets of MyoD and made their raw data files publicly available spanning 40 days post-injury.

The authors then analyzed the CEL files of Zhao *et al.* using the protocol described earlier. As a way to validate and understand the many time-point comparisons, the ontological processes were assessed to validate the pathology findings. The analysis consisted of two types of comparisons,

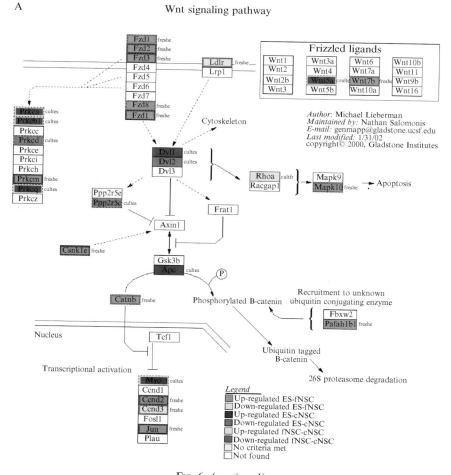

FIG. 6. (*continued*)

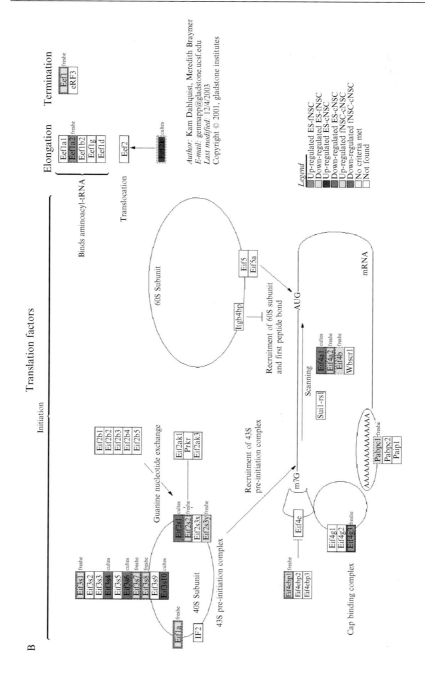

Author: Kam Dahlquist, Meredith Braymer
E-mail: genmapp@gladstone.ucsf.edu
Last modified: 12/4/2003

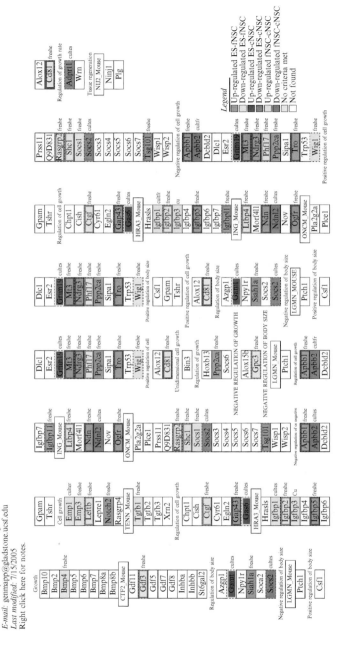

FIG. 6. Genes that were identified as being up-regulated and down-regulated on *in vivo* mouse ESC differentiation into NSCf and those that were further cultured for 5 days NSCc. (A) GenMapp Wnt pathway. (B) GenMapp translation factors pathway. (C) GenMapp growth pathway. (See color insert.)

a comparison of each time point to the control (muscle before injury) and then a comparison among multiple time-points to provide a kinetics of changes in expression over short variable time intervals. When compared with the baseline, there was a persistent down-regulation of genes involved in energy metabolism from day 1–12. This identified the multiple phases of an inflammatory response involved in healing and regeneration: there was a persistent elevation of "MHC class I receptor activity," an increase in "chemotaxis" and at days 1 and 2, "extracellular matrix structural constituent" at day 10, "cytokine activity" and "chemokine activity" at day 12, "defense/immunity protein activity" at day 30. A cell proliferation response was identified in their pathology slides at day 4, whereas the GeneChip data identified an increase in the number of cell cycle transcripts at day 2, peaking at day 4 but remaining elevated to day 10. In addition, a number of genes involved in myogenesis and neurogenesis were identified from day 3 to 5 and an increase in angiogenic genes from day 10–12.

To identify whether the *in vivo* regeneration response uses stemness and differentiation, the authors intersected the stemness genes identified above with those that were identified in the *in vivo* regeneration model. The data set containing the genes that were down-regulated at day 2 had the most in common with the differentiation genes, and the genes that were up-regulated at day 3 had the most in common with the stemness genes. These data demonstrate that 2 days after injury, the muscle down-regulates differentiation genes and on day 3 turns on stemness genes. Those genes that were identified in the differentiation data set and were down-regulated at day 2 were clustered on the basis of their ontology and identified cell differentiation as a GO Biological theme ($p = 0.0466$). Of the genes that were present in this data set were Zic1 (that had the second greatest fold change on ESC differentiation into fNSC [up-regulated 32x] and was also down-regulated after 2 days in the *in vivo* regeneration model). Others have shown that this gene acts as an inhibitor of differentiation by preserving the neuronal progenitor state (Aruga *et al.*, 2002; Brewster *et al.*, 1998; Ebert *et al.*, 2003), and its down-regulation in the *in vivo* model is indicative of regeneration. Thus, the genes that were identified as stemness and up-regulated in the day 3 data set are probably responsible for regeneration. Clustering on the basis of their GO Biological Process identified themes such as "cell proliferation" ($p = 0.00024$) and "cytoplasm organization and biogenesis" ($p = 0.0186$). This data set identified Wnt ligand Sfrp1 as the gene with the greatest up-regulation at day 3. SOX11 was the stemness gene with the greatest fold difference and could represent a novel transcriptional factor involved in regeneration.

This integration of stemness GeneChip data with *in vivo* biological models of regeneration will not only yield novel insights into the genetics of stemness and differentiation but will also provide the genetic "blue-prints" of regeneration.

Cell Screening

GeneChip can be used as a screening tool to monitor the gene expression of cellular populations as a quality control to assess ESCs throughout the stages of expansion and differentiation. A GeneChip analysis of ESCs to measure gene expression and genomic alternations could also predict which lines and passages would have the best differentiation potential. Furthermore, because there are a limited number of tissue-specific genetic markers, a GeneChip analysis comparing a differentiated derivative with its *in vivo* counterpart could potentially predict if and when clinical transplantation could occur.

Screening Differentiation Derivatives

hESC-Derived Retinal Pigmented Epithelia

In a more clinically applicable manner, GeneChips were used as a screening tool to assess differentiation. Klimanskaya *et al.* (2004) differentiated HESC into retinal pigmented epithelial cells (hESC–RPE). After determining the expression of many known molecular markers by RT-PCR, immunostaining Western blots and functional studies such as phago-cytosis of latex beads, a GeneChip analysis was run and compared with publicly available RPE GeneChip data from the lines ARPE19 and D407 (Rogojina *et al.*, 2003). A publicly available bronchial epithelial data set was selected as a control because of its similar epithelial origin but lack of RPE specific genes (Wright *et al.*, 2004). Genetic signatures were created by identifying those genes identified as Present in each cell type and then compared. This analysis not only identified many more RPE genes but demonstrated the genetic similarity between hESC–RPE and RPE cell lines. A GeneChip was then run on freshly isolated human fetal RPE (feRPE), a resource currently used in transplantation therapies and then compared with the RPE cell lines and hESC–RPE. It was demonstrated that the transcriptional profile of hESC–RPE was more similar to feRPE than to both ARPE19 and D407. Importantly, ARPE-19 has been shown to attenuate the loss of visual function in animal transplantation studies (Lund *et al.*, 2001).

There was a subset of genes (784) that were present in hESC–RPE and not in the RPE cell lines or feRPE. Because the retention of "stemness" genes could result in teratomas, we created a signature of "stemness" genes by selecting those genes Present in four hESC lines (3806 genes) using publicly available data (Abeyta *et al.*, 2004; Sato *et al.*, 2003). There were only 36 genes in common, none of which have been shown to be hESC specific such as OCT4, SOX2, and TDGF1. In conclusion, the authors believe that screening and comparing ESC derivatives with GeneChips is a valuable way to assess differentiation.

Screening hESCs for Gene Expression Variability

Using Human Affymetrix Genechips, Abeyta *et al.* (2004) studied the variability in gene expression of HESCs. They profiled hESC lines HSF6 (p46-female), HSF1 (p36-female), and H9 (p51-male) using the HG-U133 GeneChip. They used MAS5 for call detection and identified 7385 genes present in all three lines, and after analyzing with RMA, 52% of these genes had a greater than a twofold difference. They also identified 2279 present only in H9, 337 present only in HSF1, and 641 present only in HSF6. Because all three lines were grown and handled in a similar manner, Abeyta *et al.* asserted that the difference in results could be attributed to DNA sequence variability.

Screening for Genetic Mutations

Unlike the GeneChips described previously that measure RNA expression, GeneChip Mapping Arrays differ in that they identify mutations in genomic DNA (Matsuzaki *et al.*, 2004) (www.affymetrix.com). Like the GeneChips described earlier, they contain 25-bp probes, but these probes complement regions of DNA that have high sequence variability—called single nucleotide polymorphisms (SNPs). These GeneChips can screen about 100,000 SNPs in the forward and reverse direction by varying the 13th base of the probe to screen for all four possible genotypes (A, T, G, C).

These GeneChips experiments begin with the isolation of DNA rather than RNA, which is then digested with either *Xba*I or *Hind*III restriction enzymes. PCR is then performed to amplify the fragments that are then labeled and hybridized to the GeneChip (Affymetrix, 4 A.D.). Files can then be analyzed with GeneChip DNA analysis software (GDAS3.0) (Affymetrix, 4 A.D.) and Affymetrix GeneChip Chromosome Copy number analysis tool version 2.0 (Huang *et al.*, 2004) to generate genotypes and identify DNA copy numbers. A similar GeneChip has also been designed to screen for mutations in mitochondrial genes (MitoChip) (Maitra *et al.*, 2004). The MitoChip uses the basis of the same principles described earlier and screens the entire mitochondrial genome (16,569 bp). In addition, the MitoChip can detect mutations present in as few as 2% of the cells (Maitra *et al.*, 2005b).

Maitra *et al.* (2005d) used both the HU 100,000K SNP GeneChip and MitoChip to analyze nine different early (p11–59) and late (p39–147) passage

HESC lines for genomic and mitochondrial DNA mutations. SNP differences were only detected between early and late passages in the HESC line SA002/ 2.5 (240, majority on chromosome 13). The lack of SNP differences between early and late passage in the other eight hESC lines also verified their common genetic origin (Maitra *et al.*, 2005a). Four of the nine lines had changes in DNA copy number that had accumulated over passaging. These alterations were also confirmed with fluorescence *in situ* hybridization (FISH) or genomic quantitative PCR (Q-PCR). The MitoChip identified mitochondrial DNA mutations in two of the nine HESC lines that were also confirmed by dideoxy sequencing (Maitra *et al.*, 2005c).

This technology enables detailed and quantitative analysis of genomic and mitochondrial DNA. In the future, it can be used to screen populations before and after differentiation. By correlating these data with functional outcomes, one can determine mutations that are harmful or benign.

Integration and Meta-Analysis of GeneChip and Microarray Data

The ability to link GeneChip data with other data sets generated using similar high-throughput gene expression technology can serve as a *in silico* validation and a way to "biologically" filter large data sets. The difficulty in performing such experiments for a biologist is in extracting the data, importing and exporting between the different databases, filtering out the genes that were not screened by the GeneChip, and then interpreting the large data set generated. This can be accomplished with the GUI programs EASE, MS ACCESS, and Excel.

Sperger *et al.* (2003) profiled HESC lines 1.1, 7, 9, 13, 14 and compared them with a common "differentiated" reference pool of RNA using a custom dual-channel cDNA platform that screened >44,000 cDNA (~30,300 unique genes). They identified 1760 cDNA (~1163 genes) genes that were up-regulated in ESCs relative to somatic cells. The authors then took Gene Symbols present in their list and converted them to their Affymetrix probeset IDs using the EASE "Annotation" function. Using the "Refine" function in EASE, only those genes that were also present on the HU-133a GeneChip were selected. The genes present on the HU-133a GeneChip were used to standardize the type of genes being assessed. Because multiple probesets can exist for a single gene, these probesets were converted back to their Gene Symbols, and Excel was used to filter for unique genes, removing duplicated genes. This list was then imported into MS ACCESS for comparisons. This method identified 948 genes that were enriched in HESC and 480 genes down-regulated in hESC. Using MS ACCESS, these genes were compared with the data sets identified earlier. Of the 948 genes that were up-regulated in HESC, there were 197 genes in common with the Sato *et al.* hESC stemness genes identified earlier, and 144 in common with the stemness genes identified in PGESC from above (Fig. 7).

Brandenberger *et al.* (2004) created and compared EST sequence libraries from pooled HESC cell lines 1, 7, and 9 to HESC that have undergone differentiation into EB, pre-hepatocytes, and pre-neurons (2004). They identified 32,000 ESTs in HESC, 16,000 of which matched to known genes. They reported 532 genes as being up-regulated and 140 genes as down-regulated in hESC. The authors then took the NCBI Accession numbers, converted them to Affymetrix probesets with EASE, selected only those probesets present on the HU-133a GeneChip, converted these to Gene Symbols and removed duplicate genes; 406 of the 532 genes "stemness" genes and 126 of the 140 "differentiation" genes were also screened by the HU-133A GeneChip. Of the 406, there were 87 in common with the "stemness" genes identified by Sato *et al.* (2003), 96 by Sperger *et al.* (2003) and 54 from the PGESC data set from above (Fig. 7).

Boyer *et al.* (2005) used microarrays to identify genes bound to ESC-specific transcription factors. They performed a chromatin immunoprecipitation (ChIP) followed by DNA array analysis to identify genes that are bound to SOX2, Oct4, and NANOG. hESCs were fixed, sonicated, and precipitated with an antibody against SOX2, OCT4, or NANOG. The DNA was then amplified by PCR with random primers, labeled, and hybridized to an Agilent chip. The microarray was composed of probes that screened the region of -8 kb to $+2$ kb relative to the transcriptional start sites for 17,917 annotated human genes. They identified 3081 genes bound to SOX2, OCT4, or NANOG, and 353 genes that were bound to all three transcription factors. Of these 3081 and 353 genes, they identified 1346 and 210 present on the HU-133a GeneChip.

In an analogous manner described by Boyer *et al.* (2005), the authors compared the stemness and differentiation data sets identified earlier to the list of genes that were found to bind to SOX2, OCT4, NANOG, or all three. Using MS ACCESS, the four data sets (Brandenberger *et al.*, 2004; Sato *et al.*, 2003; Sperger *et al.*, 2003) were summarized to create a "master" list of genes and then intersected with the Boyer *et al.* data set; 307 of the stemness genes were found to be in common with the genes that bind to either SOX2, OCT4, or NANOG; 64 of these genes bind to all three transcription factors (these numbers differ slightly from summarizing the columns in the table because of duplicity of genes within the data sets). These likely represent stemness genes that are directly induced by the ESC specific transcription factors SOX2, OCT4, and NANOG (Fig. 6). Of the "master" list of differentiation genes, 208 were in common with the genes that bind to either SOX2, OCT4, or NANOG; 64 of these genes bind to all three transcription factors (Fig. 6). This analysis allows one to define the

A

	Sperger et al.	Sato et al.	PGESC	Brandenberger et al.	Boyer et al. 3/3	Boyer et al. 1/3
Sperger et al.	948	197	144	96	35	160
Sato et al.	197	612	122	87	22	108
PGESC	144	122	506	54	19	85
Brandenberger et al.	96	87	54	406	20	73
Boyer et al. 3/3	35	22	19	20	210	210
Boyer et al. 1/3	160	108	85	73	210	1346

B

	Sperger et al.	Sato et al.	PGESC	Brandenberger et al.	Boyer et al. 3/3	Boyer et al. 1/3
Sperger et al.	480	76	52	3	7	46
Sato et al.	76	920	170	45	13	109
PGESC	52	170	514	13	16	68
Brandenberger et al.	3	45	13	126	2	29
Boyer et al. 3/3	7	13	16	2	210	210
Boyer et al. 1/3	46	109	68	29	210	1346

FIG. 7. Genes that were up-regulated (A) and down-regulated (B) in the Sperger *et al.*, Sato *et al.*, PGESC *et al.*, Brandenberger *et al.*, and in the Boyet *et al.* (SOX2-NANOG-OCT4), and Boyet *et al.* (SOX2 or NANOG or OCT4) data sets were intersected.

subnetworks of stemness and differentiation genes that are directly under the control of known ESC-specific transcription factors. When these genes were clustered with EASE, the predominant genetic themes identified in the repressed data set were "Development," "Transcription," and "ECM" and in the induced data set were "Development," "Transcription," "Cell cycle," and "Wnt."

GenMapp Analysis

To gain further insight into these numerous and complex data sets, the authors used the program GenMapp to screen hundreds of premade pathways. Affymetrix probesets from Fig. 7 were loaded into GenMapp and color coded according to their expression pattern. This allowed for the identification of shared or uniquely expressed pathways involved in ESC growth and differentiation (Fig. 8) such as the complex genetic regulation of chromatin involved in ESC differentiation (Fig. 8A).

With the *in vitro* differentiation of ESCs as a model for organogenesis, it is not surprising to find many genes differentially regulated in the GenMapp pathways "Extracellular matrix" and "Growth" (Fig. 8B, C). These targets are of particular interest, because they could easily be manipulated to improve the efficiency and quality of differentiation. One potential application would be in the creation of novel scaffolds to guide the differentiation of ESCs.

This analysis demonstrates that the true potential of ESC GeneChip experiments lies in the *in silico* analysis—the integration and comparison of data generated by similar and different cell types and platforms. It is at this stage, *in silico,* where the biology is brought back into the GeneChip analysis, and the biological questions become the driving force in the analysis.

Applications to Cancer

Because of the similarities between cancer and stem cells, many believe that cancer is a dedifferentiation of a somatic cell back into a stem cell (Al-Hajj *et al.*, 2004; Pardal *et al.*, 2003). Not only do cancers and stem cells have similar growth properties, but germ cell tumors such as embryonal carcinomas (Andrews, 1998) and benign ovarian teratomas (Linder *et al.*, 1975) are even capable of differentiating into tissues of different germ layers. Therefore, insights into the genetic mechanisms of stem cell growth and differentiation might provide information for designing therapeutics for cancer.

A benign ovarian teratoma, a germ cell tumor, is the result of the "activation" of a diploid (Meioses II arrested) oocyte through an unknown mechanism. What is unusual about this tumor is its pluripotentiality. Not

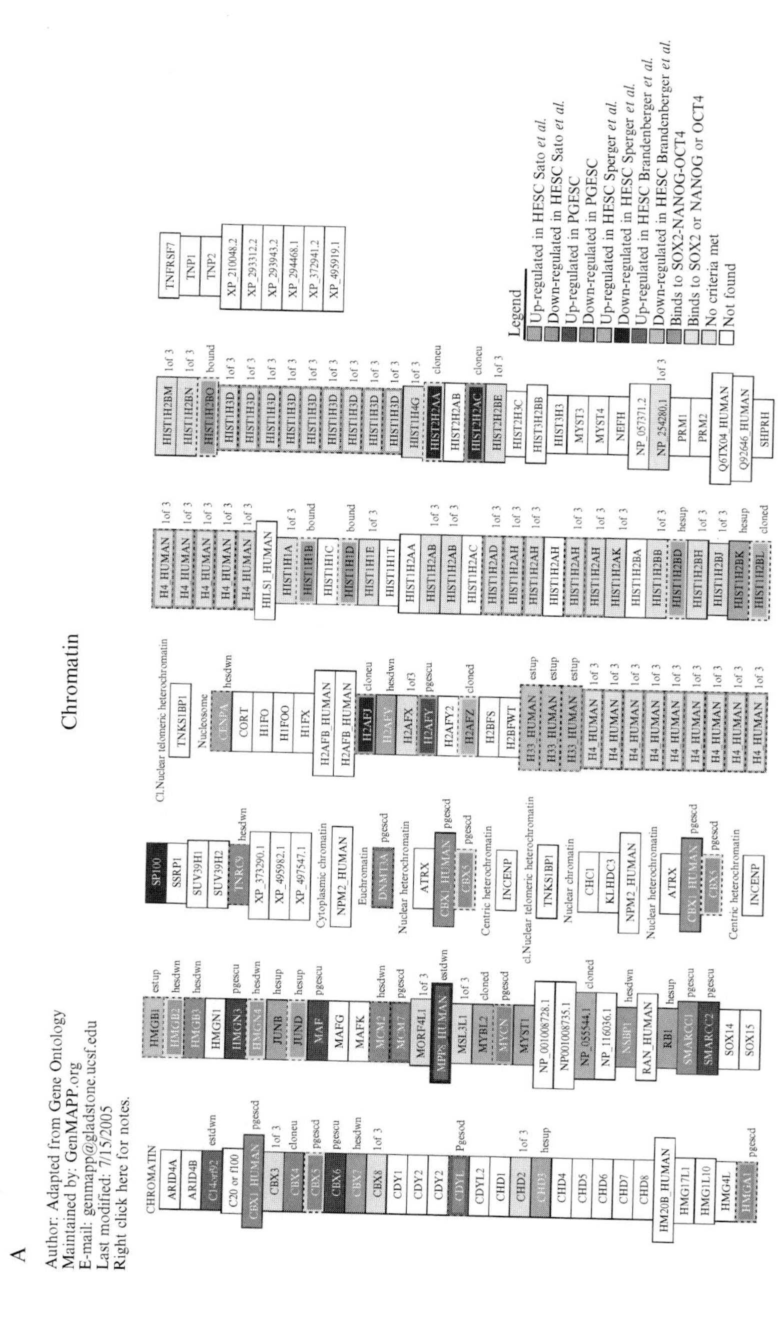

Chromatin

A

Author: Adapted from Gene Ontology
Maintained by: GenMAPP.org
E-mail: genmapp@gladstone.ucsf.edu
Last modified: 7/15/2005
Right click here for notes.

Legend

- Up-regulated in HESC Sato et al.
- Down-regulated in HESC Sato et al.
- Up-regulated in PGESC
- Down-regulated in PGESC
- Up-regulated in HESC Sperger et al.
- Down-regulated in HESC Sperger et al.
- Up-regulated in HESC Brandenberger et al.
- Down-regulated in HESC Brandenberger et al.
- Binds to SOX2-NANOG-OCT4
- Binds to SOX2 or NANOG or OCT4
- No criteria met
- Not found

FIG. 8. (*continued*)

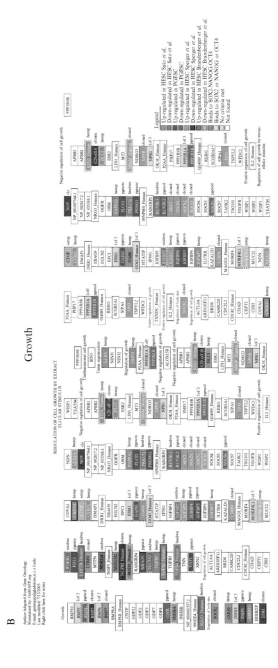

Growth

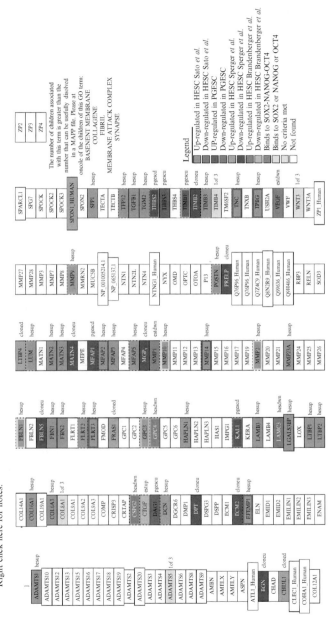

FIG. 8. Genes that were up-regulated and down-regulated in the Sperger *et al.*, Sato *et al.*, PGESC *et al.*, Brandenberger *et al.* data sets, and in the Boyet *et al.* (SOX2-NANOG-OCT4), and Boyet *et al.* (SOX2 or NANOG or OCT4) data sets. (A) GenMapp chromatin pathway. (B) Genmapp growth pathway. (C) GenMapp extracellular matrix pathway. (See color insert.)

only have many different tissue types been identified within the tumor, but they can sometimes result in a homunculus (Latin for "little man") (Abbot *et al.*, 1984). Thus, it seems that an oocyte alone is capable of differentiating into all three germ layers and can form the proper three-dimensional tissue structures and architecture.

This effect has been mimicked *in vitro* with the use of monkey oocytes, as demonstrated earlier (Cibelli *et al.*, 2002; Vrana *et al.*, 2003). The activation of oocytes in this context is referred to as parthenogenesis. Many lower species such as bees, fish, serpents, monotremes, but not eutharians, are capable of this form of reproduction. However, when mammalian oocytes are activated, they usually do not progress past the blastocyst stage, when stem cells can be isolated from their inner cell mass (ICM). These cells express ESC markers and are capable of differentiating into all three germ layers. Furthermore, injection of PGESC into the peritoneum of SCID mice results in a benign teratoma. Last, when patients with benign ovarian teratomas are treated with chemotherapy, the prognosis grading is made on the basis of the percentage of neuronal tissue contained within the teratoma. A predominance for the neuronal lineage is also seen in their *in vitro* differentiation. Thus, it seems that the induction of cell cycle arrest results in a default differentiation into neurons; however, the difference between a benign ovarian teratoma and a parthenogenetic stem cell is that the former is "activated" *in vivo*, whereas the latter is activated *in vitro*.

Regarding the question of whether a "cancer stem cell" exists, it is hypothesized that PGESC are the stem cells of benign ovarian teratomas. The advantage of studying PGESC instead of benign ovarian teratomas is that PGESC represent a single cell in which one can study its self-renewal and differentiation. An understanding of these genetic mechanisms will not only give a unique insight into cancer but also provide potential therapeutic targets. Genes that are unique to PGESC (i.e., PGESC-specific stemness genes) can serve as therapeutic targets. Comparing undifferentiated PGESC with those that have undergone neuronal differentiation as described earlier created a signature of 658 genes that could be used as tumor antigen targets.

How does one apply this GeneChip to designing new cancer therapies? Successful approaches have involved the creation of small molecule inhibitors (often associated with side effects), monoclonal antibodies to genes such as Her2/Neu (Hereptin) (Cobleigh *et al.*, 1999; Tripathy *et al.*, 2004; Vogel *et al.*, 2001, 2002), or siRNA to knock down "cancer" or stemness genes. Another option would be to create a cancer vaccine that uses a patient's own cytotoxic T cells (CTLs) to kill tumors (Rosenberg *et al.*, 2004a). CTLs are the T cells responsible for the cell-mediated immune response, and they lyse tumor cells on the basis of the expression of specific peptide sequences bound to major histocompatability type I (MHC-I). Therefore, one could potentially stimulate a specific subset of CTL to lyse tumor cells by targeting stemness genes coexpressed with MHC-I. Although the field is currently limited by the number of tumor-specific antigens, the advantage of this approach is in its specificity and ability to target micrometastasis.

In a previous study, peptides were identified from the enzyme telomerase (responsible for maintaining telomeric ends), and CTLs were generated from patients with prostate cancer to recognize and lyse 7/8 different types of tumor lines with one peptide sequence and 7/8 lines of another peptide sequence, nonoverlapping (Minev et al., 2000). This antigen was chosen on the basis of the idea that cancer cells must overexpress to replicate indefinitely. Although other cells such as bone marrow and skin cells express telomerase, it was shown that the expression level is not significant enough to generate an immune response. Parthenogenetic stemness genes and other stemness genes identified from other stem cell data sets could serve as targets in this manner. Furthermore, screening of these antigens against different cancer types (breast, lung, or melanoma) could be used to create a cocktail of tumor-specific antigens.

Conclusion

Future Direction

The interpretation of data is the most challenging task of a GeneChip experiment. Trying to ascribe ESC functions or understanding their differentiation from gene lists is analogous to explaining the difference between a car and a train by comparing their parts. These GeneChip data files contain a genetic parts list of the cell's signaling networks. Understanding the genetic networks of stem cells is analogous to a computer chip. This becomes further complicated by differentiation that allows it to alter its "motherboard." Because there are more than 300 cell types in the body, there are potentially more than 300 types of "motherboards" responsible for their lineage-directed differentiation.

To begin to address this goal, investigators are drawing on multiple comparisons among disparate stem cells to identify those genes that are conserved or uniquely expressed (Hipp et al., 2004). Future experiments will need to profile stem cell differentiation in a lineage- and temporal-specific manner that will enable one to dissect out the genetic wiring of differentiation and its commitment to a lineage. To accomplish this goal will require a collaborative effort among many laboratories to provide the critical mass of data necessary.

Summary

The goal of this chapter was to discuss the many components involved in a GeneChip experiment and the application of GeneChip technology to ESC biology. A protocol for GeneChip analysis that requires minimal computer skills is efficient, reliable, quick, inexpensive, and results in meaningful data is described.

The application of GeneChip data to regenerative medicine is discussed. GeneChips can be used to understand the genetics of ESC growth and differentiation. They can also be used as a screening tool to assess differentiation and variability among lines and to identify genomic and mitochondrial mutations. We assert that the true potential of GeneChip technology lies in the *in silico* analysis—their integration and comparison of diverse data sets, where the biological questions are the driving force in the analysis.

Appendix 1

Sample Analysis

RGui, affylmGUI, EASE

    1. CEL files→Folder
    2. Create Hybridization File (Fig. A)

RGui

    3. Open RGui (Fig. B)
    4. Increase memory size (Fig. C):
       Type >memory.limit(size = 4000)
    5. Open affylmGUI (Fig. E):
       Type >library(affylmGUI)

AffylmGUI

    6. Import CEL files
       Click File→Open→select folder where CEL files are located→Then select txt file
    7. Normalize data
       Click Normalization→Normalize→RMA or GCRMA
    8. Compute Linear Model
       Click Linear Model→Compute Linear Model
    9. Select the types of Contrasts
       Click Linear Model→Compute Contrasts→Select comparisons (Fig. I)
    10. Calculate comparison between groups

11. Click TopTable→Table of gene ranked in order of differential expression→select the number of genes to output into Table, how to rank list, and how to adjust the p value (Fig. J)
12. Save file to computer

Excel

13. Open in EXCEL
14. Select those genes B > 0
15. Create a column for fold change (Fig. M)
    In the cel, type = 2^(then click on the corresponding M value)
16. Sort data on the basis of fold change
    Select all data→click Data→Sort

EASE

17. Open EASE (Fig. N)
18. Paste in probe sets that were identified as differentially expressed
19. Click select categorical system
20. Select the ontological database in which to cluster the probe sets
21. Click on Find Overrepresented Gene Categories
22. Paste in list of probesets used for analysis (Fig. P,Q):
    Click from a population file→select type of GeneChip used→Run basic analysis
    This creates an HTML file
23. Select those genes that had an EASE score >0.05
24. To identify genes present in a particular ontology/process, select the probesets at the far right of the column (Fig. R)
25. Paste these probesets into Input genes
26. Click on select annotation fields
27. Select the different parameters/definitions→click Add
28. Click Annotate genes.

This creates an HTML file (Fig. O).

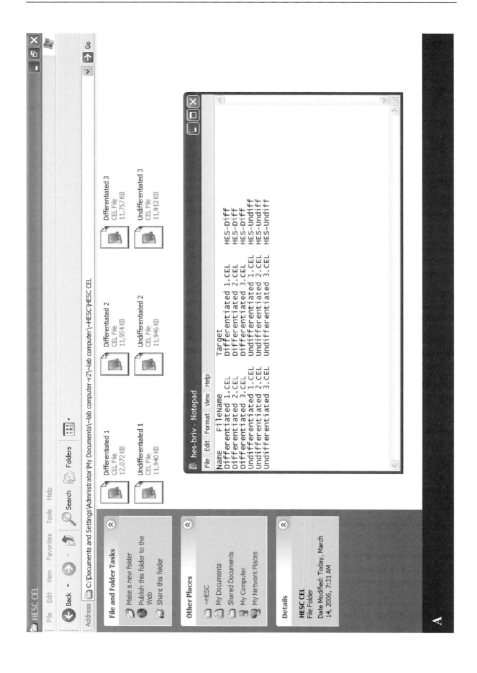

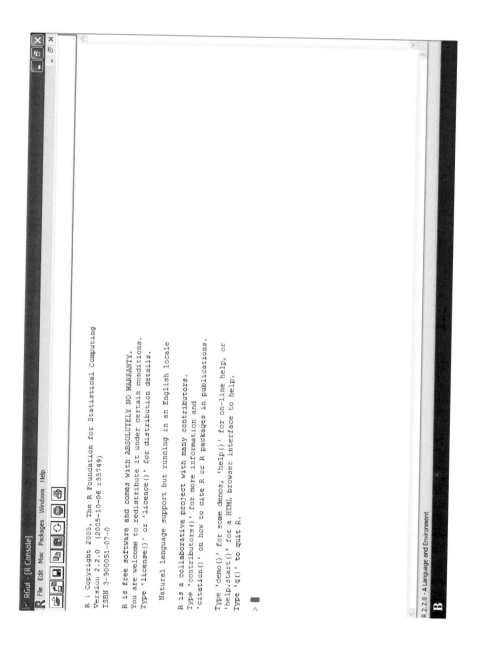

R : Copyright 2005, The R Foundation for Statistical Computing
Version 2.2.0 (2005-10-06 r35749)
ISBN 3-900051-07-0

R is free software and comes with ABSOLUTELY NO WARRANTY.
You are welcome to redistribute it under certain conditions.
Type 'license()' or 'licence()' for distribution details.

Natural language support but running in an English locale

R is a collaborative project with many contributors.
Type 'contributors()' for more information and
'citation()' on how to cite R or R packages in publications.

Type 'demo()' for some demos, 'help()' for on-line help, or
'help.start()' for a HTML browser interface to help.
Type 'q()' to quit R.

>

R 2.2.0 - A Language and Environment

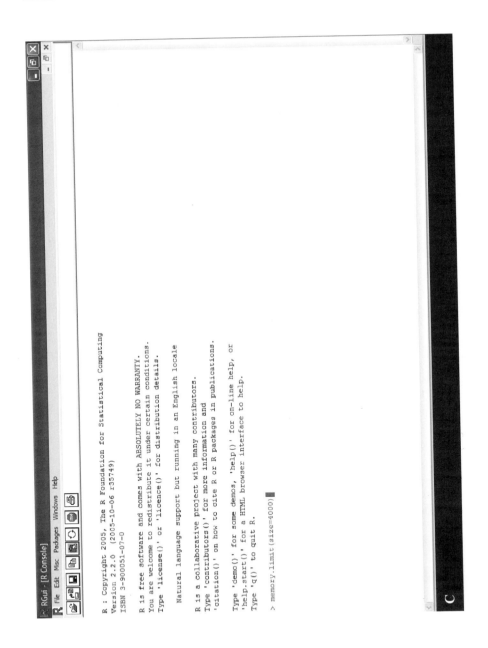

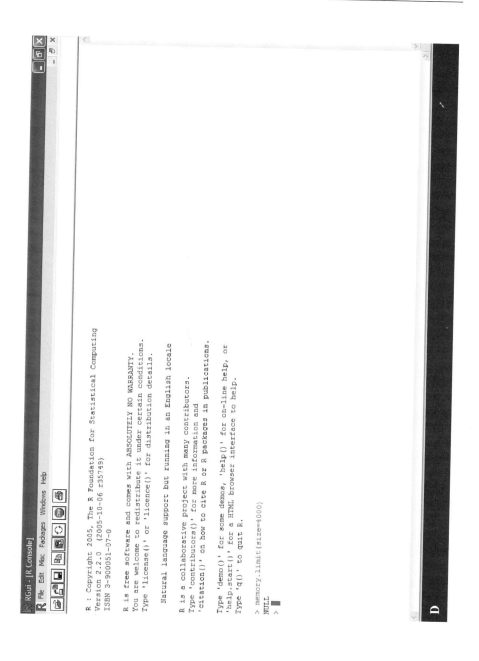

```
RGui - [R Console]
R File Edit Misc Packages Windows Help

R : Copyright 2005, The R Foundation for Statistical Computing
Version 2.2.0  (2005-10-06 r35749)
ISBN 3-900051-07-0

R is free software and comes with ABSOLUTELY NO WARRANTY.
You are welcome to redistribute it under certain conditions.
Type 'license()' or 'licence()' for distribution details.

  Natural language support but running in an English locale

R is a collaborative project with many contributors.
Type 'contributors()' for more information and
'citation()' on how to cite R or R packages in publications.

Type 'demo()' for some demos, 'help()' for on-line help, or
'help.start()' for a HTML browser interface to help.
Type 'q()' to quit R.

> memory.limit(size=4000)
NULL
>
```

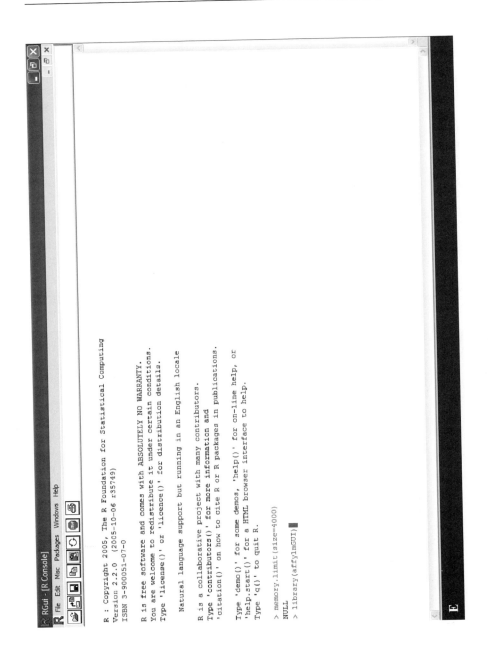

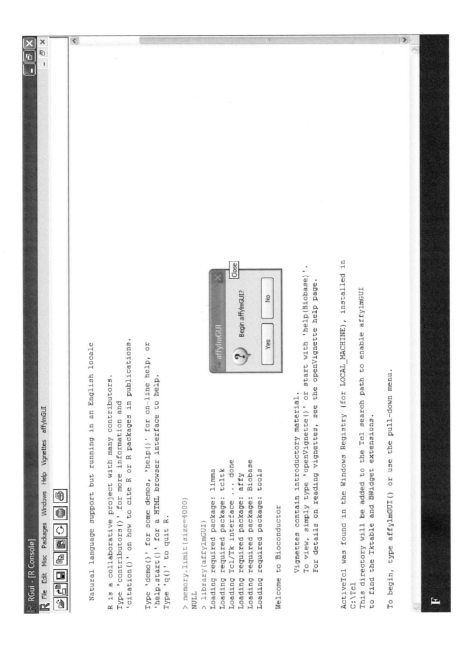

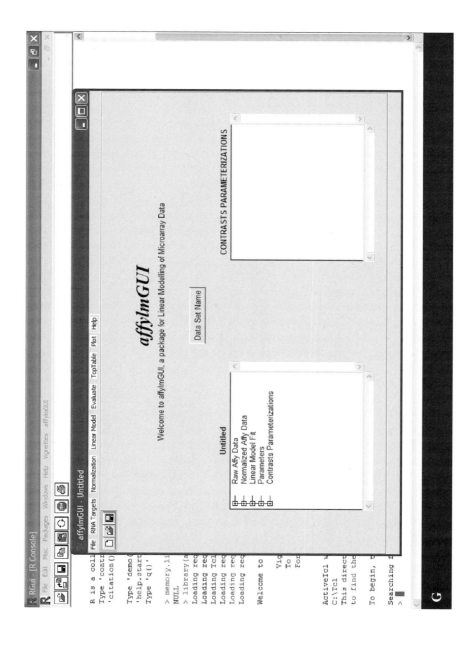

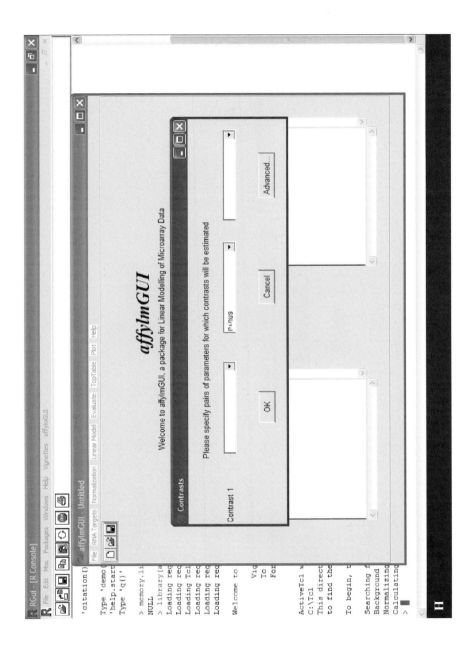

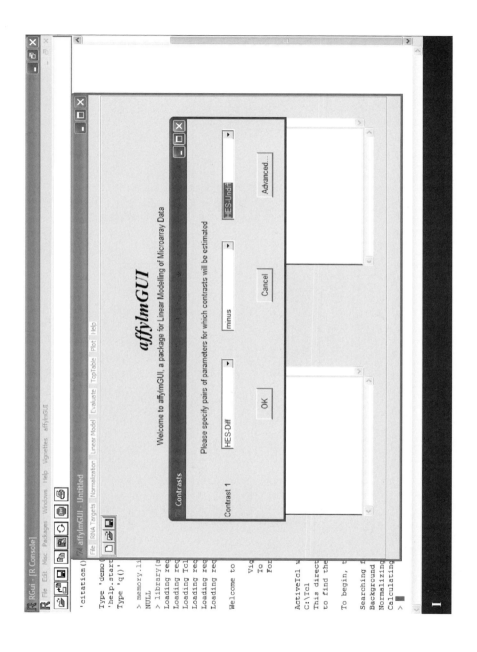

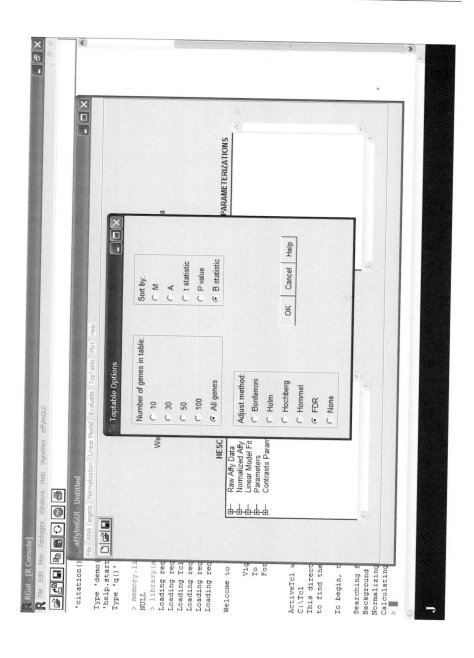

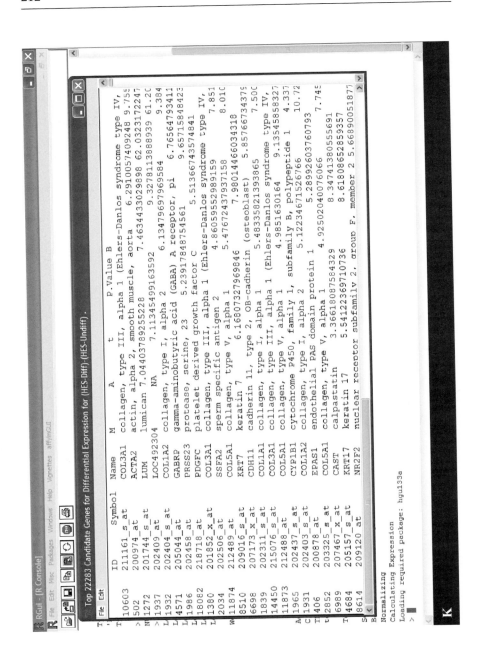

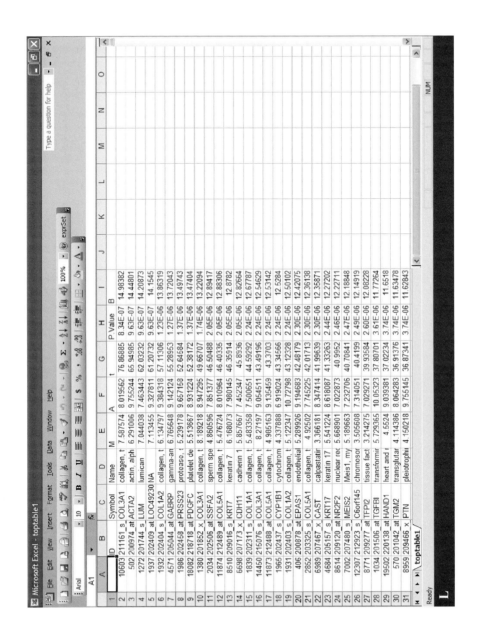

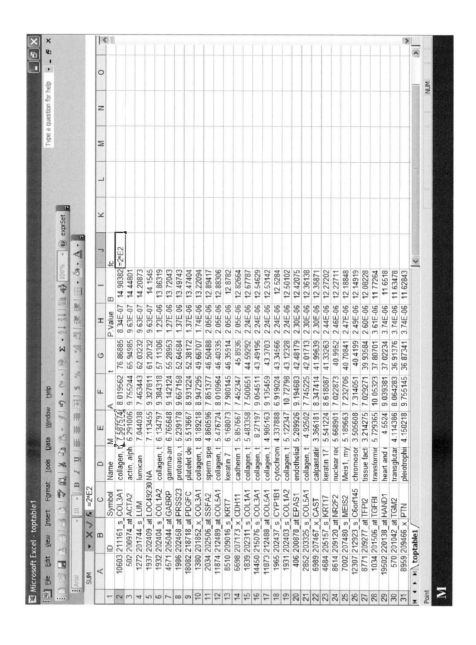

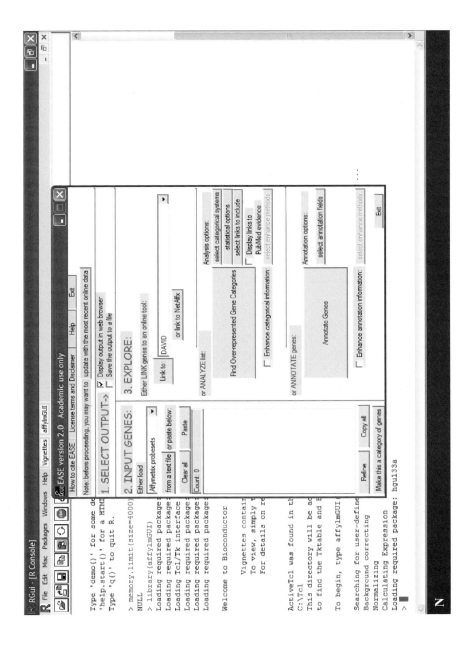

Affymetrix probesets	Gene identifiers	Chromosomal Location	GO Biological Process	GO Molecular Function	Gene Name
215076_s_at	1281	2q31	circulation;histogenesis and organogenesis;organogenesis	collagen;extracellular matrix structural constituent conferring tensile strength	collagen, type III, alpha 1 (Ehlers-Danlos syndrome IV, autosomal dominant)
201852_x_at	1281	2q31	circulation;histogenesis and organogenesis;organogenesis	collagen;extracellular matrix structural constituent conferring tensile strength	collagen, type III, alpha 1 (Ehlers-Danlos syndrome IV, autosomal dominant)
211161_s_at					
202409_at					
201744_s_at	4060	12q21.3-q22	cartilage condensation;vision	extracellular matrix structural constituent	lumican
202310_s_at	1277	17q21.3-q22.1	epidermal differentiation;skeletal development	extracellular matrix structural constituent;structural constituent of bone	collagen, type I, alpha 1
205044_at	2568	5q33-q34	ion transport;synaptic transmission	GABA-A receptor activity;extracellular ligand-gated ion channel activity	gamma-aminobutyric acid (GABA) A receptor, pi
201163_s_at	3490	4q12	negative regulation of cell proliferation;regulation of cell growth	insulin-like growth factor binding	insulin-like growth factor binding protein 7
200974_at	59	10q23.3	muscle development	motor activity;structural constituent of cytoskeleton;structural constituent of muscle	actin, alpha 2, smooth muscle, aorta
200016_x_at	3655	12q13-q13	cytoskeleton organization and biogenesis	structural molecule activity	laminin 7

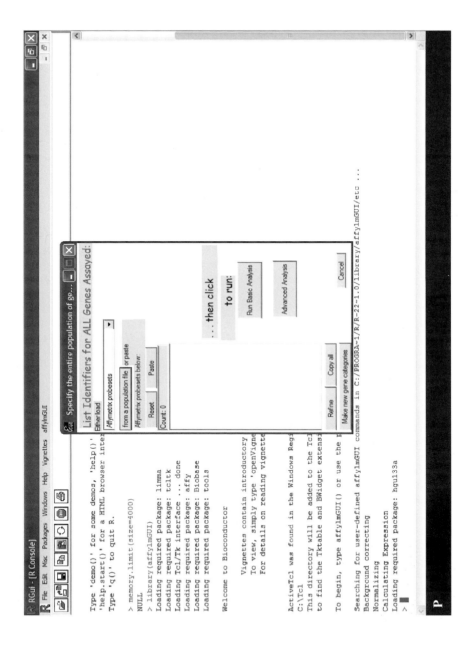

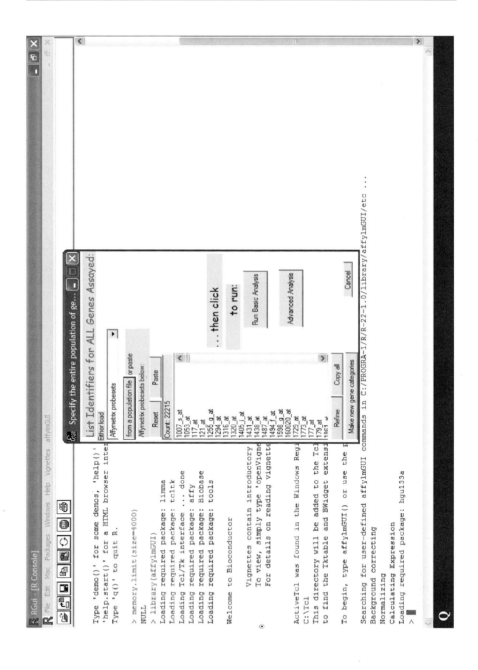

Process									
GO Biological Process	imprinting	2	815	5	10910	3.21e-001	1.00e+000	3481; 7262	209803_S_AT; 210881_S_AT
GO Biological Process	eye morphogenesis (sensu Vertebrata)	2	815	5	10910	3.21e-001	1.00e+000	1545; 2139	202435_S_AT; 202436_S_AT; 202437_S_AT; 209692_AT
GO Biological Process	growth	6	815	51	10910	3.31e-001	1.00e+000	3481; 3624; 5653; 7040; 7042; 29967	203085_S_AT; 204733_AT; 204926_AT; 209909_S_AT; 210511_S_AT; 210881_S_AT; 219631_AT; 220253_S_AT
GO Biological Process	regulation of cell shape	3	815	16	10910	3.38e-001	1.00e+000	9659; 23085; 26115	208425_S_AT; 214129_AT; 214130_S_AT; 215606_S_AT
GO Biological Process	embryonic morphogenesis	3	815	16	10910	3.38e-001	1.00e+000	1545; 2139; 4154	201152_S_AT; 201153_S_AT; 202435_S_AT; 202436_S_AT; 202437_S_AT; 209692_AT
GO Biological Process	protein amino acid alkylation	3	815	16	10910	3.38e-001	1.00e+000	3275; 23281; 57509	202098_S_AT; 212096_S_AT; 214961_AT
GO Biological Process	hydrogen ion homeostasis	3	815	16	10910	3.38e-001	1.00e+000	527; 8671; 51022	200954_AT; 203908_AT; 219933_AT
									202136_AT; 202484_S_AT

Acknowledgments

The authors thank those who made their data and computer programs publicly available. Because of space limitations, we apologize for not discussing other GeneChip and microarray studies.

References

Abbot, T. M., Hermann, W. J., and Scully, R. E. (1984). Ovarian fetiform teratoma (homunculus) in a 9-year-old girl. *Int. J. Gynecol. Pathol.* **4,** 392–402.

Abeyta, M. J., Clark, A. T., Rodriguez, R. T., Bodnar, M. S., Pera, R. A., and Firpo, M. T. (2004). Unique gene expression signatures of independently-derived human embryonic stem cell lines. *Hum. Mol. Genet.* **13,** 601–608.

Affymetrix. (2001). Microarray Suite User Guide. Version 5.

Affymetrix. (2005). Statistical algorithms description document. Technical report.

Al-Hajj, M., Becker, M. W., Wicha, M., Weissman, I., and Clarke, M. F. (2004). Therapeutic implications of cancer stem cells. *Curr. Opin. Genet. Dev.* **14,** 43–47.

Andrews, P. W. (1998). Teratocarcinomas and human embryology: Pluirpotent human EC cell lines. *Acta Pathol. Microbiol. Immunol. Scand.* **106,** 158–167.

Aruga, J., Tohmonda, T., Homma, S., and Mikoshiba, K. (2002). Zic1 promotes the expansion of dorsal neural progenitors in spinal cord by inhibiting neuronal differentiation. *Dev. Biol.* **244,** 329–341.

Ashburner, M., Ball, C. A., Blake, J. A., Botstein, D., Butler, H., Cherry, J. M., Davis, A. P., Dolinski, K., Dwight, S. S., Eppig, J. T., Harris, M. A., Hill, D. P., Issel-Tarver, L., Kasarskis, A., Lewis, S., Matese, J. C., Richardson, J. E., Ringwald, M., Rubin, G. M., and Sherlock, G. (2000). Gene ontology: Tool for the unification of biology. The Gene Ontology Consortium. *Nat. Genet.* **25,** 25–29.

Ball, C. A., Awad, I. A., Demeter, J., Gollub, J., Hebert, J. M., Hernandez-Boussard, T., Jin, H., Matese, J. C., Nitzberg, M., Wymore, F., Zachariah, Z. K., Brown, P. O., and Sherlock, G. (2005). The Stanford Microarray Database accommodates additional microarray platforms and data formats. *Nucleic Acids Res.* **33,** D580–D582.

Barrett, T., Suzek, T. O., Troup, D. B., Wilhite, S. E., Ngau, W. C., Ledoux, P., Rudnev, D., Lash, A. E., Fujibuchi, W., and Edgar, R. (2005). NCBI GEO: Mining millions of expression profiles—database and tools. *Nucleic Acids Res.* **33,** D562–D566.

Beechey, C. V., Cattanach, B. M., Blake, A., and Peters, J. (2005). World Wide Web Site—Mouse Imprinting Data and References (http://www.mgu.har.mrc.ac.uk/research/imprinting/.) MRC Mammalian Genetics Unit, Harwell, Oxfordshire.

Benjamini, Y., and Hochberg, Y. (1995). Controlling the false discovery rate: A practical and powerful approach to multiple testing. *J. R. Stat. Soc. Series B* **57,** 289–300.

Bolstad, B. M. (2005). affyPLM: Fitting Probe Level Models, Document 5–18.

Bolstad, B. M., Collin, F., Simpson, K. M., Irizarry, R. A., and Speed, T. P. (2004). Experimental design and low-level analysis of microarray data. *Int. Rev. Neurobiol.* **60,** 25–58.

Bolstad, B. M., Irizarry, R. A., Astrand, M., and Speed, T. P. (2003). A comparison of normalization methods for high density oligonucleotide array data based on variance and bias. *Bioinformatics* **19,** 185–193.

Boyer, L. A., Lee, T. I., Cole, M. F., Johnstone, S. E., Levine, S. S., Zucker, J. P., Guenther, M. G., Kumar, R. M., Murray, H. L., Jenner, R. G., Gifford, D. K., Melton, D. A., Jaenisch, R., and Young, R. A. (2005). Core transcriptional regulatory circuitry in human embryonic stem cells. *Cell* **122,** 947–956.

Brandenberger, R., Khrebtukova, I., Thies, R. S., Miura, T., Jingli, C., Puri, R., Vasicek, T., Lebkowski, J., and Rao, M. (2004). MPSS profiling of human embryonic stem cells. *BMC. Dev. Biol.* **4**, 1–10.

Brewster, R., Lee, J., and Altaba, A. (1998). Gli/Zic factors pattern the neural plate by defining domains of cell differentiation. *Nature* **393**, 579–583.

Brivanlou, A. H., Gage, F. H., Jaenisch, R., Jessell, T., Melton, D., and Rossant, J. (2003). Stem cells. Setting standards for human embryonic stem cells. *Science* **300**, 913–916.

Chen, J., Zhao, P., Massaro, D., Clerch, L. B., Almon, R. R., DuBois, D. C., Jusko, W. J., and Hoffman, E. P. (2004). The PEPR GeneChip data warehouse, and implementation of a dynamic time series query tool (SGQT) with graphical interface. *Nucleic Acids Res.* **32**, D578–D581.

Cibelli, J. B., Grant, K. A., Chapman, K. B., Cunniff, K., Worst, T., Green, H. L., Walker, S. J., Gutin, P. H., Vilner, L., Tabar, V., Dominko, T., Kane, J., Wettstein, P. J., Lanza, R. P., Studer, L., Vrana, K. E., and West, M. D. (2002). Parthenogenetic stem cells in nonhuman primates. *Science* **295**, 819.

Cobleigh, M. A., Vogel, C. L., Tripathy, D., Robert, N. J., Scholl, S., Fehrenbacher, L., Wolter, J. M., Paton, V., Shak, S., Lieberman, G., and Slamon, D. J. (1999). Multinational study of the efficacy and safety of humanized anti-HER2 monoclonal antibody in women who have HER2-overexpressing metastatic breast cancer that has progressed after chemotherapy for metastatic disease. *J. Clin. Oncol.* **17**, 2639–2648.

Cope, L. M., Irizarry, R. A., Jaffee, H. A., Wu, Z., and Speed, T. P. (2004). A benchmark for Affymetrix GeneChip expression measures. *Bioinformatics* **20**, 323–331.

Cowan, C. A., Atienza, J., Melton, D. A., and Eggan, K. (2005). Nuclear reprogramming of somatic cells after fusion with human embryonic stem cells. *Science* **309**, 1369–1373.

D'Amour, K. A., and Gage, F. H. (2003). Genetic and functional differences between multipotent neural and pluripotent embryonic stem cells. *Proc. Natl. Acad. Sci. USA* **100** (Suppl 1), 11866–11872.

Dahlquist, K. D., Salomonis, N., Vranizan, K., Lawlor, S. C., and Conklin, B. R. (2002). GenMAPP, a new tool for viewing and analyzing microarray data on biological pathways. *Nat. Genet.* **31**, 19–20.

Dennis, G., Jr., Sherman, B. T., Hosack, D. A., Yang, J., Gao, W., Lane, H. C., and Lempicki, R. A. (2003). DAVID: Database for annotation, visualization, and integrated discovery. *Genome Biol.* **4**, 0–3.

Doniger, S. W., Salomonis, N., Dahlquist, K. D., Vranizan, K., Lawlor, S. C., and Conklin, B. R. (2003). MAPPFinder: Using Gene Ontology and GenMAPP to create a global gene-expression profile from microarray data. *Genome Biol.* **4**, R7.

Ebert, P. J., Timmer, J. R., Nakada, Y., Helms, A. W., Parab, P. B., Liu, Y., Hunsaker, T. L., and Johnson, J. E. (2003). Zic1 represses Math1 expression via interactions with the Math1 enhancer and modulation of Math1 autoregulation. *Development* **130**, 1949–1959.

Fortunel, N. O., Otu, H. H., Ng, H. H., Chen, J., Mu, X., Chevassut, T., Li, X., Joseph, M., Bailey, C., Hatzfeld, J. A., Hatzfeld, A., Usta, F., Vega, V. B., Long, P. M., Libermann, T. A., and Lim, B. (2003). Comment on "'stemness': Transcriptional profiling of embryonic and adult stem cells" and "a stem cell molecular signature". *Science* **302**, 393.

Hipp, J., Cibelli, J. B., Mitalipov, S., Wolf, D. P., Studer, L., Wininger, J. D., Vrana, K. E., Grant, K. A., and Mychaleckyj, J. C. (2004). "Traansciptional Profiling of Monkey Parthenognetic Stem Cells and Their Progeny." Keystone Symposia Stem Cells Keystone, Colorado.

Hipp, J. D., Siddiqui, M. M., Hipp, J. A., Atala, A., and Soker, S. (2004). "Transcriptional Profiling of Pluriportent Progenitor cells from Human Amniotic Fluid." International Society of Differentiation Honolulu, Hawaii.

Hosack, D. A., Dennis, G., Jr., Sherman, B. T., Lane, H. C., and Lempicki, R. A. (2003). Identifying biological themes within lists of genes with EASE. *Genome Biol.* **4**, R70.

Huang, J., Wei, W., Zhang, J., Liu, G., Bignell, G. R., Stratton, M. R., Futreal, P. A., Wooster, R., Jones, K. W., and Shapero, M. H. (2004). Whole genome DNA copy number changes identified by high density oligonucleotide arrays. *Hum. Genomics* **1,** 287–299.

Irizarry, R. A., Bolstad, B. M., Collin, F., Cope, L. M., Hobbs, B., and Speed, T. P. (2003a). Summaries of Affymetrix GeneChip probe level data. *Nucleic Acids Res.* **31,** e15.

Irizarry, R. A., Hobbs, B., Collin, F., Beazer-Barclay, Y. D., Antonellis, K. J., Scherf, U., and Speed, T. P. (2003b). Exploration, normalization, and summaries of high density oligonucleotide array probe level data. *Biostatistics* **4,** 249–264.

Irizarry, R. A., Wu, Z., and Jaffee, H. A. (2005). Comparison of Affymetrix GeneChip expression measures. *Bioinformatics* **1,** 1–7.

Ivanova, N. B., Dimos, J. T., Schaniel, C., Hackney, J. A., Moore, K. A., and Lemischka, I. R. (2002). A stem cell molecular signature. *Science* **298,** 601–604.

Jirtle, R. L. (2004). IGF2 loss of imprinting: A potential heritable risk factor for colorectal cancer. *Gastroenterology* **126,** 1190–1193.

Klimanskaya, I., Hipp, J., Rezai, K. A., West, M., Atala, A., and Lanza, R. (2004). Derivation and comparative assessment of retinal pigment epithelium from human embryonic stem cells using transcriptomics. *Cloning Stem Cells* **6,** 217–245.

Larkin, J. E., Frank, B. C., Gavras, H., Sultana, R., and Quackenbush, J. (2005). Independence and reproducibility across microarray platforms. *Nat. Methods* **2,** 337–344.

Li, C., and Wong, W. H. (2001). Model-based analysis of oligonucleotide arrays: Expression index computation and outlier detection. *Proc. Natl. Acad. Sci. USA* **98,** 31–36.

Linder, D., McCaw, B. K., and Hecht, F. (1975). Parthenogenic origin of benign ovarian teratomas. *N. Engl. J. Med.* **292,** 63–66.

Lipshutz, R. J., Fodor, S. P., Gingeras, T. R., and Lockhart, D. J. (1999). High density synthetic oligonucleotide arrays. *Nat. Genet.* **21,** 20–24.

Lockhart, D. J., Dong, H., Byrne, M. C., Follettie, M. T., Gallo, M. V., Chee, M. S., Mittmann, M., Wang, C., Kobayashi, M., Horton, H., and Brown, E. L. (1996). Expression monitoring by hybridization to high-density oligonucleotide arrays. *Nat. Biotechnol.* **14,** 1675–1680.

Lund, R. D., Adamson, P., Sauve, Y., Keegan, D. J., Girman, S. V., Wang, S., Winton, H., Kanuga, N., Kwan, A. S., Beauchene, L., Zerbib, A., Hetherington, L., Couraud, P. O., Coffey, P., and Greenwood, J. (2001). Subretinal transplantation of genetically modified human cell lines attenuates loss of visual function in dystrophic rats. *Proc. Natl. Acad. Sci. USA* **98,** 9942–9947.

Maitra, A., Arking, D. E., Shivapurkar, N., Ikeda, M., Stastny, V., Kassauei, K., Sui, G., Cutler, D. J., Liu, Y., Brimble, S. N., Noaksson, K., Hyllner, J., Schulz, T. C., Zeng, X., Freed, W. J., Crook, J., Abraham, S., Colman, A., Sartipy, P., Matsui, S., Carpenter, M., Gazdar, A. F., Rao, M., and Chakravarti, A. (2005d). Genomic alterations in cultured human embryonic stem cells. *Nat. Genet.* **37,** 1099–1103.

Maitra, A., Arking, D. E., Shivapurkar, N., Ikeda, M., Stastny, V., Kassauei, K., Sui, G., Cutler, D. J., Liu, Y., Brimble, S. N., Noaksson, K., Hyllner, J., Schulz, T. C., Zeng, X., Freed, W. J., Crook, J., Abraham, S., Colman, A., Sartipy, P., Matsui, S., Carpenter, M., Gazdar, A. F., Rao, M., and Chakravarti, A. (2005a). Genomic alterations in cultured human embryonic stem cells. *Nat. Genet.* **37,** 1099–1103.

Maitra, A., Arking, D. E., Shivapurkar, N., Ikeda, M., Stastny, V., Kassauei, K., Sui, G., Cutler, D. J., Liu, Y., Brimble, S. N., Noaksson, K., Hyllner, J., Schulz, T. C., Zeng, X., Freed, W. J., Crook, J., Abraham, S., Colman, A., Sartipy, P., Matsui, S., Carpenter, M., Gazdar, A. F., Rao, M., and Chakravarti, A. (2005b). Genomic alterations in cultured human embryonic stem cells. *Nat. Genet.* **37,** 1099–1103.

Maitra, A., Arking, D. E., Shivapurkar, N., Ikeda, M., Stastny, V., Kassauei, K., Sui, G., Cutler, D. J., Liu, Y., Brimble, S. N., Noaksson, K., Hyllner, J., Schulz, T. C., Zeng, X., Freed, W. J., Crook, J., Abraham, S., Colman, A., Sartipy, P., Matsui, S., Carpenter, M.,

Gazdar, A. F., Rao, M., and Chakravarti, A. (2005c). Genomic alterations in cultured human embryonic stem cells. *Nat. Genet.* **37,** 1099–1103.

Maitra, A., Cohen, Y., Gillespie, S. E., Mambo, E., Fukushima, N., Hoque, M. O., Shah, N., Goggins, M., Califano, J., Sidransky, D., and Chakravarti, A. (2004). The Human MitoChip: A high-throughput sequencing microarray for mitochondrial mutation detection. *Genome Res.* **14,** 812–819.

Matsuzaki, H., Dong, S., Loi, H., Di, X., Liu, G., Hubbell, E., Law, J., Berntsen, T., Chadha, M., Hui, H., Yang, G., Kennedy, G. C., Webster, T. A., Cawley, S., Walsh, P. S., Jones, K. W., Fodor, S. P., and Mei, R. (2004). Genotyping over 100,000 SNPs on a pair of oligonucleotide arrays. *Nat. Methods* **1,** 109–111.

Minev, B., Hipp, J., Firat, H., Schmidt, J. D., Langlade-Demoyen, P., and Zanetti, M. (2000). Cytotoxic T cell immunity against telomerase reverse transcriptase in humans. *Proc. Natl. Acad. Sci. USA* **97,** 4796–4801.

Morison, I. M., Paton, C. J., and Cleverley, S. D. (2001). The imprinted gene and parent-of-origin effect database. *Nucleic Acids Res.* **29,** 275–276.

Murphy, S. K., and Jirtle, R. L. (2003). Imprinting evolution and the price of silence. *Bioessays* **25,** 577–588.

Pardal, R., Clarke, M. F., and Morrison, S. J. (2003). Applying the principles of stem-cell biology to cancer. *Nat. Rev. Cancer* **3,** 895–902.

Parkinson, H., Sarkans, U., Shojatalab, M., Abeygunawardena, N., Contrino, S., Coulson, R., Farne, A., Lara, G. G., Holloway, E., Kapushesky, M., Lilja, P., Mukherjee, G., Oezcimen, A., Rayner, T., Rocca-Serra, P., Sharma, A., Sansone, S., and Brazma, A. (2005). ArrayExpress—a public repository for microarray gene expression data at the EBI. *Nucleic Acids Res.* **33,** D553–D555.

Perez-Iratxeta, C., Palidwor, G., Porter, C. J., Sanche, N. A., Huska, M. R., Suomela, B. P., Muro, E. M., Krzyzanowski, P. M., Hughes, E., Campbell, P. A., Rudnicki, M. A., and Andrade, M. A. (2005). Study of stem cell function using microarray experiments. *FEBS Lett.* **579,** 1795–1801.

Ramalho-Santos, M., Yoon, S., Matsuzaki, Y., Mulligan, R. C., and Melton, D. A. (2002). "Stemness": Transcriptional profiling of embryonic and adult stem cells. *Science* **298,** 597–600.

Rao, R. R., Calhoun, J. D., Qin, X., Rekaya, R., Clark, J. K., and Stice, S. L. (2004). Comparative transcriptional profiling of two human embryonic stem cell lines. *Biotechnol. Bioeng.* **88,** 273–286.

Rao, R. R., and Stice, S. L. (2004). Gene expression profiling of embryonic stem cells leads to greater understanding of pluripotency and early developmental events. *Biol. Reprod.* **71,** 1772–1778.

Rogojina, A. T., Orr, W. E., Song, B. K., and Geisert, E. E., Jr. (2003). Comparing the use of Affymetrix to spotted oligonucleotide microarrays using two retinal pigment epithelium cell lines. *Mol. Vis.* **9,** 482–496.

Rosenberg, S. A., Yang, J. C., and Restifo, N. P. (2004a). Cancer immunotherapy: Moving beyond current vaccines. *Nat. Med.* **10,** 909–915.

Rosenberg, S. A., Yang, J. C., and Restifo, N. P. (2004b). Cancer immunotherapy: Moving beyond current vaccines. *Nat. Med.* **10,** 909–915.

Saha, S., Sparks, A. B., Rago, C., Akmaev, V., Wang, C. J., Vogelstein, B., Kinzler, K. W., and Velculescu, V. E. (2002). Using the transcriptome to annotate the genome. *Nat. Biotechnol.* **20,** 508–512.

Sarkans, U., Parkinson, H., Lara, G. G., Oezcimen, A., Sharma, A., Abeygunawardena, N., Contrino, S., Holloway, E., Rocca-Serra, P., Mukherjee, G., Shojatalab, M., Kapushesky, M., Sansone, S. A., Farne, A., Rayner, T., and Brazma, A. (2005). The ArrayExpress gene expression database: A software engineering and implementation perspective. *Bioinformatics* **21**, 1495–1501.

Sato, N., Sanjuan, I. M., Heke, M., Uchida, M., Naef, F., and Brivanlou, A. H. (2003). Molecular signature of human embryonic stem cells and its comparison with the mouse. *Dev. Biol.* **260**, 404–413.

Smyth, G. K. (2004). Linear models and empirical Bayes methods for assessing differential expression in microarray experiments. *Stat. Appl. Genet. Mol. Biol.* **3**.

Smyth, G. K. (2005). Limma: Linear models for microarray data. *In* "Bioinformatics and Computational Biology Solutions using R and Bioconductor." (R. Gentleman, V. Carey, S. Dudoit, R. Irizarry, and W. Huber, eds.), pp. 397–420. Springer, New York.

Sperger, J. M., Chen, X., Draper, J. S., Antosiewicz, J. E., Chon, C. H., Jones, S. B., Brooks, J. D., Andrews, P. W., Brown, P. O., and Thomson, J. A. (2003). Gene expression patterns in human embryonic stem cells and human pluripotent germ cell tumors. *Proc. Natl. Acad. Sci. USA* **100**, 13350–13355.

Stein, L. D. (2004). Human genome: End of the beginning. *Nature* **431**, 915–916.

Suarez-Farinas, M., Noggle, S., Heke, M., Hemmati-Brivanlou, A., and Magnasco, M. O. (2005). Comparing independent microarray studies: The case of human embryonic stem cells. BMC. *Genomics* **6**, 99.

Tripathy, D., Slamon, D. J., Cobleigh, M., Arnold, A., Saleh, M., Mortimer, J. E., Murphy, M., and Stewart, S. J. (2004). Safety of treatment of metastatic breast cancer with trastuzumab beyond disease progression. *J. Clin. Oncol.* **22**, 1063–1070.

Velculescu, V. E., Zhang, L., Vogelstein, B., and Kinzler, K. W. (1995). Serial analysis of gene expression. *Science* **270**, 484–487.

Vogel, C. L., Cobleigh, M. A., Tripathy, D., Gutheil, J. C., Harris, L. N., Fehrenbacher, L., Slamon, D. J., Murphy, M., Novotny, W. F., Burchmore, M., Shak, S., and Stewart, S. J. (2001). First-line Herceptin monotherapy in metastatic breast cancer. *Oncology* **61**(Suppl 2), 37–42.

Vogel, C. L., Cobleigh, M. A., Tripathy, D., Gutheil, J. C., Harris, L. N., Fehrenbacher, L., Slamon, D. J., Murphy, M., Novotny, W. F., Burchmore, M., Shak, S., Stewart, S. J., and Press, M. (2002). Efficacy and safety of trastuzumab as a single agent in first-line treatment of HER2-overexpressing metastatic breast cancer. *J. Clin. Oncol.* **20**, 719–726.

Vrana, K. E., Hipp, J. D., Goss, A. M., McCool, B. A., Riddle, D. R., Walker, S. J., Wettstein, P. J., Studer, L. P., Tabar, V., Cunniff, K., Chapman, K., Vilner, L., West, M. D., Grant, K. A., and Cibelli, J. B. (2003). Nonhuman primate parthenogenetic stem cells. *Proc. Natl. Acad. Sci. USA* **100** (Suppl 1), 11911–11916.

Wettenhall, J. M. (2004). affylmGUI Package Vignette Document. 4–6.

Wettenhall, J. M., and Smyth, G. K. (2004). limmaGUI: A graphical user interface for linear modeling of microarray data. *Bioinformatics* **20**, 3705–3706.

Wright, J. M., Zeitlin, P. L., Cebotaru, L., Guggino, S. E., and Guggino, W. B. (2004). Gene expression profile analysis of 4-phenylbutyrate treatment of IB3-1 bronchial epithelial cell line demonstrates a major influence on heat-shock proteins. *Physiol. Genomics* **16**, 204–211.

Wu, Z., and Irizarry, R. A. (2005). Stochastic models inspired by hybridization theory for short oligonucleotide arrays. *J. Comput. Biol.* **12**, 882–893.

Zhao, P., Iezzi, S., Carver, E., Dressman, D., Gridley, T., Sartorelli, V., and Hoffman, E. P. (2002). Slug is a novel downstream target of MyoD. Temporal profiling in muscle regeneration. *J. Biol. Chem.* **277**, 30091–30101.

Further Reading

Affymetrix (2004). GeneChip Expression Analysis Technical Manual.

[10] Microarray Analysis of Stem Cells and Differentiation

By HOWARD Y. CHANG, JAMES A. THOMSON, and XIN CHEN

Abstract

Microarrays have revolutionized molecular biology and enabled biologists to perform global analysis on the expression of tens of thousands of genes simultaneously. They have been widely used in gene discovery, biomarker determination, disease classification, and studies of gene regulation. Microarrays have been applied in stem cell research to identify major features or expression signatures that define stem cells and characterize their differentiation programs toward specific lineages. Here we provide a review of the microarray technology, including the introduction of array platforms, experimental designs, RNA isolation and amplification, array hybridization, and data analysis. We also detail examples that apply microarray technology to address several of the main questions in stem cell biology.

Introduction

For the past several decades, biologists have only been able to analyze one or a few genes at a time. However, the advent of complete genomic sequences of more than 800 organisms (including the human and mouse genomes) and the development of microarray technology have revolutionized molecular biology. Microarrays enable biologists to perform global analysis on the expression of tens of thousands of genes simultaneously, and they have been widely used in gene discovery, biomarker determination, disease classification, and studies of gene regulation (Brown and Botstein, 1999; Butte, 2002; Chung *et al.*, 2002; Gerhold *et al.*, 2002). Expression profiling using microarrays is generally considered "discovery research," although it can also be a powerful approach to test defined hypotheses. One advantage of microarray experiments is that at the outset, microarray experiments need not be hypothesis driven. Instead, they allow biologists a means to gather gene expression data on an unbiased basis and can help to identify genes that may be further tested as the targets in hypothesis-driven studies.

Overview of Microarray Technology

Two major microarray platforms have been widely used: cDNA microarrays and oligonucleotide microarrays.

METHODS IN ENZYMOLOGY, VOL. 420
Copyright 2006, Elsevier Inc. All rights reserved.

0076-6879/06 $35.00
DOI: 10.1016/S0076-6879(06)20010-7

cDNA Microarrays

The principle of cDNA microarray is illustrated in Fig. 1. cDNA clones, which generally range from several hundred base pairs to several kilobases, are printed on a glass surface, either by mechanical or ink jet microspotting. Sample RNA and a reference RNA are differentially labeled with fluorescent Cy5 or Cy3 dyes, respectively, using reverse transcriptase. The subsequent cDNA are hybridized to the arrays overnight. The slides are washed and scanned with a fluorescence laser scanner. The relative abundance of the transcripts in the samples can be determined by the red/green ratio on each spotted array element.

One of the limitations of cDNA microarray has been that it required relatively large amounts of total RNA ($\geq 10\ \mu g$) for hybridization. However, significant progress has recently been made for linear amplification of RNA, generally on the basis of Eberwine's protocol (Wang *et al.*, 2000). In this case, RNA is converted into cDNA with oligo dT primers that contain T7

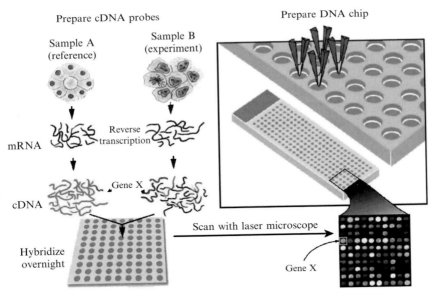

Fig. 1. Principle of cDNA microarrays. PCR products are printed onto glass slides to produce high-density cDNA microarrays. RNA is extracted from experimental samples and reference samples and differentially labeled with Cy5 and Cy3, respectively, by reverse transcriptase. The subsequent cDNA probes are mixed and hybridized to cDNA microarray overnight. The slides are washed and scanned with fluorescence laser scanner. The relative red/green ratio of gene X indicates the relative abundance of gene X in experimental samples versus reference. (See color insert.)

RNA polymerase promoter sequence at its 5′ end. The cDNA can be subsequently used as the template for T7 RNA polymerase to transcribe into anti-sense RNA. The linear amplification protocol can produce 10^6 fold of amplification. Therefore, only very small amounts of samples are required in modern microarray experiments.

There are several advantages to using cDNA microarray. The two-color competitive hybridization can reliably measure the difference between two samples, because variations in spot size or amount of cDNA probe on the array will not affect the signal ratio. cDNA microarrays are relatively easy to produce. In fact, the arrayer can be easily built and allow the micro-arrays to be manufactured in university research laboratories. Also, cDNA microarrays are in general less expensive than oligonucleotide arrays and are affordable to most research biologists.

There are also some disadvantages with this system. One is that the production of cDNA microarray requires the collection of a large set of sequenced clones. The clones, however, may be misidentified or contaminated. Second, genes with high sequence similarity may hybridize to the same clone and generate cross hybridization. To avoid this problem, clones with 3′ end untranslated regions, which, in general, are much more divergent compared with the coding sequences, should be used in producing the microarrays.

Oligonucleotide Arrays

The most widely used oligonucleotide arrays are GeneChips produced by Affymetrix, which uses photolithography-directed synthesis of oligo-nucleotides on glass slides. Affymetrix GeneChip measures the absolute levels for each transcript in the sample. The principle of the Affymetrix GeneChip is shown in Fig. 2. In general, for each transcript, approximately 20 distinct and minimally overlapped 25-mer oligonucleotides are selected and synthesized on the array. For each oligonucleotide, there is also a paired mismatch control oligonucleotide, which differs from the perfect match probe by one nucleotide in the central position. Comparison of the hybridi-zation signals from perfect match oligonucleotide with the paired mismatch oligonucleotide will allow automatic subtraction of background.

Because the sequences of oligonucleotide arrays are determined by sequencing information from the database and synthesized *de novo* for the arrays, there is no need to validate cDNA clones or PCR products that are used to print cDNA microarrays. The use of multiple oligonucleotides for each transcript also allows for the detection of splice variants and helps to distinguish genes with high sequence similarities.

The major disadvantage to oligonucleotide arrays is that they can only be produced by commercial manufacturers, and these prefabricated

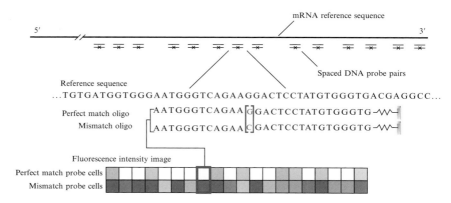

Fɪɢ. 2. Principle of Affymetrix GeneChip. For each gene, approximately 20 distinct and minimally overlapped 25-mer oligonucleotides are selected and synthesized on the array. For each oligonucleotide, there is also a paired mismatch control oligonucleotide probe, which differs from the perfect match probe by one nucleotide in the central position. Comparison of the hybridization signals from perfect match oligonucleotide with the paired mismatch oligonucleotide allows automatic subtraction of background. (Figure is kindly provided by Affymetrix, Santa Clara, CA.)

GeneChips are still very expensive. Besides GeneChips from Affymetrix, several other companies produce oligo arrays: Most use long oligos and two-color comparisons that are more similar to cDNA arrays. These companies include Agilent Technologies (Palo Alto, CA), NimbleGen Systems (Madison, WI), and CombiMatrix Corporation (Mukilteo, WA).

Systematic comparison of different microarray platforms showed that standardized protocols for microarray hybridization and data processing, rather than array platform, seemed to be more important in achieving reproducibility among different investigators (Irizarry *et al.*, 2005; Larkin *et al.*, 2005).

Next, we will describe basic procedures and protocols for microarray experiments, including experimental design, RNA isolation and amplification, array labeling and hybridization, data analysis, and gene validation. Our discussion will focus on cDNA microarrays, but most of the general principles can be applied to both cDNA microarrays and oligonucleotide arrays.

Experimental Design

cDNA microarrays use two-color competitive hybridization; therefore, the design of experiments (i.e., which samples are labeled for each color) is very important in the subsequent data interpretation. There are two commonly used experimental designs, and in this chapter, we refer to them as "type I" or "type II" designs.

In the type I experimental design, the sample RNA (for example, drug-treated cells, diseased tissues) is labeled with one dye, and another sample RNA (for example, mock treated cells, normal tissues) is labeled with another dye. The two sample cDNA probes are mixed and cohybridize to microarray. The data analysis for the type I design can be quite straightforward. The relative red/green ratio represents the relative up regulation or downregulation of each gene. This design is most suited for experiments with a few perturbations; for example, to identify genes' responses to certain stimulus or genes affected by a genetic mutation. However, it is difficult to apply this pairwise type I design to a complicated system. For example, to identify genes differentially expressed in a disease and normal tissues, it may not be appropriate to compare diseased tissues with corresponding normal tissues from the sample patients. Gene expression patterns in normal and diseased tissues are affected by many factors, including patient variation (ethnicity, sex, age, genetic background), sample variation (proximity to disease, anatomical location, and developmental range), as well as heterogeneity of cell populations within the samples. In the simple pairwise type I design, it is impossible to distinguish all these variations within both normal and diseased tissues. Another drawback of the type I experiment is that it cannot accurately measure the relative abundance of a transcript that is not expressed or is expressed at very low levels in Cy3 labeling, because this would produce a green channel signal very close to the background signal.

The type II experimental design avoids most of the problems associated with the simple pairwise type I design. In the type II design, a common reference is used in Cy3 channel labeling, and each sample is compared with the same common reference. The two most important criteria for selection of common reference are gene coverage ("light up" most of the spots on the array) and reproducibility (can be relatively easily reproduced with minimum batch to batch variation). In most cases, the reference pool RNA is derived from a mixture of tumor cell lines (Perou et al., 2000), and they are commercially available from Strategene and Clontech. Cell lines from different histological origins ensure the complex of the reference. This provides relatively good coverage of the spots on the array. Cell lines can be recultured to produce more reference RNA; however, growth conditions need to be tightly controlled to reduce batch-to-batch variation. The greatest advantage of the type II experimental design is that it allows the cross comparison of many samples collected over long periods of time, by different persons, as well as samples from different sources.

Another situation in which type II designs are widely used is in the time series experiments (i.e., to study gene expression variations in response to a stimulus, for example, drug treatment, growth factor stimulation) (Boldrick *et al.*, 2002; Diehn *et al.*, 2002). A simple pairwise type I design using treated cells against untreated cells may be quite straightforward. However, some of the genes that are induced by the stimulus may not be expressed in the untreated cells. It is difficult to obtain an accurate description of the expression profile changes over time for these genes. A better design is a type II design in which the cells from different time points are mixed and used as reference. All the samples, including untreated cells ($t = 0$), can then be compared with this reference. This average $t = 0$ measurement can then be subtracted from each subsequent time point measurement to depict the temporal response patterns of expression relative to $t = 0$ as the baseline. Such a design ensures that all the transcripts present in the different time points are represented in the reference RNA and, therefore, accurately describe the temporal changes in response to the stimulus.

Although there are many advantages with the type II design, this design may make the experiments more complicated and sometimes inefficient. In the analysis, the baseline reference signals have to be subtracted to extract biologically meaningful data. This undoubtedly will add more data variations. Thus the proper selection of experimental design is one of the most important steps toward the success of experiments.

Total RNA Isolation and Clean-Up

Trizol extraction is the most widely used method for isolation of total RNA. Because RNA is prone to RNase degradation, it is very important to work in an RNase-free area and use DEPC-treated water. Following is the protocol for isolating RNA from tissues. Note that when isolating RNA from tissues, it is best to handle the tissues when they are frozen. Also, before or between uses of the homogenizer, rinse the probe with DEPC-water.

1. Place 100 mg tissue into 2 ml of Trizol reagent (1 ml of Trizol per 50–100mg of tissue), and homogenize tissue at high speed for 1 min, then incubate the homogenized samples for 5 min at room temperature.
2. Add 0.2 ml of chloroform per ml of Trizol reagent used in step 1. Shake by hand for 15 sec and incubate for 2–3 min. Centrifuge for 10 min at 14,000 rpm at 4°.
3. Remove the upper colorless aqueous phase containing RNA to a fresh tube. Precipitate RNA with 0.5 ml isopropanol per 1 ml of Trizol. Centrifuge at 14,000 rpm for 10 min at 4°.
4. Carefully remove the supernatant. Wash the pellet with 75% ethanol, and centrifuge at 14,000 rpm for 5 min at 4°.

5. Again carefully remove all the supernatant and air dry for 5–10 min.
6. Dissolve RNA in appropriate amount of RNase-free water. In some cases, total RNA may need to be incubated at 55–60° for 5 min before it can be dissolved.
7. Take 1 μl of total RNA for quality and quantity measurement, and store the rest of the total RNA at −80°.

It is important to obtain high-quality total RNA for microarray labeling or amplification. Several methods can be used to estimate the quality of RNA extracted. For example, when measuring the RNA concentration using UV spectrophotometer, A_{260}/A_{280} ratio should be between 1.9 and 2.1. Another method is to run the RNA on an agarose gel and look for two clear bands: one 18S (0.9 kb) and the other 28S (2 kb) rRNA. Alternately, a Bioanalyzer chip (Agilent Technologies) can be used to properly assay the quality of total RNA.

If a sufficient amount (15–50 μg) of total RNA is obtained, the RNA may be used directly for labeling. However, in most cases, further purification may be required before the labeling. One method is to reprecipitate RNA. Add 1/10 volume of 3 M sodium acetate (pH 5.2) and 2.5 volumes of 100% ethanol. Mix and incubate at −20° for at least 1 h. Centrifuge at 14,000 rpm for 30 min at 4°. Remove the supernatant, wash the pellet with 70% ethanol, air dry, and dissolve in RNase-free water. Take 1 μl of total RNA for quality and quantity measurement. Another method is to use the RNeasy Mini Kit (Qiagen) and follow the manufacturer's protocol. Up to 100 μg of total RNA can be purified at a time. If DNA-free RNA is desired, the RNase-free DNase Set (Qiagen) provides a convenient and efficient on-column digestion of DNA during RNA purification using the RNeasy kit.

RNA Amplification

If a small amount (<10 μg) of total RNA is isolated, amplification may be necessary before labeling and microarray hybridization. Several commercially available kits, for example MessageAmp kit from Ambion or RiboAmp Amplification kit from Arctur, have been widely used. Most of these protocols are based on of Eberwine's protocol for linear amplification (Van Gelder *et al.*, 1990). Following is a protocol based on the publication by Zhao *et al.* (2002):

   I. First strand cDNA synthesis:
     I. Mix total RNA (0.5–5 μg) with 1 μl of Eberwine primer (1 μg/μl) together with RNase-free water to total 9 μl. Incubate at 70° for 3 min and cool on ice for 2 min. The sequence of Eberwine primer is 5′-AAA

CGA CGG CCA GTG AAT TGT AAT ACG ACT CAC TAT AGG CGC-3′.

I.2. Briefly spin the tube. Add 4 μl of 5× first-strand buffer, 2 μl of 0.1 M DTT, 1 μl of RNasin, 2 μl of 10 mM dNTP mix, and 2 μl of Superscript II (Invitrogen) to a total volume of 20 μl. Mix the contents, and incubate at 42° for 90 min.

II. Second-strand cDNA synthesis:

II.1. Add the following contents to the first-strand synthesis reaction: RNase-free water 106 μl, 10X Advantage PCR buffer 15 μl, 10 mM dNTP mix, 3 μl, RNase H (2 U/μl) 1 μl, and Advantage Polymerase Mix (Clontech) 3 μl.

II.2. Incubate at 37° for 5 mins, 94° for 2 min, 65° for 1 minute, and 75° for 30 mins. Stop the reaction by adding 7.5 ml of 1 M NaOH with 2 mM EDTA, and incubate at 65° for 10 min.

III. Ds cDNA clean-up:

III.1. Add 150 μl of phenol/chloroform/isoamyl alcohol (25:24:1) and mix by vortexing. Spin at 14,000 rpm for 5 min.

III.2. Transfer the aqueous layer to a new tube. Add 1 μl liner acrylamide (0.1 μg/μl), 70 μl of 7.5 M NH$_4$Ac, 1 ml 100% ethanol. Spin at 14,000 rpm for 20 min at room temperature.

III.3. Wash pellet with 500 μl of 75% ethanol, spin at 14,000 rpm for 5 min. Carefully remove all the supernatant and air dry for 3 min. Suspend the pellet in 16 μl of RNase-free water.

IV. *In vitro* transcription:

IV.1. Mix the cDNA from Step III with 10× reaction buffer, 75 mM NTP mix, and T7 enzyme mix (from T7 MEGAscript kit of Ambion).

IV.2. Incubate at 37° for 5–6 h.

aRNA cleanup:

V. Qiagen RNeasy Mini Kit was used in the aRNA cleanup.

V.1. Transfer the reaction from step IV into a new tube. Add 60 μl RNase-free water and 350 μl buffer RLT (add β-mercaptoethanol to RLT before use). Mix by pipetting. Add 250 μl 100% ethanol and mix well.

V.2. Apply the sample to the RNeasy column. Spin at 14,000 rpm for 15 sec at room temperature. Transfer column to a new collection tube.

V.3. Add 500 μl buffer RPE. Spin at 14,000 rpm for 15 sec. Discard flow through. Add 500 μl buffer RPE, spin at 14,000 rpm for 2 min.

V.4. Transfer column to new collection tube. Add 30 μl RNase-free water to the membrane. Let stand for 1 min, and spin at 14,000 rpm for 1 min.

V.5. Measure aRNA yield using a UV spectrometer.

Amplified RNA or isolated total RNA can be used in the labeling reaction for microarray hybridization. Two methods are commonly used for labeling. One is called *direct labeling*, which uses Cy3 or Cy5 coupled with dUTP in the reaction. The second method is generally referred as indirect labeling, in which aminoallyl-dUTP is used in the reverse transcription reaction. Cy3 or Cy5 dye will then need to be coupled with aminoallyl-dUTP. In general, direct labeling is faster and convenient but may require more starting materials. Indirect labeling, on the other hand, tends to be more sensitive and, therefore requires less RNA for labeling. In the following, we will provide general protocols for both methods.

Direct Labeling of RNA for Microarray Hybridization

Before starting the labeling reaction, unlabeled dNTPs will need to be made that include 25 mM dATP, 25 mM dCTP, 25 mM dGTP, and 10 mM dTTP.

1. For total RNA, mix 50–100 μg of total RNA with 4 mg of anchored oligo-dT primer (5′-TTT TTT TTT TTT TTT TTT TTV N-3′) in a total volume of 15.4 μl. For aRNA, use 3–5 μg of aRNA and mix with 10 mg of random hexamer primer (dN$_6$). Heat to 65° for 10 min and cool on ice.
2. Add to the reaction from step 1, 6 μl of 5× first-strand buffer, 3 μl of 0.1 M DTT, 0.6 μl unlabeled dNTP, 3 μl of 1 mM Cy3 or Cy5-dUTP, and 2 μl of Superscript II (Invitrogen) to total reaction of 30 μl.
3. Incubate at 42° for 1 h.
4. Add 1 μl of Superscript II to each sample. Incubate for an additional 0.5–1 h.
5. Degrade RNA and stop the reaction by adding 15 μl of 0.1 N NaOH, 2 mM EDTA, and incubate at 65–70° for 10 min. Neutralize by addition of 15 μl of 0.1 N HCl.
6. Use the MicroconYM-30 (Millipore) to clean up. Add 380 μl of TE (10 mM Tris, 1 mM EDTA) to the Microcon column. Combine the Cy5 and Cy3 probes, and add to the column. Spin the column for 7–8 min at 14,000 rpm. Discard the flow-through and add 450 μl of TE and spin for 7–8 min at 14,000 rpm.
7. Remove flow-through and add 450 μl of TE, 2 μl of Cot1 human DNA (10 μg/μl), 2 μl of polyA RNA (10 μg/μl) and 2 μl tRNA (10 μg/μ Spin 7–10 min at 14,000 rpm so that the probe on the column is less than 28 μl.
8. Invert the Microcon into a clean tube and spin at 14,000 rpm for 1 min to recover the probe.

9. Adjust the probe volume to 28 μl. Add 5.95 μl of 20× SSC and 1.05 μl of 10% SDS to total of 35 μl. Denature probe by heating for 2 min at 100°, and spin at 14,000 rpm for 15–20 min. The probe is now ready for hybridization.

Indirect Labeling of RNA for Microarray Hybridization

Before the reaction, make a 50× dNTP solution to include 25 mM dATP, 25 mM dCTP, 25 mM dGTP, 5 mM dTTP, and 20 mM aminoallyl-dUTP. Monofunctional NHS-ester Cy3 or Cy5 dye (Amersham) is supplied as dry pellet. Before use, add 16 μl of DMSO to each dye tube.

1. For total RNA, mix 10–15 μg of total RNA with 4 μg of anchored oligo-dT primer (5′-TTT TTT TTT TTT TTT TTT TTV N-3′) in a total volume of 14.5 μl. For aRNA, use 1–1.5 μg of aRNA and mix with 1.25 μg of random hexamer primer (dN$_6$). Heat to 72° for 10 min and cool on ice.

2. Add to the reaction from step 1, 3 μl of 10× StrataScript buffer, 0.6 μl AA-dNTPs, 3 μl of 0.1 M DTT, 2 μl of Stratascript RT, and 5.9 μl of DEPC water to total 30 μl. Incubate at 42° for 2 h.

3. Add 10 μl of 1 M NaOH and 10 μl of 0.5 M EDTA to each tube. Incubate for 15 min at 65°. Neutralize the reaction by adding 15 μl of 1 M HEPES (pH7.4).

4. Use the MicroconYM-30 (Millipore) to clean up. Add 450 μl of DEPC water to the column, and add the probes. Spin at 14,000 rpm for 8 min. Discard the flow-through. Add again 450 μl of DEPC water to the column, and spin at 14,000 rpm for 8 min. Discard the flow-through.

5. Invert the Microcon into a clean tube and spin at 14,000 rpm for 1 min to recover the probe.

6. Speed vac the samples until dry.

7. Resuspend cDNA in 9 μl of 50 mM NaOH (pH9.0), and stand at room temperature for 15 min.

8. Add 1.25 μl of Cy3 or Cy5 to the appropriate reaction tube, and incubate for 1–2 h at room temperature in the dark.

9. Add 4.5 μl 4 M hydroxylamine to each sample, incubate for 15 min in dark. Add 70 μl of DEPC water and 8.5 μl of Cot-1 DNA to the sample.

10. Clean up the reaction using the QiaQuick PCR-purification kit (Qiagen). Add 500 μl of buffer PB to the reaction from step 9, mix well. Transfer to the QiaQuick column. Spin at 14,000 rpm for 1 min and discard the flow-through. Add 700 μl buffer PE, spin at 14,000 rpm for 1 min, and discard the flow-through. Spin for an

additional 1 min to dry the column. Transfer the column to a new collection tube. Add 30 μl EB to the center of the filter, incubate for 2 min. Spin at 14,000 rpm for 1 min to collect the labeled cDNA.

11. Mix the corresponding Cy3 and Cy5 tubes, and speed vac to dry the samples.

12. Dissolve the sample in 25.375 μl of DEPC water, 5.25 μl of 20$\times$ SSC, 0.875 μl of 1 M HEPES (pH = 7), 2.625 μl of PolyA and 0.9 μl of 10%SDS. Denature the probe by heating for 2 min at 100°, cool for 1 min. The probe is now ready for hybridization.

Microarray Hybridization

Before the microarray slides can be used in hybridization, it generally requires postprocessing to reduce array background and denature the cDNA on the arrays. The procedure for postprocessing varies, depending on the glass surface. The following protocol was developed using the UltraGAPS slides (Corning).

1. Mark boundaries of the array on the back of the slide using a diamond scriber, because the array spots will become invisible after postprocessing.
2. UV crosslink the DNA to the slide with 150–300 mJoules.
3. Incubate arrays in 35–45% formamide, 5$\times$ SSC, 0.1% SDS, 0.1 mg/ml BSA at 42° for 30–60 min.
4. Rinse arrays briefly with water, then denature DNA on the slide by transferring into a dish of boiling water for 2 min.
5. Wash briefly with 95% ethanol and dry arrays by centrifugation.

For hybridization, add the labeled probes onto microarray slides and cover with a proper cover slip. Incubate the slide chamber in a water bath for 16 h at 65°.

For washing microarray slides, prepare the following solution: Wash 1A: 2$\times$ SSC and 0.03%SDS; Wash 1B: 2$\times$ SSC; Wash 2: 1$\times$ SSC, and Wash 3: 0.2$\times$ SSC. Take the slides out of the slide chamber and wash for 5 min in Wash 1A solution. Then, rinse briefly in Wash 1B, which minimizes the transfer of SDS to Wash 2. Wash the slides for 5 min in Wash 2, followed by 5 min in Wash 3. Spin dry the slide by centrifugation.

The microarray slides can be scanned. Before the arrays can be loaded into the database for analysis, array images generally need to be analyzed to exclude weak or bad spots, a process that is referred as *gridding*. The most widely used array image analysis software include Scanalyze, Genepix, and SpotReader.

Array-Based Comparative Genomic Hybridization (Array CGH)

In addition to quantifying the mRNA expression level, microarrays can be used to detect DNA copy number and other genomic aberrations in a high-throughput fashion, which is generally referred as *array CGH*. Array CGH has been widely used in cancer research to identify chromosomal aberration in cancer cells (Albertson and Pinkel, 2003; Pinkel and Albertson, 2005). Genomic DNA of stem cells can be compared with reference DNA from somatic cells (e.g., normal blood) by two-color labeling and competitive hybridization in an analogous fashion as mRNA expression arrays. This application is particularly valuable for verifying the genomic integrity of stem cells that may be used for therapeutic purposes (Maitra *et al.*, 2005). For both basic research and clinical applications, it is essential to verify that the stem cells of interest have not acquired oncogenic or other genetic abnormalities in tissue culture. The high density of probes on microarrays can enable detection of small deletions and amplifications (Ishkanian *et al.*, 2004).

Array CGH can be performed using either cDNA array or, more commonly, BAC clone–based arrays (Pinkel *et al.*, 1998; Pollack *et al.*, 1999; Snijders *et al.*, 2001). Following is the protocol for BAC clone based array CGH.

> I. Preparation of probe
> I.1. Mix DNA (0.2–1 μg) with 10 μl of 2.5× random primer (Invitrogen Bioprime random prime kit) together with water to total 21 μl.
> I.2. Briefly spin the tube. Denature the DNA mixture at 100° for 10 min and immediately cool on ice.
> I.3. Briefly spin the tube. Add 2.5 μl of dNTP (mixture of 4 mM each of dATP, dCTP, dGTP and dTTP in TE) mix together with Cy3 or Cy5-dCTP, and 0.5 μl of Klenow. Mix the contents and incubate at 37° overnight.
> I.4. Place the MicroSpin G-50 column (Amersham) into Eppendorf tube. Spin at 770 rcf for 1 min to remove excess liquid. Place the columns into a new Eppendorf tube and apply 25 μl of test probe and 25 μl of reference probe to the column. Spin at 770 rcf for 2 min. Collect the flow-through.
> II. Hybridization
> II.1. Add 50 μl of Human Cot-1 DNA, 10 μl of 3 M sodium acetate and 250 μl of ethanol into the probe mixture. Precipitate the probe at 14000 rpm for 20 min at 4°. Carefully remove the supernatant.
> II.2. Dissolve the pellet in 5 μl of water, 10 μl of 20% SDS, and 35 μl of Master Mix. Master Mix is produced by mixing 1 g of dextransulfate, 5 ml of formamide, 1 ml of 20× SSC and 1 ml of

water. Resuspend the pellet with pipette tip by stirring. Denature the hybridization solution at 73° for 10 min and incubate at 37° for 30–to 60 min.

II.3. Apply the hybridization mixture to the arrays. Incubate the slide at 37° for 48–72 h.

III. Washing and scanning

III.1. Disassemble the slide assembly and rinse the hybe solution from the slide in a room temp stream of PN (0.1 M sodium phosphate with 0.1% NP-40). Wash slides in wash solution (50% formamide, $2\times$ SSC, pH 7) at 45° for 15 min. Finally, wash slides in PN at room temperature for another 15 min.

III.2. Apply DAPI mix (90% glycerol, 10% $1\times$ PBS, 1 μl DAPI (Sigma), pH 8) on top of the array. Place cover slip on top of the array and remove excess DAPI mix.

III.3. The single color intensity image for each channel (Cy3, Cy5 and DAPI) can be collected using a charge coupled device camera.

Data Analysis

Microarray experiments produce large amounts of data; for example, 20,000 genes $\times$ 100 samples will generate 2 million data points. Data analysis may be one of the most challenging issues facing biologists in microarray experiments. Microarray data are often noisy and not normally distributed and usually with missing values in its matrix. During the past several years, with the combined efforts of biologists, statisticians, and computer scientists, there has been great progress in bioinformatics techniques that can be used for the analysis of genome-wide expression data (Sherlock, 2001; Slonim, 2002). However, there is no standard or one-size-fits-all solution for interpretation of microarray data. Here we highlight several useful methods and provide links to freely available resources (Table I).

Current methods for microarray data analysis can be divided into two major categories: supervised and unsupervised methods. Supervised approaches try to identify gene expression patterns that fit a predetermined pattern. Unsupervised approaches characterize expression components without prior input or knowledge of the predetermined pattern.

Supervised Analysis

The purpose of supervised analysis is to identify genes that are differentially expressed between groups of samples and to find genes that can be used to accurately predict the characteristics of groups.

TABLE I

INFORMATION RESOURCES ON THE INTERNET

Tool	Function	Web Site
Cluster	Performs hierarchical clustering. Genes and samples in microarray experiments are organized by similarity.	http://rana.lbl.gov/EisenSoftware.htm
GenePattern	Analysis and data visualization software from Broad Institute at MIT. Performs sequence and microarray analysis, including GSEA test. Curated gene sets are also available for download and analysis.	http://www.broad.mit.edu/cancer/software/genepattern/
Genomica	1. Implements Gene Module Map. 2. Identifies enriched transcription factor binding sites in the promoters of gene modules. 3. Implements module networks.	http://genomica.weizmann.ac.il/index.html
Gene Ontology Term Finder	Gene Ontology classifies each gene in the genome using a controlled vocabulary. Tool identifies enriched GO terms within groups of select genes.	http://search.cpan.org/dist/GO-TermFinder/
GeneHopping	Identifies sets of coregulated genes between organisms and provides visualization of modules.	http://barkai-serv.weizmann.ac.il/Software/GeneHopping/Hopping.html
Onto-Tools	Web-based program to (1) identify GO term enrichment, (2) map probes among different array platforms, (3) retrieve annotations of specific genes.	http://vortex.cs.wayne.edu:8080/ontoexpress/servlet/UserInfo
GenMapp	For visualizing gene expression data along pathways, creating new pathways, and identifying global biological data associated with an expression dataset.	http://www.genmapp.org/

Many statistical tests have been developed for identification of differentially expressed genes in microarray data, for example, the t test for detecting significant changes between repeated measurements of a variable in two groups and the ANOVA F statistic for detecting significant changes in multiple groups. All these tests involve two parts: calculating a test statistic and determining the false discovery rate (FDR) or the significance of the test statistic. Here are some commonly used statistical methods for two group comparisons.

Nonparametric t Test (Dudoit and Fridlyand, 2002)

In the nonparametric t test, the statistical significance of each gene is calculated by computing a p value for it without assuming specific parametric form for the distribution of the test statistics. To determine the p value, a permutation procedure is used in which the class labels of the samples are permuted (10,000–500,000 times), and for each permutation, t statistics are computed for each gene. The permutation p value for a particular gene is the proportion of the permutations in which the permuted test statistic exceeds the observed test statistic. A p value cutoff can be chosen for the dataset. The FDR = number of genes test × cutoff p value/ gene declared to be significant.

Wilcoxon (or Mann–Whitney) Rank Sum Rest (Troyanskaya et al., 2002)

This test rank transforms the data and looks for genes with a skewed distribution of ranks. The rank transform smoothes the data by reducing the effect of outliers. This method is proven to be superior for decidedly non-normal data. In general, the Wilcoxon rank sum test has been shown to be the most conservative, with the lowest FDR.

Ideal Discriminator Method (Park et al., 2001; Troyanskaya et al., 2002)

This method is based on the similarity of gene expression patterns on the array to a theoretical pattern that clearly discriminates between two groups. It potentially allows more flexibility in defining more complex theoretical patterns of behavior.

Significant Analysis of Microarray (SAM) (Tusher et al., 2001)

SAM uses a statistic that is similar to a t statistic. However, it introduces a "fudge factor" at the denominator when calculating the t statistic; therefore, it underweights those genes that have relatively small magnitude of differences and small variation within groups. It also permutes the whole dataset and sets a threshold for a FDR, instead of assigning an individual p value to each gene.

Overall, each statistical method has its own advantages. Each biologist may need to choose proper tests for his or her own dataset, and in some cases, try different statistical tests. In a situation where the most reliable list of genes is desirable, the best approach may be to examine the intersection of genes identified by different statistical tests or by the more conservative rank sum test and nonparametric t test. However, if a more inclusive list of genes is desired, a higher p value cutoff or SAM may be more appropriate.

Unsupervised Analysis

Users of unsupervised analysis try to find internal structure in the data set without any prior input knowledge. Here are some widely used analytical methods.

Hierarchical Clustering (Eisen et al., 1998)

Hierarchical clustering is a simple but proven method for analyzing gene expression data by building clusters of genes with similar patterns of expression. This is done by iteratively grouping genes that are highly correlated in their expression matrix. As the result, a dendrogram is generated. Branches in the dendrogram represent the similarities among the genes; the shorter the branch, the greater similarity of the gene expression pattern. Hierarchical clustering is also popular because it helps to visualize the overall similarities of expression profiles. The number and size of expression patterns within a data set can be quickly estimated by biologists.

Self-Organizing Maps (SOM) (Tamayo et al., 1999; Toronen et al., 1999)

In SOM, each biological sample is considered as a separate partition of the space, and after partitions are defined, genes are plotted using expression matrix as coordinate. To initiate SOM, the number of partitions to use must first be defined by the users as an input parameter. A map is set with the centers of each partition to be (known as centroids) arranged in an initially arbitrary way. As the algorithm iterates, the centroids move toward randomly chosen genes at a decreasing rate. The method continues until there is no further significant movement of these centroids. The advantage of SOM is that it can be used to partition the data with easy two-dimensional visualization of expression patterns. It also reduces computational requirements compared with other methods. The drawbacks of the method are that the number of partitions has to be user-defined, and genes can only belong to a single partition at a time.

Singular Value Decomposition (SVD) (Alter et al., 2000; Raychaudhuri et al., 2000)

SVD is also known as *principle components analysis* by statisticians. SVD transforms the genome-wide expression data into diagonalized "eigengenes" and "eigenarrays" space, in which the eigengenes (or eigenarrays) are the unique orthogonal superpositions of the genes (or arrays). Sorting the gene expression data according to the eigengenes and eigenarrays will reduce the features of the data to their principal components and may help to identify the main patterns within the data. Importantly, SVD is also a powerful technique to capture any patterns within the data that may be due to experimental artifacts. For example, array hybridization on different days or hybridization on different batches of arrays occasionally gives slight differences in gene expression patterns. SVD can also remove the artifacts without removing any genes or arrays from the dataset.

Gene Module Analysis

Gene module analysis is based on the simple idea that genes typically work together in groups, such as in enzymatic pathways or regulatory cascades. Thus, the unit of analysis in a microarray experiment should be groups of functionally related genes, termed *modules*, and one assigns more significance to a group of genes having coordinate regulation than just one member of a group being regulated in the experiment (Mootha *et al.*, 2003; Segal *et al.*, 2004). Using previous biological knowledge, gene modules can be defined by sets of genes that are members of the same biological pathway, have a shared structural motif, are expressed in a specific tissue, or are induced by a specific stimulus. A biological pathway is typically defined by two gene modules: one for the upregulated genes in the pathway and one for the downregulated genes. Gene modules can have different numbers of member genes, and each gene can belong to multiple modules. In a microarray experiment, gene module analysis searches for coordinate regulation of genes that belong to these *a priori* defined gene modules; a statistical test is performed for each module relative to all other genes on the microarray to calculate whether the degree of coordinate regulation is more than one would expect by chance.

The gene module approach has several advantages over our current gene-by-gene methods of analysis. First, coordinated small magnitude regulation of gene expression of many genes in the same pathway can be biologically more important than a large magnitude change that is discordant with other members of the pathway; however, this type of regulation is often missed by the gene-by-gene approach. Moreover, the large number of genes examined in the gene-by-gene approach necessitates significant penalties for multiple hypothesis testing; many biologically meaningful changes can be missed. Gene module analysis takes advantage of the power of groups of genes to detect those genes that have biologically significant, albeit subtle, expression changes. Second, because modules are defined by groups of genes known to share certain biological functions or characteristics, defining the unit of analysis by modules improve the investigator's mechanistic interpretation of the biology underlying the gene expression changes. For example, modules can consist of groups of genes previously found to be coordinately regulated in other microarray experiments. In this way, gene module analysis allows one to compare each new microarray experiment to every previously performed experiment to identify commonalities and unifying mechanisms. By analogy with sequence searches in which a newly cloned gene is compared with genes in the database for blocks of sequence similarity, gene module analysis allows one to discover features of gene expression patterns that have been observed in other microarray experiments.

In one instantiation of this strategy, Mootha *et al.* (2003) pioneered a type of gene module analysis (which they termed *gene set enrichment* analysis or GSEA) to discover the biological pathways underlying type II diabetes mellitus. They compared global gene expression patterns of skeletal muscle biopsy specimens from individuals with normal glucose tolerance, impaired glucose tolerance, and type II diabetes mellitus. After rigorous statistical tests on a gene-by-gene basis (and suffering the concomitant multiple hypothesis testing penalty), they found no single gene with a significant difference in expression. However, Mootha *et al.* noticed that many genes that showed the most consistent changes encoded enzymes involved in mitochondrial oxidative phosphorylation. To test the significance of this observation, the authors implemented gene module analysis by constructing 149 modules of various metabolic pathways or coregulated genes. The authors sorted all genes on the microarray into a ranked list, from the one best able to distinguish diabetes versus normal to the least informative. They then asked whether the distribution of genes on this list is surprising given the membership of genes in modules.

Specifically, the authors applied the Kolmogorov–Smirnov running sum statistic: Beginning with the gene at the top of the ranked list, the running sum increases when a gene that is a member of the gene set is encountered and decreases otherwise. The maximum enrichment score is the greatest positive deviation of the running sum across all genes. To determine the statistical significance of the maximum enrichment score and validate that the results are unlikely to arise by chance alone, permutation testing is performed, comparing the maximum enrichment score using the actual data to that seen in each of 1000 permuted data sets.

GSEA revealed that a module of genes involved in oxidative phosphorylation was significantly down-regulated in patients with diabetes. Each gene in the oxidative phosphorylation gene module was transcriptionally downregulated by roughly only 20% and thus was not clearly detected at the individual gene level. Independent work by Shulman and colleagues using magnetic resonance spectroscopy confirmed that defective mitochondrial oxidative phosphorylation is strongly associated with glucose intolerance and seems to be a strong predictor for development of diabetes (Petersen *et al.*, 2003).

In addition to looking at whether each gene module is significantly regulated in the experiment, gene module analysis also examines which particular genes within a module are contributing to the regulation. This information can refine the gene module and lead to additional mechanistic insight. For instance, Mootha *et al.* noticed that not all genes in the oxidative phosphorylation modules were equally down-regulated in diabetes mellitus; the subset of genes that were down-regulated consisted of many known targets of the transcriptional coactivator PGC-1α in muscle cells (Mootha *et al.*, 2003). Analysis of shared promoter elements of genes that comprise the refined oxidative phosphorylation module has identified two transcription factors, estrogen receptor related α and GA-repeat binding protein, as key regulators that cooperate with PGC-1α to regulate expression of this gene module and cellular energy metabolism (Mootha *et al.*, 2004). Thus, gene module analysis has generated a model for impaired glucose tolerance and diabetes mellitus in which down-regulation of PGC-1α function in skeletal muscle results in the down-regulation of genes involved in oxidative phosphorylation.

Second, gene module analysis has also been used for exploratory discovery of the shared biological pathways that underlie different human cancers. Using a strategy termed *Gene Module Map*, Segal *et al.* (2004) performed a comprehensive analysis of 1975 previously published microarrays with 2849 gene modules. These gene modules included tissue-specific genes, coregulated genes, and genes that function in the same process, act in the same pathway or share similar subcellular localization. Each microarray experiment was also annotated using a controlled vocabulary for several hundred biological and clinical conditions that it represents, including tumor type, stage, and clinical outcomes. For each gene module and each array, they calculated the fraction of genes from that module that was induced or repressed in that array and asked whether this fraction of enrichment was surprising on the basis of chance alone, estimated using the hypergeometric distribution. A similar algorithm was applied to the clinical annotations, and clinical annotations that were enriched for each gene module were identified.

In this fashion, the large number of microarray experiments and their associated clinical information was distilled to a core set of relationships that defined each cancer by a specific combination of gene modules, many of which provide insight into molecular mechanisms underlying cancer phenotypes. For example, poorly differentiated tumors of many histological types were found to share an activation of the spindle checkpoint and M phase modules, which have been previously associated with chromosomal instability and aneuploidy. Many modules that were specific to particular types of cancer or even stages of the same disease were also identified, such as deactivation of a growth inhibitory module of dual specificity phosphatases in acute lymphoblastic leukemia and repression of an intermediate filament module in breast cancers (Segal *et al.*, 2004). Although it is impressive that many of the newly described relationships between gene modules and their respective cancers can be supported by the literature, the significance of most gene modules in human cancers awaits experimental validation.

Regulatory Networks

In many biological studies, we are interested in identifying causal relationships (i.e., gene A is upstream of gene B and induces B). Several investigators have applied probabilistic graphical models, specifically Bayesian networks, to identify regulatory relationships from static views of global gene expression patterns (Beer and Tavazoie, 2004; Segal *et al.*, 2003). Bayesian networks are a particularly useful type of model because they organize a set of variables into a hierarchical model of conditional probabilities; the value of the daughter variables is the joint conditional probability of the parent variables. Typically, the model is used to evaluate many combinations of specific variables, and particular models that produce good fit of the data are validated by additional computational and experimental tests (Friedman, 2004).

For example, because microarray data provide a global view of mRNA abundance, the underlying regulatory network could be the set of active transcription factors or the set of promoter and enhancer elements that produced the genome-wide transcriptional pattern. Segal *et al.* (2003) approached this problem by reasoning that many transcription factors and signal transducers are under transcriptional control themselves; thus, a regulatory model may be constructed by relating the expression pattern of genes that encode transcription factors to that of all other genes. Segal *et al.* developed a probabilistic Bayesian algorithm, termed *module networks*, to identify the correlations between the expression level of a manually curated set of genes encoding transcription factors and signaling proteins, termed *regulators*, and, separately, all other transcribed genes (Segal *et al.*, 2003). Transcribed genes were grouped into modules on the basis of the expression changes of the regulators, and regulators were allowed to combine into hierarchical patterns that were conditional, additive, or antagonistic. Thus, unlike hierarchical clustering that only identifies genes with similar patterns of expression, regulatory programs allowed logical operations such as *and, or, if*, and *but*. An iterative process of regulatory tree building and gene module assignment is performed to optimize both predictions. In each iteration, the procedure learns the best regulation program for each module and, given the inferred regulation programs, reassigns each gene to the module whose program best predicts its behavior. These two steps are iterated until convergence is reached. This method has the advantage of generating testable hypotheses about gene modules and their regulatory programs in a single analysis. However, this method is limited by current biological knowledge, because it relies on compiling a list of candidate regulators. In addition, although this strategy can accommodate heterologous data such as proteomic or enzyme activity profile data, currently most high-throughput data of regulators are transcriptional analysis. Thus, the predicted regulatory trees can be wrong, because they fail to take into account posttranscriptional and post-translational regulation.

To demonstrate the power of this strategy, Segal *et al.* used a set of 466 candidate regulators and a set of 173 arrays that measure responses of *S. cerevisiae* to various stresses, which resulted in 50 modules with regulation trees. It should be noted that this type of algorithm would always produce a regulatory tree; the key assessment is the quality of the regulatory trees and gene modules that are produced. A good regulatory tree will encompass transcription factors that are known to act or interact with one another, and the gene modules will have member genes that can be shown to have shared functions. Segal *et al.* found that 31 of the 50 modules had more than 50% of its genes that had the same functional annotation, 30 of the 50 modules included genes previously known to be regulated by at least one of the module's predicted regulators, and 15 of 50 modules had a match between the *cis*-regulatory motifs in the upstream regions of the module's genes and the regulator known to bind to that motif. This is a rather remarkable feat, given that the only input information was gene expression data; no biochemical, genetic, or sequence data were used to make the predictions. To further validate this strategy, Segal *et al.* chose three novel regulatory relationships predicted by the regulatory network model, mutated each regulator, and performed global gene expression analysis. In all three cases, the deletion mutants selectively affected the gene modules that they were predicted to regulate. Thus, module networks are a useful method for generating hypotheses that can accurately predict regulators, the processes that they regulate, and the conditions under which they are active.

Hypotheses of regulatory mechanisms can also be generated from shared *cis*-regulatory DNA elements in the upstream regions of the genes in each module. Beer and Tavazoie (2004) demonstrate a computational modeling method for building regulatory networks on the basis of these regulatory DNA elements on a genome-wide scale. They used a similar Bayesian probabilistic model to identify the upstream DNA motifs that predict the expression pattern of each gene module under different conditions. Beer and Tavazoie demonstrate that prediction with DNA elements requires complex rules because the expression level of a gene is controlled by the occupancy states of multiple upstream binding sites. They validated their regulatory network models by demonstrating that they correctly predicted the expression patterns of 73% of the genes using 20% leave-out analysis. Although this *cis*-regulatory DNA elements method would not reliably predict genes that are regulated by more distant DNA elements or that have alternative regulatory mechanisms such as chromatin modification, they demonstrate that local upstream DNA sequence can predict gene expression patterns of a large portion of genes, at least in *S. cerevisiae*.

The large number of hypotheses generated from regulatory networks analysis or *cis*-regulatory DNA elements analysis can be validated in a high-throughput fashion using chromatin-immunoprecipitation followed by microarray analysis (ChIP-chip). ChIP-chip uses antibodies specific to a candidate regulator for genome-scale chromatin-immunoprecipitation combined with microarrays spotted with intergenic sequences to identify their bound targets. For example, Odom *et al.* (2004) demonstrate the use of antibodies to HNF1α, HNF4α, and HNF6 to identify all genes that are bound by these transcription factors in human liver and pancreas tissues and hybridized the immunoprecipitated chromatin fragments to a custom microarray of more than 10,000 human promoter sequences. These results revealed that a surprisingly large percentage of genes transcribed in the liver and pancreas were bound by HNF4α, providing a molecular explanation for the role of HNF4α mutations and polymorphisms in hereditary and sporadic forms of diabetes mellitus. In addition, as mentioned previously, regulator networks also can be validated by expression profiling of mutants of the regulator to see whether its signature recapitulates the effect on the genes in the module that it was predicted to regulate.

Confirmation Studies

It is important to independently verify array observations. There are two approaches: *in silico* analysis and experimental validation.

The *in silico* method compares array results with information available in the literature or other independent array expression database. Agreement between array results from other groups, especially using different array platforms, will validate the general performance of the system and provide confidence in the overall data.

Experimental validation uses an independent experimental method to assay the expression levels of genes of interest, preferably on a sample set other than the samples that have been used in the microarray analysis. The methods that have been used widely depend on the specific scientific questions. Commonly used techniques include at the mRNA level: semiquantitative RT-PCR, real time RT-PCR (Taqman, Applied Biosystems), Northern blot, *in situ* hybridization (ISH); and at protein level: Western blot, fluorescence-activated cell sorting, enzyme-linked immunoabsorbent assays, immunofluorescence, and immunohistochemistry (IHC). Both ISH and IHC can be performed in a high-throughput manner by tissue arrays. In addition, both methods provide additional information on the anatomical relationship and cellular origin of gene expression programs.

Examples of Microarray Experiments for Stem Cell Biology and Differentiation

Classically, *differentiation* is defined by the expression of lineage-specific markers, appearance of unique cell morphologies, or acquisition of specific biologic functions (e.g., hemoglobin synthesis in red blood cells). From a genomic perspective, differentiation can be considered as sets of gene expression programs; these gene expression programs may be self-reinforcing, sequential, or mutually exclusive depending on the specific biological context. Thus, the biological state of stem cells and their subsequent differentiated states are highly amenable to microarray analysis. In exploring stem cell biology expression profiling offers a decided advantage as an experimental approach, because no specific assumptions are necessary at the outset. By observing the activity of the entire genome, one can determine what major features define stem cells and characterize their differentiation programs toward specific lineages. Here we highlight several examples in the literature that apply microarray technology to tackle several of the main questions in stem cell biology.

Identification of Stemness

Stem cells share certain biological properties—the capacity for self-renewal and multipotency. What are the molecular programs that underlie these properties? Several investigators have approached this problem by comparing the gene expression profiles of several embryonic and adult stem cells. By comparing the intersection of the relatively enriched genes in stem cells, a set of genes that are shared by several stem cells has been identified (Ivanova *et al.*, 2002; Ramalho-Santos *et al.*, 2002). It is reassuring that traditional markers of stem cells (e.g., CD34 for marrow-derived hematopoietic stem cells) were also found to be enriched in the stem cell transcriptome by microarray analysis (Ramalho-Santos *et al.*, 2002). In addition, these results provide several candidate pathways that may be involved in regulating maintenance of stem cell fate (Ramalho-Santos *et al.*, 2002). Intriguingly, it was observed that a large fraction of stem cell–enriched genes are genes or expressed sequence tags with no previously ascribed function and that in the mouse an unexpected larger percentage of stem cell–enriched genes reside on chromosome 17 (Ramalho-Santos *et al.*, 2002). Similar chromosomal domains of muscle-specific transcription has been observed in *C. elegans* (Roy *et al.*, 2002), and transcriptional profiling of *Drosophila* in a variety of conditions revealed significant correlation of the expression patterns for chromosomally adjacent genes (Spellman and Rubin, 2002). The large number and precise quantitative nature of gene expression measurements make microarray analysis particularly attractive to analyze the relationship between chromosomal clustering of genes and differentiation.

After publication of the initial studies, additional analyses have raised important questions regarding the gene expression markers associated with "stemness." For one, comparison of the genes identified in the two initial studies demonstrated little overlap in genes, and additional studies following the same strategy of intersecting stem cell–enriched genes from multiple tissue types failed to identify a core set of conserved genes (Evsikov and Solter, 2003; Fortunel *et al.*, 2003; Vogel, 2003). These conflicting findings raised the importance of cross-validation in microarray studies; that is, demonstrating the validity of a finding in multiple sample or data sets. The complexity and subtlety of putative stemness programs that may be evident in several types of stem cells may be better approached using gene module approach rather than analyses focused on individual genes.

Differentiation

The excitement about stem cells arises from their ability to differentiate into many lineages and cell types, but on a practical level, the pluripotency of stem cells present experimental difficulties in guiding and assessing their development into particular lineages *in vitro* and *in vivo*. Traditionally, one may rely on certain well-established markers of the cell types in question, and in some instances, one may verify the ability of one or more stem cells to repopulate a compartment by reconstitution experiments (e.g., reconstitution of peripheral blood cells by transplantation of hematopoietic stem cells [HSCs]). However, these approaches rely on a relatively small number of protein markers or are laborious and time-consuming. The specificity of lineage markers has been explored to a limited extent in many cases, and many cell types of biological and medical interest do not have well-defined markers. For instance, CD34, the classical marker for HSC, is also present in a number of other cell types and neoplasms (e.g., endothelial cells and the fibrohistiocytic tumor dermatofibrosarcoma protuberans). Expression profiling of stem cells and their differentiated derivatives can help to identify the direction and progress of the differentiation program and the interrelationships of the possible differentiation states with one another.

In a prime example of this strategy, Xu *et al.* observed that exposure of hESCs to bone morphogenetic protein 4 (BMP4) induced a substantial number of trophoblast markers, including the placental hormone human chorionic gonadotropin (Xu *et al.*, 2002). Thus, BMP4 is probably a key molecular switch that guides the first differentiation event of embryonic stem cells toward this extraembryonic lineage, and BMP4-treated ESCs provide a simple system to derive human trophoblastic cells for studying maternal–fetal interactions. In another powerful use of microarray technology, cell surface markers can also be identified in a high-throughput fashion by isolating messenger RNA associated with membrane-bound polysomes (Diehn *et al.*, 2000); hybridization of such selected RNAs to microarrays allows rapid identification of membrane proteins that are likely to be useful lineage markers and receptors that respond to environmental stimuli. More recently, Eggan and colleagues used gene expression profiling to demonstrate that fusion of fibroblasts with embryonic stem cells reprogrammed the fibroblast genome to express genes in a pattern similar to ESCs on a genome-wide scale (Cowan *et al.*, 2005).

Stem Cell Niches

One of the central questions in stem cell biology is the molecular features of the niches that govern the behavior of fetal and adult tissue-specific stem cells. Although some of these key molecules have been identified genetically in amenable organisms (Watt and Hogan, 2000), many of the molecular details that define stem cell niches, especially in mammalian systems, are incompletely understood and may be approached by microarray analysis (Hackney *et al.*, 2002). One approach to understanding stem niches is to explore the diversity of the normal tissue compartments, especially that provided by resident stromal cells.

An illustrative demonstration of this concept is a study of global gene expression patterns of fibroblasts derived from different anatomical sites of skin. Chang *et al.* cultured fibroblasts from multiple sites of human skin, and microarray analysis of their global gene expression patterns revealed that

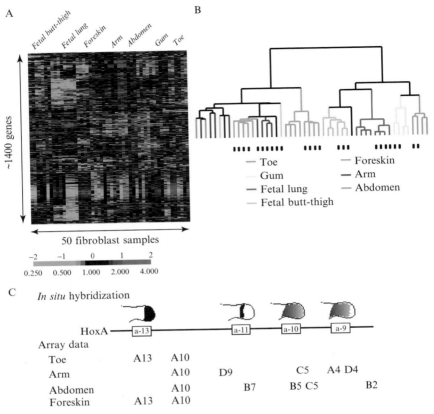

FIG. 3. Topographic differentiation of fibroblasts identified by microarray analysis. (A) Heat map of fibroblast gene expression patterns. Fibroblasts from several anatomical sites were cultured, and their mRNAs were analyzed by cDNA microarray hybridization (Chang *et al.*, 2002). Approximately 1400 genes varied by at least threefold in two samples. The fibroblast samples were predominantly grouped together on the basis of site of origin. (B) Supervised hierarchical clustering revealed the relationship of fibroblast cultures to one another. Site of origin is indicated by the color code, and high or low serum culture condition is indicated by the absence (high) or presence (low) of the black square below each branch. Because fibroblasts from the same site were grouped together irrespective of donor, passage number, or serum condition, topographic differentiation seemed to be the predominant source of gene expression variation among these cells. (C) *HOX* expression in adult fibroblasts recapitulates the embryonic Hox code. In a comparison of *HOX* expression pattern in secondary axes, schematic of expression domains of 5′ *HoxA* genes in the mouse limb bud at approximately 11.5 days after coitus is shown on top. The *HOX* genes up-regulated in fibroblasts from the indicated sites are shown below. *HoxC5* is expressed in embryonic chick forelimbs, and *HoxD9* functions in proximal forelimb morphogenesis. (Discussed in detail in Chang *et al.* [2002]). (See color insert.)

fibroblasts from different sites have distinct gene expression programs that have the stability and diversity characteristic of differentiated cell types (Fig. 3) (Chang et al., 2002). Some of the site-specific gene expression programs in fibroblasts included components of extracellular matrix and many cell fate–signaling pathways, including members of transforming growth factor β, Wnt, receptor tyrosine kinase, and G-protein–coupled receptor signaling pathways. An intriguing hint to the specification program in fibroblasts is the maintenance of key features of the embryonic Hox code (which specifies the anterior–posterior body plan) in adult fibroblasts. Thus, stromal cells such as fibroblasts are likely to encode position-specific information in a niche that specifies the developmental potential of interacting stem cell populations. In the case of fibroblasts, because their positional identities are maintained in vitro (as evidenced by the fidelity of the Hox expression patterns), it is likely that efforts using stem cells to develop artificial tissue and organs will benefit from incorporation of site-specific fibroblasts or their molecular signatures that recreate the stem cell niche. Identification of the specific stem cell niches—and specific cell fate-determining pathways—can thus be accelerated by a comprehensive description and understanding of the stromal cell diversity using microarray analysis.

Future Directions

The rapid evolution of microarray technology, bioinformatics techniques, and availability of new genome sequences in model organisms will present many opportunities for harnessing genomic information in stem cell and development research. Fuzzy clustering, a method that gives proportional weight to class assignment, is a valuable technique that may help to reveal more subtle and intricate relationships among various stem cells and their differentiated progenies (Gasch and Eisen, 2002). Additional methods of selecting mRNA or DNA fragments coupled to microarray analysis provide rapid and powerful techniques to explain protein subcellular localization or the interaction with DNA binding proteins (Diehn et al., 2000; Iyer et al., 2001; Lieb et al., 2001). Because of its versatility and ability for revealing unexpected features of biology, microarray analysis is likely to become one of the main workhorses of the stem cell biologist.

References

Albertson, D. G., and Pinkel, D. (2003). Genomic microarrays in human genetic disease and cancer. Hum. Mol. Genet. 12 Spec No 2, R145–R152.
Alter, O., Brown, P. O., and Botstein, D. (2000). Singular value decomposition for genome-wide expression data processing and modeling. Proc. Natl. Acad. Sci. USA 97, 10101–10106.

Beer, M. A., and Tavazoie, S. (2004). Predicting gene expression from sequence. *Cell* **117,** 185–198.

Boldrick, J. C., Alizadeh, A. A., Diehn, M., Dudoit, S., Liu, C. L., Belcher, C. E., Botstein, D., Staudt, L. M., Brown, P. O., and Relman, D. A. (2002). Stereotyped and specific gene expression programs in human innate immune responses to bacteria. *Proc. Natl. Acad. Sci. USA* **99,** 972–977.

Brown, P. O., and Botstein, D. (1999). Exploring the new world of the genome with DNA microarrays. *Nat. Genet.* **21,** 33–37.

Butte, A. (2002). The use and analysis of microarray data. *Nat. Rev. Drug Discov.* **1,** 951–960.

Chang, H. Y., Chi, J. T., Dudoit, S., Bondre, C., van de Rijn, M., Botstein, D., and Brown, P. O. (2002). Diversity, topographic differentiation, and positional memory in human fibroblasts. *Proc. Natl. Acad. Sci. USA* **99,** 12877–12882.

Chung, C. H., Bernard, P. S., and Perou, C. M. (2002). Molecular portraits and the family tree of cancer. *Nat. Genet.* 32 Suppl, 533–540.

Cowan, C. A., Atienza, J., Melton, D. A., and Eggan, K. (2005). Nuclear reprogramming of somatic cells after fusion with human embryonic stem cells. *Science* **309,** 1369–1373.

Diehn, M., Alizadeh, A. A., Rando, O. J., Liu, C. L., Stankunas, K., Botstein, D., Crabtree, G. R., and Brown, P. O. (2002). Genomic expression programs and the integration of the CD28 costimulatory signal in T cell activation. *Proc. Natl. Acad. Sci. USA* **99,** 11796–11801.

Diehn, M., Eisen, M. B., Botstein, D., and Brown, P. O. (2000). Large-scale identification of secreted and membrane-associated gene products using DNA microarrays. *Nat. Genet.* **25,** 58–62.

Dudoit, S., and Fridlyand, J. (2002). A prediction–based resampling method for estimating the number of clusters in a dataset. *Genome Biol.* **3,** RESEARCH0036.

Eisen, M. B., Spellman, P. T., Brown, P. O., and Botstein, D. (1998). Cluster analysis and display of genome-wide expression patterns. *Proc. Natl. Acad. Sci. USA* **95,** 14863–14868.

Evsikov, A. V., and Solter, D. (2003). Comment on " 'Stemness': transcriptional profiling of embryonic and adult stem cells" and "a stem cell molecular signature". *Science* **302,** 393; author reply 393.

Fortunel, N. O., Otu, H. H., Ng, H. H., Chen, J., Mu, X., Chevassut, T., Li, X., Joseph, M., Bailey, C., Hatzfeld, J. A., Hatzfeld, A., Usta, F., Vega, V. B., Long, P. M., Libermann, T. A., and Lim, B. (2003). Comment on " 'Stemness': transcriptional profiling of embryonic and adult stem cells" and "a stem cell molecular signature". *Science* **302,** 393; author reply 393.

Friedman, N. (2004). Inferring cellular networks using probabilistic graphical models. *Science* **303,** 799–805.

Gasch, A. P., and Eisen, M. B. (2002). Exploring the conditional coregulation of yeast gene expression through fuzzy k-means clustering. *Genome Biol.* **3,** RESEARCH0059.

Gerhold, D. L., Jensen, R. V., and Gullans, S. R. (2002). Better therapeutics through microarrays. *Nat. Genet.* 32 Suppl, 547–551.

Hackney, J. A., Charbord, P., Brunk, B. P., Stoeckert, C. J., Lemischka, I. R., and Moore, K. A. (2002). A molecular profile of a hematopoietic stem cell niche. *Proc. Natl. Acad. Sci. USA* **99,** 13061–13066.

Irizarry, R. A., Warren, D., Spencer, F., Kim, I. F., Biswal, S., Frank, B. C., Gabrielson, E., Garcia, J. G., Geoghegan, J., Germino, G., Griffin, C., Hilmer, S. C., Hoffman, E., Jedlicka, A. E., Kawasaki, E., Martinez-Murillo, F., Morsberger, L., Lee, H., Petersen, D., Quackenbush, J., Scott, A., Wilson, M., Yang, Y., Ye, S. Q., and Yu, W. (2005). Multiple-laboratory comparison of microarray platforms. *Nat. Methods* **2,** 345–350.

Ishkanian, A. S., Malloff, C. A., Watson, S. K., DeLeeuw, R. J., Chi, B., Coe, B. P., Snijders, A., Albertson, D. G., Pinkel, D., Marra, M. A., Ling, V., MacAulay, C., and Lam, W. L.

(2004). A tiling resolution DNA microarray with complete coverage of the human genome. *Nat. Genet.* **36,** 299–303.

Ivanova, N. B., Dimos, J. T., Schaniel, C., Hackney, J. A., Moore, K. A., and Lemischka, I. R. (2002). A stem cell molecular signature. *Science* **298,** 601–604.

Iyer, V. R., Horak, C. E., Scafe, C. S., Botstein, D., Snyder, M., and Brown, P. O. (2001). Genomic binding sites of the yeast cell-cycle transcription factors SBF and MBF. *Nature* **409,** 533–538.

Larkin, J. E., Frank, B. C., Gavras, H., Sultana, R., and Quackenbush, J. (2005). Independence and reproducibility across microarray platforms. *Nat. Methods* **2,** 337–344.

Lieb, J. D., Liu, X., Botstein, D., and Brown, P. O. (2001). Promoter-specific binding of Rap1 revealed by genome-wide maps of protein-DNA association. *Nat. Genet.* **28,** 327–334.

Maitra, A., Arking, D. E., Shivapurkar, N., Ikeda, M., Stastny, V., Kassauei, K., Sui, G., Cutler, D. J., Liu, Y., Brimble, S. N., Noaksson, K., Hyllner, J., Schulz, T. C., Zeng, X., Freed, W. J., Crook, J., Abraham, S., Colman, A., Sartipy, P., Matsui, S., Carpenter, M., Gazdar, A. F., Rao, M., and Chakravarti, A. (2005). Genomic alterations in cultured human embryonic stem cells. *Nat. Genet.* **37,** 1099–1103.

Mootha, V. K., Handschin, C., Arlow, D., Xie, X., St Pierre, J., Sihag, S., Yang, W., Altshuler, D., Puigserver, P., Patterson, N., Willy, P. J., Schulman, I. G., Heyman, R. A., Lander, E. S., and Spiegelman, B. M. (2004). Erralpha and Gabpa/b specify PGC-1alpha-dependent oxidative phosphorylation gene expression that is altered in diabetic muscle. *Proc. Natl. Acad. Sci. USA* **101,** 6570–6575.

Mootha, V. K., Lindgren, C. M., Eriksson, K. F., Subramanian, A., Sihag, S., Lehar, J., Puigserver, P., Carlsson, E., Ridderstrale, M., Laurila, E., Houstis, N., Daly, M. J., Patterson, N., Mesirov, J. P., Golub, T. R., Tamayo, P., Spiegelman, B., Lander, E. S., Hirschhorn, J. N., Altshuler, D., and Groop, L. C. (2003). PGC-1alpha-responsive genes involved in oxidative phosphorylation are coordinately downregulated in human diabetes. *Nat. Genet.* **34,** 267–273.

Odom, D. T., Zizlsperger, N., Gordon, D. B., Bell, G. W., Rinaldi, N. J., Murray, H. L., Volkert, T. L., Schreiber, J., Rolfe, P. A., Gifford, D. K., Fraenkel, E., Bell, G. I., and Young, R. A. (2004). Control of pancreas and liver gene expression by HNF transcription factors. *Science* **303,** 1378–1381.

Park, P. J., Pagano, M., and Bonetti, M. (2001). A nonparametric scoring algorithm for identifying informative genes from microarray data. *Pac. Symp. Biocomput.* 52–63.

Perou, C. M., Sorlie, T., Eisen, M. B., van de Rijn, M., Jeffrey, S. S., Rees, C. A., Pollack, J. R., Ross, D. T., Johnsen, H., Akslen, L. A., Fluge, O., Pergamenschikov, A., Williams, C., Zhu, S. X., Lonning, P. E., Borresen-Dale, A. L., Brown, P. O., and Botstein, D. (2000). Molecular portraits of human breast tumours. *Nature* **406,** 747–752.

Petersen, K. F., Befroy, D., Dufour, S., Dziura, J., Ariyan, C., Rothman, D. L., DiPietro, L., Cline, G. W., and Shulman, G. I. (2003). Mitochondrial dysfunction in the elderly: possible role in insulin resistance. *Science* **300,** 1140–1142.

Pinkel, D., and Albertson, D. G. (2005). Array comparative genomic hybridization and its applications in cancer. *Nat. Genet.* 37 (Suppl.), S11–S17.

Pinkel, D., Segraves, R., Sudar, D., Clark, S., Poole, I., Kowbel, D., Collins, C., Kuo, W. L., Chen, C., Zhai, Y., Dairkee, S. H., Ljung, B. M., Gray, J. W., and Albertson, D. G. (1998). High resolution analysis of DNA copy number variation using comparative genomic hybridization to microarrays. *Nat. Genet.* **20,** 207–211.

Pollack, J. R., Perou, C. M., Alizadeh, A. A., Eisen, M. B., Pergamenschikov, A., Williams, C. F., Jeffrey, S. S., Botstein, D., and Brown, P. O. (1999). Genome-wide analysis of DNA copy-number changes using cDNA microarrays. *Nat. Genet.* **23,** 41–46.

Ramalho-Santos, M., Yoon, S., Matsuzaki, Y., Mulligan, R. C., and Melton, D. A. (2002). "Stemness": transcriptional profiling of embryonic and adult stem cells. *Science* **298,** 597–600.

Raychaudhuri, S., Stuart, J. M., and Altman, R. B. (2000). Principal components analysis to summarize microarray experiments: application to sporulation time series. *Pac. Symp. Biocomput.* 455–466.

Roy, P. J., Stuart, J. M., Lund, J., and Kim, S. K. (2002). Chromosomal clustering of muscle-expressed genes in *Caenorhabditis elegans*. *Nature* **418,** 975–979.

Segal, E., Friedman, N., Koller, D., and Regev, A. (2004). A module map showing conditional activity of expression modules in cancer. *Nat. Genet.* **36,** 1090–1098.

Segal, E., Shapira, M., Regev, A., Pe'er, D., Botstein, D., Koller, D., and Friedman, N. (2003). Module networks: Identifying regulatory modules and their condition-specific regulators from gene expression data. *Nat. Genet.* **34,** 166–176.

Sherlock, G. (2001). Analysis of large-scale gene expression data. *Brief Bioinform.* **2,** 350–362.

Slonim, D. K. (2002). From patterns to pathways: gene expression data analysis comes of age. *Nat. Genet.* 32 Suppl, 502–508.

Snijders, A. M., Nowak, N., Segraves, R., Blackwood, S., Brown, N., Conroy, J., Hamilton, G., Hindle, A. K., Huey, B., Kimura, K., Law, S., Myambo, K., Palmer, J., Ylstra, B., Yue, J. P., Gray, J. W., Jain, A. N., Pinkel, D., and Albertson, D. G. (2001). Assembly of microarrays for genome-wide measurement of DNA copy number. *Nat. Genet.* **29,** 263–264.

Spellman, P. T., and Rubin, G. M. (2002). Evidence for large domains of similarly expressed genes in the *Drosophila* genome. *J. Biol.* **1,** 5.

Tamayo, P., Slonim, D., Mesirov, J., Zhu, Q., Kitareewan, S., Dmitrovsky, E., Lander, E. S., and Golub, T. R. (1999). Interpreting patterns of gene expression with self-organizing maps: methods and application to hematopoietic differentiation. *Proc. Natl. Acad. Sci. USA* **96,** 2907–2912.

Toronen, P., Kolehmainen, M., Wong, G., and Castren, E. (1999). Analysis of gene expression data using self-organizing maps. *FEBS Lett.* **451,** 142–146.

Troyanskaya, O. G., Garber, M. E., Brown, P. O., Botstein, D., and Altman, R. B. (2002). Nonparametric methods for identifying differentially expressed genes in microarray data. *Bioinformatics* **18,** 1454–1461.

Tusher, V. G., Tibshirani, R., and Chu, G. (2001). Significance analysis of microarrays applied to the ionizing radiation response. *Proc. Natl. Acad. Sci. USA* **98,** 5116–5121.

Van Gelder, R. N., von Zastrow, M. E., Yool, A., Dement, W. C., Barchas, J. D., and Eberwine, J. H. (1990). Amplified RNA synthesized from limited quantities of heterogeneous cDNA. *Proc. Natl. Acad. Sci. USA* **87,** 1663–1667.

Vogel, G. (2003). Stem cells. 'Stemness' genes still elusive. *Science* **302,** 371.

Wang, E., Miller, L. D., Ohnmacht, G. A., Liu, E. T., and Marincola, F. M. (2000). High-fidelity mRNA amplification for gene profiling. *Nat. Biotechnol.* **18,** 457–459.

Watt, F. M., and Hogan, B. L. (2000). Out of Eden: stem cells and their niches. *Science* **287,** 1427–1430.

Xu, R. H., Chen, X., Li, D. S., Li, R., Addicks, G. C., Glennon, C., Zwaka, T. P., and Thomson, J. A. (2002). BMP4 initiates human embryonic stem cell differentiation to trophoblast. *Nat. Biotechnol.* **20,** 1261–1264.

Zhao, H., Hastie, T., Whitfield, M. L., Borresen-Dale, A. L., and Jeffrey, S. S. (2002). Optimization and evaluation of T7 based RNA linear amplification protocols for cDNA microarray analysis. *BMC Genomics* **3,** 31.

[11] Purification of Hematopoietic Stem Cells Using the Side Population

By K. K. LIN and MARGARET A. GOODELL

Abstract

Hematopoietic stem cells (HSCs) primarily reside in bone marrow, are defined by their ability to maintain blood homeostasis, and replenish themselves through self-renewal. Although HSC purification schemes vary from laboratory to laboratory, the resulting cell populations are similar, if not the same. This chapter will discuss different enrichment methods for HSCs and provide a detailed protocol for staining HSC with Hoechst 33342 for the side population (SP).

Introduction

Cell Surface Markers of HSCs

Bone marrow–hematopoietic stem cell (HSC) activity has been extensively studied since the 1950s when Ford et al. (1956) discovered a robust contribution of transplanted donor bone marrow in lethally irradiated recipients. HSCs were first enriched from murine bone marrow by Weissman and colleagues via surface marker expression using fluorescent-activated cell sorting (FACS) (Spangrude et al., 1988). Thereafter, other laboratories have also modified or refined the approach with different combinations of surface markers. Of these surface markers, positive expression of c-kit (CD117), a tyrosine kinase receptor, Sca-1, a membrane glycoprotein, and lack of expression of hematopoietic differentiation ("lineage⁻") markers (CD4, CD8, B220, Mac-1, Gr-1, Ter119) are the core elements to enrich for HSCs. The c-Kit+ Sca-1+ Lineage (KSL) cells comprise ~0.1% of the whole bone marrow, and despite being highly enriched for HSCs, they are still a very heterogeneous population that includes lineage-primed multipotent progenitors, as well as short-term HSCs and long-term HSCs (Okada et al., 1992). Therefore, several additional markers to exclude differentiated progenitors such as Thy1.1 (Morrison and Weissman, 1994), CD34 (Osawa et al., 1996), and Flk-2 (Christensen and Weissman, 2001) have been used to further fractionate bone marrow KSL (Table I). Although these approaches result in highly overlapping populations, there are also slight differences, and efforts have been made to quantify the long-term repopulating activity

METHODS IN ENZYMOLOGY, VOL. 420   0076-6879/06 $35.00

TABLE I
Comparison of the Modern Canonical Purification Schemes

Purification strategy	Fraction of WBM (%)	Purity of functional HSC	References
c-kit + Sca-1 + Lin − (KSL)	0.08	+	Okada *et al.*, 1992
KSL Thy1.1 − (KTSL)	0.05	++	Morrison and Weissman, 1994
KSL CD34−	0.008	++	Osawa *et al.*, 1996
KSL Thy1.1^{lo} Flk − 2⁻	0.01	+++	Christensen and Weissman, 2001
SP (Hoechst 33342)	0.05	++	Goodell *et al.*, 1996

The resulting purity of HSCs is based on the functional assays provided by the original articles. There are no absolute number in turns of HSC purity because the calculation of enrichment power in each laboratory slightly varies.

of these purified populations using bone marrow transplantation assays. However, because the stringency of quantification varies among different groups, depending on the precise strategy for assessment, there is not yet an absolute standard to compare the power of every enrichment scheme. Ultimately, the choice of optimal enrichment scheme will also depend on the flow cytometry equipment available, the local expertise, and the reproducibility of the different methods in the hands of the particular investigators.

Other HSC Surface Markers: Tie-2, Endoglin, and the SLAM Family Receptors

Although c-Kit, Sca-1, and Lineage markers have been the canonical cell surface markers used to enrich for HSCs for more than a decade, this combination of more than eight different antibodies makes HSC purification an expensive process. Furthermore, the complexity of this scheme was incompatible with standard fluorescence microscopy, if one wanted to identify HSC *in situ*. More surface markers such as Tie-2 (Arai *et al.*, 2004) and endoglin (Chen *et al.*, 2002) have been found to be expressed in HSCs. In addition, Morrison and his colleagues recently have used markers from the SLAM family, CD150, CD244, and CD48, to distinguish HSCs from differentiated hematopoietic lineages (Kiel *et al.*, 2005). They were able to enrich for murine HSCs by fractionating bone marrow cells with SLAM family markers (CD150$^+$CD244$^-$CD48$^-$). Although, these fractionated cell populations have yet to be quantitatively compared with other enrichment strategies, the stem cell activity of Tie-2$^+$ or CD150$^+$ bone marrow population have enabled the *in situ* visualization of HSC in bone marrow, revealing putative endothelial niches.

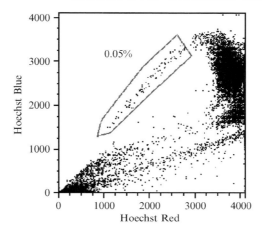

FIG. 1. SP gate of an unenriched whole bone marrow sample. To visualize the SP population, signals are displayed in a Hoechst Blue versus Hoechst Red dot plot. The FACS PMT voltages are adjusted until most of the cells are at the upper right corner while the red blood cells and debris are at the lower left corner. The SP population comprises ~0.02–0.05% of whole bone marrow cells. (This figure is generously provided by Stuart M. Chambers).

Fluorescent Dye Efflux in HSCs and the SParKLS

HSCs have been recognized to exhibit high multidrug-type efflux activity, which results in low retention of fluorescent dyes such as Hoechst 33342 and Rhodamine 123, relative to other bone marrow cells (Goodell *et al.*, 1996; Li and Johnson, 1992). This trait has been exploited in one of the most widely used HSC purification strategies, in which differential efflux of the fluorescent DNA binding dye Hoechst 33342 results in a "side population" (SP) of low staining cells that is highly enriched for HSC. The SP (Fig. 1) is highly enriched for HSC functionally and phenotypically overlaps with $c\text{-}Kit^{+}Sca\text{-}1^{+}Lin^{-}Thy1^{lo}$ $CD34^{-}Flt3^{-}$ cells (Camargo *et al.*, 2006). Although HSC purified using the SP strategy are probably one of the most pure and potent populations available, the method is sensitive to slight modifications in staining procedures, so that the resulting population is somewhat variable from person to person and laboratory to laboratory, leading to some claims that the SP is quite heterogeneous. Therefore, to ensure a successful purification of HSC using the SP, we recommend inclusion of cell surface markers, such as c-Kit, Lineage-, and Sca-1 in the purification scheme as a purity index. The resulting highly homogeneous SP cells are termed *SParKLS* (pronounced as "sparkles"), which excludes the possible contamination of precursor cells in the SP (Fig. 2).

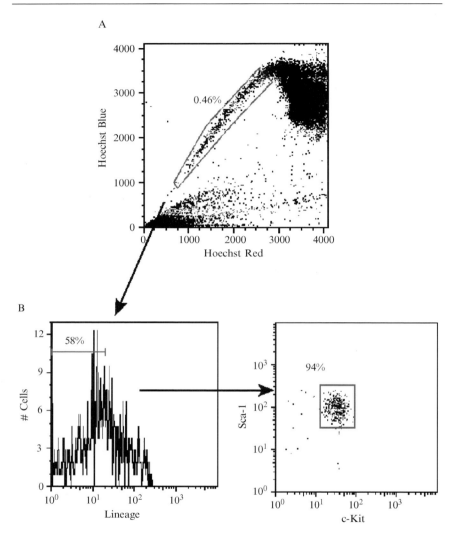

FIG. 2. The SParKLS (SP, c-Kit$^+$, Lin$^-$, Sca-1$^+$) cells. To exclude a low-level contamination of progenitor cells, we include antibodies such as c-Kit, Sca-1, and the markers of differentiated cells (lineage) during SP analysis. The resulting population is named SParKLS. This bone marrow sample was preenriched with Sca-1 antibody using magnetic sorting.

High expression of multidrug-resistant ABC transporters such as MDR-1 and ABCG2 in HSCs has been suggested to contribute to the dye efflux ability, perhaps with a natural role of efflux of differentiation factors (Goodell et al., 1996). Indeed, retroviral-mediated overexpression of human multidrug resistance-1 (MDR-1) leads to stem cell expansion (Bunting et al., 1998) and an increased SP (Bunting et al., 2000). However, loss of Mdr1 only impacts the efflux of Rhodamine dye, but not Hoechst, indicating that Mdr1 is not absolutely required for Hoechst effect. The expression of ABCG2 in murine bone marrow cells was found essential to detect the SP after Hoechst staining (Zhou et al., 2002). Nevertheless, the expression of ABCG2 does not always reflect the SP phenotype. A residual SP has been found in ABCG2-deficient murine bone marrow (Zhou et al., 2002). Although a higher expression level of ABCG2 was found in both the SPs of murine and human, some progenitors and differentiated lineages that were also found to express a detectable level of ABCG2 in the absence of a SP phenotype (Scharenberg et al., 2002; Zhou et al., 2001). Therefore, one cannot equate ABCG2 expression with SP, and antibodies against ABCG2 may not detect HSC, or other stem cells, with fidelity. It is likely that multiple multidrug-resistant transporters can contribute to the SP phenotype. Recently, a microarray gene expression study of HSC has further revealed that a number of multidrug-resistant transporters were expressed (Venezia et al., 2004).

Protocol of HSC Sorting with Hoechst 33342 Staining (SP)

Overview

After staining with Hoechst 33342, HSCs appear as SP in FACS (Fig. 1). High dye efflux ability and the quiescent cell-cycle stage of HSCs are thought to account for the SP. Reproducible staining for SP cells is dependent on careful control of various parameters such as Hoechst dye concentration, cell concentration, and staining temperature and time. Furthermore, the protocol was originally established for murine HSC from normal C57Bl/6 bone marrow, so optimization is required when staining other tissues or species. To establish the Hoechst staining procedure de novo, we strongly recommend that initial experiments be performed with murine bone marrows exactly as we describe. When proper Hoechst staining is performed, the SP comprises ~0.02–0.05% of whole bone marrow cells, which often seems low to a beginner's eyes, but this small population is very highly purified for active long-term HSC (Goodell et al., 1996). To increase the total yield, we often use a pre–enrichment scheme on the basis of magnetic enrichment of progenitors using a canonical HSC surface marker (e.g., Sca-1 or c-kit). Thus, an enrichment protocol, which gives rise to an at least 10-fold enrichment for bone marrow SP (Fig. 2), is also provided. The use of these protocols in combination can result in roughly 50,000 purified HSC when starting from 10 mice, in a ~8–10 h procedure.

Hoechst Staining Protocol

1. Prewarm DMEM + medium in a 37° circulating water bath. Ensure the temperature is precisely at 37°.

2. Using mice ~8 weeks of age, prepare bone marrow from femurs and tibias, resuspend in iced HBSS + buffer.

3. Count nucleated cells: To count nucleated cells and avoid the similarly sized red blood cells (RBC), one can lyse RBCs in an aliquot of the bone marrow removed for counting. Mix a 5-μl bone marrow aliquot with 95 μl of RBC lysis buffer (D-5001, Gentra), vortex thoroughly and take 10 μl to count under a hemacytometer. Do *not* perform RBC lysis to the whole bone marrow suspension. We typically find an average of 40–70 million nucleated cells per C57Bl/6 mouse (2 femurs and 2 tibias). Cell number is one critical parameter to a successful Hoechst staining, so count cells carefully.

4. Spin down bone marrow cells. Resuspend cells at 10^6/ml in pre-warmed DMEM+. To avoid retention of cells in tubes, polypropylene tubes must be used when Hoechst staining is performed. We find staining in 250 ml polypropylene tubes (Cat. No 430776, Corning) the most convenient when staining large volumes.

5. Add Hoechst to a final concentration of 5 μg/ml. We suggest using a 200× (1 mg/ml) stock, which is made in water by dissolving an entire bottle of Hoechst powder (B2261, Sigma), aliquoting, and storing the concentrated Hoechst solution in a −20° freezer.

6. Incubate cells in a 37° water bath and periodically mix the tubes during the exact 90-min incubation. Time and temperature are crucial to Hoechst staining, so the DMEM should be prewarmed and the tubes fully immersed in the water bath.

7. After the Hoechst stain, cells *must* be maintained at 4° to prevent further Hoechst dye efflux. No Ficoll or other extended higher temperature procedures should be performed after the Hoechst stain because this will result in dye efflux from other bone marrow cells that are *not* HSC, ultimately reducing the purity of the SP. The cells should be spun down in a 4° centrifuge and resuspended in ice-cold HBSS+.

8. Antibody staining can now be performed on ice. To ensure good HSC purification, antibodies against Sca-1, c-Kit, and one or more lineage markers are added at concentrations determined by standard antibody titration procedures, or as recommended by the manufacturer

(e.g., Becton Dickinson/Pharmingen). All staining and centrifugation should be performed at 4°.

9. At the point when cells are ready for FACS analysis, resuspend cells in cold HBSS+ with 2 μg/ml propidium iodide (PI) to distinguish dead cells. Although staining with PI is not absolutely required to see P, it is strongly recommended. Hoechst is toxic to some bone marrow cells, and PI allows the dead cells to be distinguished, simplifying the Hoechst emission plot.

10. Reagents
    a. DMEM+
       1. DMEM with high glucose (Cat No. 11965-092, Gibco Invitrogen)
       2. Penicillin/streptomycin (Cat No.15140-122, Gibco Invitrogen)
       3. 10 mM HEPES (Cat No. 15630-080, Gibco Invitrogen)
       4. 2% Fetal bovine serum/fetal calf serum
    b. HBSS+
       1. Hank's balanced salt solution (Cat. No. 14170-112, Gibco Invitrogen)
       2. 10 mM HEPES
       3. 2% Fetal bovine serum/fetal calf serum
    c. Hoechst 33342 powder (Cat. No. B2261, Sigma): 200× stock (1 mg/ml) is made first by dissolving powder in distilled water and filter sterilizing. From what we have obtained from Sigma, a bottle of powder is good for ~500 ml of Hoechst stock solution. It is strongly recommended that a large batch of Hoechst from a *whole* bottle be made at once, and frozen in small (~1 ml) aliquots. Thawed Hoechst powder may be less reliable refreezing, possibly because of acquisition of water.
    d. Propidium iodide (Cat. No. P-4170, Sigma): Working stock is 100× (200 μg/ml) in PBS, and is covered with aluminum foil in a 4° fridge. Final concentration of PI in resuspension HBSS+ should be 2 μg/ml.

Protocol For Antibody Staining and Magnetic Enrichment of Hoechst-Stained Cells

1. After Hoechst staining, resuspend cells at 1×10^8 cells/ml in iced HBSS+. For Sca-1 enrichment, incubate biotinylated Sca-1 antibody with cells at 1/100 dilution, on ice for 10 min.
2. Wash out unbound antibody with 10-fold volume of HBSS+, spin down in a cold centrifuge.
3. Label cells with magnetic beads. We obtain the anti-biotin magnetic microbeads from Miltenyi Biotech (Cat. No. 130-090-485). Incubate

cells with 20% volume of microbeads at 4° for 15 min. We have found the binding efficiency of microbeads to antibody-labeled cells very low when incubating on ice. Incubate in a 4° fridge instead.

4. Wash the cells with a 10-fold volume of HBSS+ and spin down in a cold centrifuge.
5. Resuspend cells at 2×10^8 cells/ml in iced HBSS+, and cells are ready to be loaded into autoMACs column.

FACS Analysis for Hoechst SP Cells

1. Excitation of Hoechst 33342: To view the SP, an ultraviolet laser is needed to excite the Hoechst 33342 dye and PI. A violet laser has also been used with good results (Simpson *et al.*, 2006). The Hoechst dye is excited at 350 nm. Additional lasers such as a 488 laser for FITC and PE can be used to excite additional fluorochromes.

2. Detection of Hoechst emission: The emission of Hoechst dye is measured with two detectors: Hoechst Blue and Hoechst Red. Hoechst Blue is measured with a 450/20 filter, whereas the red is measured with a 675LP filter. To separate the emission wavelength, a dichroic mirror is used (we use a 610 DMSP). Fluorescence from PI is also measured with the 675LP channel, but the positive signal is much brighter than the Hoechst red signal. The simultaneous excitation and emission of PI off the 488 lasers can be used to identify the dead cells and distinguish from red-fluorescing live Hoechst-stained cells. Although other filter sets similar to the ones we describe may work sufficiently, these are optimal.

In addition, a high-power UV laser (50–100 mW) gives the best resolution of the SP. Less power may be sufficient, but the population may not be as distinct. It is important to confirm the SP population with a transporter inhibitor, Verapamil, or antibody costaining, particularly for initial SP identification.

3. FACS Analysis: The Hoechst fluorescence is displayed on Hoechst BLUE versus RED plot, with BLUE on the vertical axis and RED on the horizontal axis, both in *linear mode*. The voltage is adjusted so that red blood cells appear in the lower left corner, whereas the dead cells that are stained with PI positive line up at the far right vertical line. Most the bone marrow cells can be seen in the center, or in the upper right quarter (Fig. 1). It is also possible to detect a major G0–G1 population with S-G2M cells going toward the upper right corner.

To be able to see the SP cells, draw a sample gate to exclude the red blood cells and dead cells. With an unenriched bone marrow sample, 50,000–100,000 events within the sample gate are needed to identify the SP. The SP region should be drawn as Fig. 1. The prevalence of SP is approximately

0.01%–0.05% of an unenriched whole bone marrow sample in the mouse. A population of SP cells in normal mouse bone marrow significantly higher in proportion than this-0.05% invariably indicates poor Hoechst staining and contamination of the SP cells with non-SP. This is readily visualized by the presence of cells in the SP that do not express the canonical HSC surface markers. If the staining is done properly, between 65 and 95% of the SP cells will have canonical HSC surface markers, and these are selected for purification.

4. Tips for operating the FACS: Because Hoechst emission is displayed under the linear mode, good CVs are critical for SP identification. To maintain good CVs, it is important to perform alignment with particles that display a tight distribution in linear mode (DNA check beads, Coulter). In addition, a low sample differential pressure is important. The maximal differential pressure for samples should not be faster than the one for calibrating with alignment particle. The bone marrow cells should be run at high concentration so as to maintain a low sample pressure.

5. Confirmation of a good SP staining
    a. Include a Verapamil-treated control to confirm the SP population in one aliquot. Verapamil (Cat. No. V-4629, Sigma) at the final concentration of 50 μM can be added throughout the entire Hoechst staining procedure. With Verapamil treatment, SP population will be blocked.
    b. Costain with antibodies. The mouse bone marrow SP population is highly enriched with HSCs. With a good Hoechst staining, 60%–80% of SP cells are Sca-1$^+$ and Lineage$^-$cells (Fig. 2).

References

Arai, F., Hirao, A., Ohmura, M., Sato, H., Matsuoka, S., Takubo, K., Ito, K., Koh, G. Y., and Suda, T. (2004). Tie2/angiopoietin-1 signaling regulates hematopoietic stem cell quiescence in the bone marrow niche. *Cell* **118,** 149–161.

Bunting, K. D., Galipeau, J., Topham, D., Benaim, E., and Sorrentino, B. P. (1998). Transduction of murine bone marrow cells with an MDR1 vector enables *ex vivo* stem cell expansion, but these expanded grafts cause a myeloproliferative syndrome in transplanted mice. *Blood* **92,** 2269–2279.

Bunting, K. D., Zhou, S., Lu, T., and Sorrentino, B. P. (2000). Enforced P-glycoprotein pump function in murine bone marrow cells results in expansion of side population stem cells *in vitro* and repopulating cells *in vivo*. *Blood* **96,** 902–909.

Camargo, F. D., Chambers, S. M., Drew, E., McNagny, K. M., and Goodell, M. A. (2006). Hematopoietic stem cells do not engraft with absolute efficiencies. *Blood* **107,** 501–507.

Chen, C. Z., Li, M., de Graaf, D., Monti, S., Gottgens, B., Sanchez, M. J., Lander, E. S., Golub, T. R., Green, A. R., and Lodish, H. F. (2002). Identification of endoglin as a functional marker that defines long-term repopulating hematopoietic stem cells. *Proc. Natl. Acad. Sci. USA* **99,** 15468–15473.

Christensen, J. L., and Weissman, I. L. (2001). Flk-2 is a marker in hematopoietic stem cell differentiation: A simple method to isolate long-term stem cells. *Proc. Natl. Acad. Sci. USA* **98**, 14541–14546.

Ford, C. E., Hamerton, J. L., Barnes, D. W., and Loutit, J. F. (1956). Cytological identification of radiation-chimaeras. *Nature* **177**, 452–454.

Goodell, M. A., Brose, K., Paradis, G., Conner, A. S., and Mulligan, R. C. (1996). Isolation and functional properties of murine hematopoietic stem cells that are replicating *in vivo*. *J. Exp. Med.* **183**, 1797–1806.

Kiel, M. J., Yilmaz, O. H., Iwashita, T., Yilmaz, O. H., Terhorst, C., and Morrison, S. J. (2005). SLAM family receptors distinguish hematopoietic stem and progenitor cells and reveal endothelial niches for stem cells. *Cell* **121**, 1109–1121.

Li, C. L., and Johnson, G. R. (1992). Rhodamine123 reveals heterogeneity within murine Lin-, Sca-1+ hemopoietic stem cells. *J. Exp. Med.* **175**, 1443–1447.

Morrison, S. J., and Weissman, I. L. (1994). The long-term repopulating subset of hematopoietic stem cells is deterministic and isolatable by phenotype. *Immunity* **1**, 661–673.

Okada, S., Nakauchi, H., Nagayoshi, K., Nishikawa, S., Miura, Y., and Suda, T. (1992). *In vivo* and *in vitro* stem cell function of c-kit- and Sca-1-positive murine hematopoietic cells. *Blood* **80**, 3044–3050.

Osawa, M., Hanada, K., Hamada, H., and Nakauchi, H. (1996). Long-term lymphohematopoietic reconstitution by a single CD34-low/negative hematopoietic stem cell. *Science* **273**, 242–245.

Scharenberg, C. W., Harkey, M. A., and Torok-Storb, B. (2002). The ABCG2 transporter is an efficient Hoechst 33342 efflux pump and is preferentially expressed by immature human hematopoietic progenitors. *Blood* **99**, 507–512.

Simpson, C., Pearce, D. J., Bonnet, D., and Davies, D. (2006). Out of the blue: A comparison of Hoechst side population (SP) analysis of murine bone marrow using 325, 363 and 407 nm excitation sources. *J. Immunol. Methods* **310**, 171–181.

Spangrude, G. J., Heimfeld, S., and Weissman, I. L. (1988). Purification and characterization of mouse hematopoietic stem cells. *Science* **241**, 58–62.

Venezia, T. A., Merchant, A. A., Ramos, C. A., Whitehouse, N. L., Young, A. S., Shaw, C. A., and Goodell, M. A. (2004). Molecular signatures of proliferation and quiescence in hematopoietic stem cells. *PloS. Biol.* **2**, e301.

Zhou, S., Morris, J. J., Barnes, Y., Lan, L., Schuetz, J. D., and Sorrentino, B. P. (2002). Bcrp1 gene expression is required for normal numbers of side population stem cells in mice, and confers relative protection to mitoxantrone in hematopoietic cells *in vivo*. *Proc. Natl. Acad. Sci. USA* **99**, 12339–12344.

Zhou, S., Schuetz, J. D., Bunting, K. D., Colapietro, A. M., Sampath, J., Morris, J. J., Lagutina, I., Grosveld, G. C., Osawa, M., Nakauchi, H., and Sorrentino, B. P. (2001). The ABC transporter Bcrp1/ABCG2 is expressed in a wide variety of stem cells and is a molecular determinant of the side-population phenotype. *Nat. Med.* **7**, 1028–1034.

[12]   Cellular Reprogramming

By SADHANA AGARWAL

Abstract

The concept of reprogramming a cell is very intriguing and has immense therapeutic potential. Examples from physiology and developmental biology suggest that it may well be possible. Experimental approaches are beginning to suggest this also, in particular the initially astonishing accomplishment of somatic cell nuclear transfer and cloning. This chapter reviews current strategies and describes emerging methods for the proposition of reprogramming cells with cell extracts.

Introduction

Stem cells hold great promise for regenerative medicine and, as indicated by the previous chapters, an intense scientific effort to isolate, characterize, and differentiate them into various cell types for therapeutic applications has, and continues to, ensue. Concomitantly, however, inspired by evidence for the plasticity of cell fate, small but increasing attention is being paid to exploring the possibility of an alternative to harvesting stem cells: that of reprogramming somatic cells *in vitro*, instead. Reprogramming involves the conversion of one differentiated cell type into another, a process that at its core entails the reinstruction of the gene expression profile of a cell (Collas and Hakelien, 2002; Hochedlinger and Jaenisch, 2006; Pomerantz and Blau, 2004; Raff, 2003). This process could theoretically be applied *in vitro* to reversing the differentiated state of a cell to an embryonic or progenitor state (also referred to as *dedifferentiation*), and these early-stage cells could then be differentiated to a desired cell type. Alternately, one differentiated cell type could perhaps be induced to convert to another desired differentiated cell type (also called *transdifferentiation*).

Besides being of fundamental biological interest, the prospect of reprogramming has great therapeutic possibilities. Although still in its infancy, it could also possibly obviate some of the currently outstanding issues surrounding the clinical use of embryonic or adult stem cells. Since it proposes transforming a patient's own cells into a desired cell type that needs replacement, reprogramming would permit the generation of autologous, genetically matched cells that would not be subject to immune rejection on transplantation (a concern during the use of embryonic stem cell derivatives).

METHODS IN ENZYMOLOGY, VOL. 420   0076-6879/06 $35.00
                DOI: 10.1016/S0076-6879(06)20012-0

The approach of generating embryonic stem cells after somatic cell nuclear transfer (SCNT) of patient-specific nuclei into enucleated oocytes (also called *therapeutic cloning* and itself a form of reprogramming), could address this problem (Gurdon and Byrne, 2003). However, SCNT is as yet technically challenging for human cells; like all derivations of human embryonic stem cells, raises ethical objections from some (involves the destruction of embryos); and has the logistical problem of the availability of enough human oocytes. Reprogramming techniques that could bypass the use of oocytes completely are, therefore, sought. The use of patient-specific adult stem cells could also offer a solution around these issues; however, so far they have been generally difficult to obtain and expand in large numbers and/or can, unlike embryonic stem cells, usually be differentiated into only a limited range of cell types (Pomerantz and Blau, 2004; Raff, 2003). Thus, the impetus to explore reprogramming strategies is, thus, significant.

Many examples of the plasticity of the differentiated state appear in development and physiology *in vivo* (Li *et al.*, 2005; Pomerantz and Blau, 2004; Raff, 2003). In *Drosophila*, regenerating imaginal disks, larval structures that are committed to form specific fly structures, can alter fate in response to homeotic gene expression changes in a process called *transdetermination* (Lawrence and Morata, 1983; Wei *et al.*, 2000). In lower vertebrates, there are examples of dedifferentiation and redifferentiation during limb regeneration in urodeles (Brockes and Kumar, 2002) and in zebra fish (Poss *et al.*, 2003). Newt lens regeneration is studied as an example of transdifferentiation (Okada, 1991), and retinal pigment epithelial cells can dedifferentiate and then form lens or neural retina both *in vivo* and in culture, in urodeles as well as avians (Eguchi and Kodama, 1993). Recently, in a study of tail regeneration in axolotls, spinal cord glial cells were found to dedifferentiate and give rise to mesodermal (as well as expected neural and ectodermal) cells, in an example of naturally occurring germ layer switching (Echeverri and Tanaka, 2002). In a mammalian rodent model, similar to limb regeneration in urodeles, severing a peripheral nerve causes Schwann cells to dedifferentiate, proliferate, and redifferentiate (Brockes and Kumar, 2002). During normal mammalian development, transdifferentiation from smooth muscle cells to skeletal muscle cells occurs in the esophagus (Kablar *et al.*, 2000; Patapoutian *et al.*, 1995) and has also been described for adult organs like the liver, thyroid, mammary gland, and kidney (Hay and Zuk, 1995; Strutz and Muller, 2000). Transdifferentiation is also reported during pathological conditions in humans: for example, during wound healing, when bone formation has been seen in scars and muscles; and, during the development of Barrett's metaplasia, a condition in which esophageal epithelium switches from stratified squamous to intestinal-type columnar epithelium and leads to a predisposition to esophageal adenocarcinoma (Haggitt *et al.*, 1978). Finally, more recently, adult stem cells have been reported to be capable of being reprogrammed and giving rise to cells outside of their normal developmental lineage—although the mechanism by which they do so (response to extracellular stimuli or cell fusion) has been controversial and is being clarified on a case-by-case basis (Pomerantz and Blau, 2004; Raff, 2003). Collectively, these (and other) examples indicate that the differentiation state of a cell is not irreversible. In fact, reprogramming is a naturally occurring process wherein, under certain conditions, a differentiated cell can alter its gene expression pattern considerably in response to its environment (presumably through alterations in the signaling pathways regulating it and resulting epigenetic changes) and adopt a new or under-differentiated state.

Key elements in reprogramming, then, would seem to be environmental cues or factors that cause and/or maintain the new reprogrammed state and resulting signaling networks that lead to the activation/repression of critical transcription factors and to epigenetic modifications in DNA/chromatin conformation that determine whether a gene is transcribed. These elements together, presumably, bring about the expression of a specific repertoire of genes that defines the new reprogrammed cell's identity. Several experimental approaches that apply these elements to engineer reprogramming *in vitro* are being investigated (Collas and Hakelien, 2003; Hochedlinger and Jaenisch, 2006; Li *et al.*, 2005; Pomerantz and Blau, 2004). Successful application of these approaches, in turn, provides further evidence for the plasticity of a cell. The most dramatic illustration of the possibility and power of reprogramming is the development of nuclear transfer technology (Gurdon and Byrne, 2003), as first captured in the cloning of Dolly, the sheep (Wilmut *et al.*, 1997). Subsequently, cloning in various species, including cloning of mice using nuclear transfer from terminally differentiated cells (Eggan *et al.*, 2004; Gurdon and Byrne, 2003; Hochedlinger and Jaenisch, 2002) and derivation of embryonic stem cells after somatic cell nuclear transplantations into enucleated oocytes (Cibelli *et al.*, 1998; Munsie *et al.*, 2000; Wakayama *et al.*, 2001) showed that nuclei of even the most differentiated and committed cells can be reprogrammed to pluripotency. The implication is that the oocyte contains the microenvironment and factors that are able to erase previously imposed developmental programming of the nucleus and redirect it to a pluripotent state.

Altering the extracellular microenvironment has been shown to change the fate of intact cells also; for example, pancreatic progenitor cells can convert to hepatocytes on transplantation to the liver (Dabeva *et al.*, 1997; Shen *et al.*, 2003), and endothelial cells can change to cardiomyocytes on injection into the damaged area of the heart (Condorelli *et al.*, 2001). In cell culture, cocultivation of endothelial cells with neonatal cardiomyocytes promotes their transdifferentiation to beating cardiomyocytes (Condorelli *et al.*, 2001). Cell culture in appropriate growth factors, including FGF2, has been shown to elicit the switching of primordial germ cells (PGCs) which normally give rise only to germ cells, oocytes, and spermatozoa, to embryonic stem (ES) cell–like "embryonic germ (EG)" cells that are pluripotent (Andrews, 2002). ES-like cells have also been reported to be generated from neonatal and adult testis cells in specific growth factor conditions (Guan *et al.*, 2006; Kanatsu-Shinohara *et al.*, 2004). In addition, ectopic expression of specific key transcription factors can also induce dramatic cell-type conversions. Examples include conversion of pancreatic cells to hepatic cells on expression of C/EBP-β (Shen *et al.*, 2003); transdifferentiation of hepatocytes to pancreatic cells on expression of PDX-1 (Ferber *et al.*, 2000) and of myoblasts to adipocytes by PPAR-γ and C/EBP-α (Hu *et al.*, 1995).

While the examples just cited rely on trying to alter the programming of a cell by means of specific growth conditions or transcription factors, two more "comprehensive" experimental approaches that do not require prior knowledge of specific factors have also been explored. Formation of heterokaryons by cell–cell fusion and reprogramming cells by exposing them to whole cell extracts of a different cell have both been reported to achieve reprogramming (Blau and Blakely, 1999; Collas and Hakelien, 2003; Hakelien *et al.*, 2002). Experimental fusion (usually mediated by polyethylene glycol, PEG) of two distinct cells to generate a single cell with two nuclei (a heterokaryon) results in changes in gene expression such that the pattern of one fusion partner is usually dominant, suggesting that transacting factors in the cytoplasm, or those emanating from the dominant nucleus, are capable of reprogramming the second nucleus (Blau and Baltimore, 1991; Blau *et al.*, 1985). Earlier examples of such studies include the fusion of rat myoblasts with chicken erythrocytes (Ringertz and Savage, 1976) and that of mouse muscle cells with a variety of nonmuscle human cell partners, wherein each human nucleus was induced to express previously repressed muscle genes (Blau *et al.*, 1983, 1985; Chiu and Blau, 1984, 1985). Fusion between pluripotent embryonic carcinoma (EC) cells and thymocytes resulted in heterokaryons that exhibited attributes of the EC cell partner, including pluripotency and tumor formation (Miller and Ruddle, 1976). Similar, more recent reports of deprogramming of a differentiated somatic cell to an embryonic state on fusion with pluripotent mouse ES cells (Tada *et al.*, 2001, 2003), with mouse embryonic germ (EG) cells (Tada *et al.*, 1997, 2003) and with human ES cells (Cowan *et al.*, 2005) demonstrate further that these pluripotent stem cells, like oocytes, can reset the developmental transcriptional state of fully committed cells, albeit that the efficiency of this approach remains low (Cowan *et al.*, 2005; Surani, 2005). The question remains as to whether the nucleus or the cytoplasm (or both) of the embryonic cell are required for this reprogramming activity, with one study (Do and Scholer, 2004) reporting that the nucleus is essential and another (Strelchenko *et al.*, 2006) implicating the cytoplasm. In addition, to indisputably ascertain the reprogramming of the somatic cell genome, the embryonic cell genome needs to be eliminated from the hybrid, a challenging technicality that would be required for the therapeutic use of such reprogrammed cells as well (Cowan *et al.*, 2005; Surani, 2005). Further study and development of this method will clearly be addressing such questions.

The methods described in this chapter pertain to the approach of directing the reprogramming of permeabilized somatic cells by exposing them to nuclear and cytoplasmic extracts of the cell type desired *in vitro* (Alberio *et al.*, 2005; Collas and Hakelien, 2003; Hakelien *et al.*, 2002; Hansis *et al.*, 2004). The working hypothesis in this approach is that every given cell type contains the key regulatory factors that determine its gene expression profile and hence, identity; and that exposing a second permeabilized distinct cell to this defined milieu of regulatory factors (such that it takes up critical components, as in cell fusion) can redirect the gene expression pattern, and hence, identity, of the second cell type toward that of the first. If realized, this method would undoubtedly be very powerful, with the clear advantages of being applicable to many cell types even in the absence of complete knowledge of their specific regulatory factors; not involving the complication of tetraploidy inherent in the cell fusion approach; and being scalable because it would use relatively easily available cells in culture. Emerging reports suggest that this could be plausible (see later). However, like other reprogramming strategies, this approach is also at early stages of development, and extensive characterization, optimization, and maturing is forthcoming.

Meanwhile, several researchers have been exploring the use of cellular extracts in obtaining reprogramming, with encouraging results. Incubation of terminally differentiated mouse myotubes in extracts from regenerating newt limbs was found to induce the dedifferentiation of the myotubes to mononucleated cells with a loss of expression of muscle differentiation markers (McGann *et al.*, 2001). Subsequently, a transcriptional repressor, msx1, which is expressed in early regenerating newt limbs, was found to also be able to initiate this dedifferentiation process (Odelberg *et al.*, 2000), indicating that specific factors in cellular extracts can, indeed, initiate reprogramming. Permeabilized human cells (primary leukocytes and the embryonic kidney cell line, 293T) were induced to express the pluripotency markers, the transcription factor Oct 4, and germ cell alkaline phosphatase (GCAP) by exposure to extracts of *Xenopus laevis* eggs and early embryos in a process that seems to involve chromatin remodeling (Hansis *et al.*, 2004). Nuclear lamina remodeling of permeabilized primary bovine somatic cells was also observed on incubation with *Xenopus* egg and oocyte extracts (Alberio *et al.*, 2005). In an impressive body of work using mammalian cell extracts, the Collas group has reported the reprogramming of a variety of reversibly permeabilized mammalian cells including that of the human 293T cell line with T-cell extracts (Hakelien *et al.*, 2002, 2005), neuronal precursor cell extracts (Hakelien *et al.*, 2002), and embryonal carcinoma (EC) cell extract (Taranger *et al.*, 2005); of human primary skin fibroblasts with T-cell extracts (Hakelien *et al.*, 2002); of primary fetal rat fibroblasts with extracts of an insulinoma cell line (Hakelien *et al.*, 2004); of human adipose stem cells with rat cardiomyocyte extracts (Gaustad *et al.*, 2004); of mouse embryonic stem cells with murine pneumocyte extracts (Qin *et al.*, 2005); and of mouse NIH 3T3 cells with mouse ES cell extracts (Taranger *et al.*, 2005). Depending on the study, a variety of assays were used to test for reprogramming. For instance, 293T cells exposed to T-cell extracts were reported to exhibit T-cell characteristics such as expression of T cell–specific genes and cell surface receptors, interleukin-2 (IL-2) secretion, and IL-2 receptor assembly in response to T-cell stimulation agents (Hakelien *et al.*, 2002, 2005). Similarly, 293T cells exposed to EC cell extracts were reported to have attained EC cell–like features such as up-regulation of pluripotency-associated genes Oct 4, Sox 2, and Nanog; down-regulation of differentiation markers such as Lamin A; epigenetic modification (DNA demethylation) in the Oct 4 promoter; and EC-cell–like ability to differentiate into various lineages (Taranger *et al.*, 2005). Although remarkable, the effects obtained were sometimes low, transient (Gaustad *et al.*, 2004; Hakelien *et al.*, 2004), or partial (Hakelien *et al.*, 2002, 2005), and issues remain regarding the long-term stability of the changes seen, the karyotype of resulting cells, and the ability to obtain similar effects with primary cells. Future development of this strategy will hopefully clarify some of these uncertainties.

We have been experimenting with the described strategy above. It can be used, conceivably, to convert an adult differentiated somatic cell to an embryonic or progenitor state (using embryonic stem cell or adult stem cell reprogramming cell extracts) or to another defined differentiated cell type (using extracts from differentiated cells). We present here details of our current protocol that involves the reversible permeabilization of cells using the bacterial toxin Streptolysin O and exposure of these cells to reprogramming cell extracts. Similar methods have been described (Hakelien *et al.*, 2002, 2004, 2006; Walev *et al.*, 2001), and our procedures are adapted from previous publications, on the basis of our optimizing experiences.

Streptolysin O–Mediated Cell Permeabilization and Uptake of Reprogramming Cell Extracts

Streptolysin O (SLO) is a cholesterol binding, thiol-activated, calcium-sensitive bacterial cytotoxin that can form pores in the plasma membrane of mammalian cells up to the size of 35 nm, a process that is generally lethal to the cell (Bhakdi *et al.*, 1985; Walev *et al.*, 2001). Clever exploitation of its properties in the laboratory has, however, provided a powerful way of delivering macromolecules like anti-sense oligonucleotides and functional proteins into a cell (Fawcett *et al.*, 1998; Walev *et al.*, 2001). Limited and transient exposure of cells to low doses of SLO in the absence of calcium ions allows the formation of membrane pores that are large enough to allow the passive diffusion of proteins up to the size of 100 kDa, but not large enough for organelles (Walev *et al.*, 2001). Subsequently, reversal of this membrane permeabilization by adding calcium ions allows the membrane to repair itself, and the resealed cells are viable and can proliferate (Walev *et al.*, 2001).

The reprogramming strategy described here relies on SLO-mediated transient permeabilization of the plasma membrane of the cell to be reprogrammed (referred to here as the *target cell*). During the permeabilization process, the target cell is incubated with whole cell extracts of a defined and different cell type in the presence of permeabilization/reprogramming promoting agents such as an energy-generating system. The whole cell extract provides regulatory factors that are taken up by the permeabilizing target cell. The plasma membrane is then resealed, the cells are allowed to recover, and cultured further. Ideally, components taken up from the cell extracts direct an alteration in the gene expression pattern of the target genome. This is assayed over time.

In this system, efficient permeabilization and uptake of regulatory extract components are clearly crucial to obtaining reprogramming. Optimization of the procedure for a particular cell type is, therefore, highly recommended and may be necessary sometimes. The inclusion of fluorescently conjugated proteins (such as 70 kDa rhodamine-dextran or 68 kDa rhodamine albumin) during the cell and extract incubation provides a convenient way to monitor the efficiency of the process by fluorescence microscopy. On examining various parameters, we find that the efficiency of SLO-mediated membrane permeabilization and uptake of proteins is very sensitive to several factors, including the density of the cells, use of adherent versus suspension cell cultures, the concentration of SLO, SLO activation, length of exposure to SLO and exogenous proteins, the quality of the cell extracts, and time given for resealing of membrane pores and recovery. The most efficient results require striking a balance between maximum exposure to the streptolysin O toxin and the health and recovery of the cells after treatment. The following sections outline details of our optimized conditions in a stepwise fashion.

Cell Permeabilization and the Reprogramming Reaction

As mentioned previously, on the basis of our optimizing experiments, we perform incubations of target cells with reprogramming cell extracts and other reaction ingredients at the same time as we permeabilize them with SLO. The following steps are presented in the order in which they should be performed on the day of the experiment and include a description of the materials needed at each step. Preparation of the reprogramming cell extracts should have been done earlier and is presented in a separate section below. Because these are cell-based manipulations, all materials and supplies must be maintained in a tissue culture sterile manner.

Streptolysin O Activation

Like other toxins of its family, streptolysin O is reversibly inactivated by atmospheric oxygen and requires the presence of a reducing agent for maximum activity (Bhakdi *et al.*, 1985). We routinely activate our working aliquot of SLO by incubation with a reducing agent just before use.

Materials

- Streptolysin O (Sigma-Aldrich, St. Louis, MO; Catalog No. S 0149): Stock solution 25 units/μl in sterile Milli-Q water; stored in single-use 20-μl aliquots at $-20°$.
- Dithiothreitol (DTT; Sigma-Aldrich; Catalog No. D 5545): Stock solution 1M, in Milli-Q water (sterile filtered); aliquoted and stored at $-20°$.
- Hank's balanced salt solution without calcium and magnesium (HBSS; Mediatech, Inc., Herndon, VA; Catalog No. 21–022-CV).

Protocol

1. Thaw one 20-μl aliquot of the stock SLO solution (25 units/μl).
2. Add 5 μl of 1 M DTT (final concentration 5 mM) and 975 μl of HBSS. Mix well (final SLO concentration 0.5 units/μl).
3. Incubate at $37°$ for 2 h.

Preparation of the Cells to be Permeabilized (Target Cells)

Materials

- Growth and passaging reagents specific to the target cell type (cell culture media, phosphate-buffered saline [PBS], trypsin-ethylenediaminetetraacetic acid [Trypsin-EDTA]).

Protocol

1. Seed and grow the target cells in their regular growth conditions such that healthy, exponentially growing cultures are available on the day of the experiment.

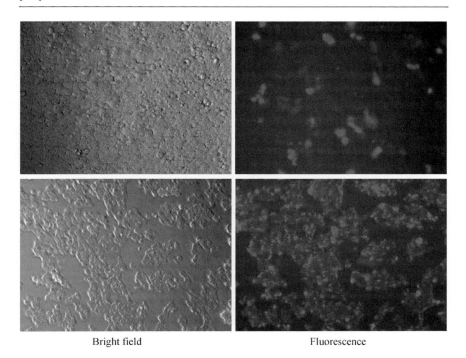

Bright field						Fluorescence

FIG. 1. Comparison of Streptolysin-O (SLO)-mediated permeabilization and uptake of fluorescently labeled marker proteins in adherent and suspension cell cultures. Adherent *(top row)* or suspension *(bottom row)* cultures of human embryonic kidney 293T cells were permeabilized using SLO in the presence of rhodamine-conjugated 70-KDa dextran. Left panels, bright field images; Right panels, fluorescence views of the same corresponding fields. Original magnification, ×20.

2. In the case of adherent cells, detach them from the cell culture dish (usually by trypsinization as per their passaging protocol) and bring into suspension. The efficiency of SLO-mediated permeabilization and uptake of proteins from the cell extracts is much higher in suspension cell cultures than in attached cells grown in monolayers (Fig. 1), presumably because of the difference in the cell surface area exposed to SLO and the extracts. As shown in Fig. 1, this can be a difference of 10–20% of the cells taking up protein in adherent cultures versus 90–100% of the cells in suspension cultures. This aspect can make a very large difference in the extent of reprogramming obtained.

3. Wash the cells in HBSS (calcium and magnesium free) two times, sedimenting them in a swinging bucket rotor at 1000 rpm for 5 min at room

temperature. This is important to eliminate any serum proteins or calcium ions that could interfere with the permeabilization reaction.

4. Count the cells using a hemacytometer.

5. Aliquot $1–3 \times 10^5$ cells per reaction in sterile 1.5-ml Eppendorf tubes. The number of cells per reaction is cell type–dependent for one given concentration of SLO. In general, lower numbers of larger sized cells are optimal. To set up several identical reactions (to assay them at different times post the reprogramming reaction, for instance), multiple reactions can be set up together in bulk to a limited extent, as long as the cells are not found to start clumping.

Assembly of Permeabilization and Reprogramming Reaction

Materials

- EDTA (Sigma-Aldrich; Catalog No. E 6758): Stock solution 0.5 M, pH 8.5, in Milli-Q water (sterile filtered); stored at room temperature (RT).
- Magnesium chloride ($MgCl_2$; Sigma-Aldrich; Catalog No. M 8266): Stock solution 0.1 M in Milli-Q water (sterile filtered); stored at RT.
- Nucleotide triphosphate (NTP) set (Roche, Basel, Switzerland; Catalog No. 1277057): Stock mix of each NTP at 25 mM, aliquoted, and stored at $-20°$.
- Creatine kinase (Viral Therapeutics, Inc., Ithaca, NY; Catalog No. CKMB2): Stock 1.5 mg/ml, aliquoted, and stored at $-80°$.
- Phosphocreatine (Sigma-Aldrich; Catalog No. P 7936): Stock 1 M in Milli-Q water (sterile filtered), aliquoted, and stored at $-20°$.
- ATP (Sigma-Aldrich; Catalog No. A 3377): Stock 100 mM in Milli-Q water (sterile filtered), aliquoted, and stored at $-20°$.
- GTP (Sigma-Aldrich; Catalog No. G 8752): Stock 10 mM in Milli-Q water (sterile filtered), aliquoted, and stored at $-20°$.
- Cytochalasin B (Sigma-Aldrich; Catalog No. C 6762): Stock 2 mg/ml in dimethyl sulfoxide (DMSO), aliquoted, and stored at $-20°$.
- Rhodamine-conjugated dextran 70,000 MW (Invitrogen-Molecular Probes, Carlsbad, CA; Catalog No. D 1819): Stock 5 mg/ml in sterile Milli-Q water, aliquoted, and stored at $-20°$.
- Rhodamine-conjugated albumin (Invitrogen-Molecular Probes, Carlsbad,CA; Catalog No. A 23016): Stock 5 mg/ml in sterile Milli-Q water, aliquoted, and stored at $-20°$.

Protocol

1. Sediment the prepared target cell aliquots ($1–3 \times 10^5$ cells per reaction) in a swinging bucket rotor at 1000 rpm for 5 min at RT.

2. To each cell pellet add, in order:
   a. Reprogramming cell extract/ control extract (1.5–6 μg/l): 73 μl
   b. 0.5 M EDTA: 2 μl (final concentration: 10 mM)
   c. 0.1 M MgCl$_2$: 5 μl (final concentration: 5 mM)
   d. 25 mM NTP stock mix: 4 μl (final concentration: 1 mM each NTP)
   e. 1.5 mg/ml Creatine kinase: 1.5 μl (final concentration: 25 μg/ml)
   f. 1 M Phosphocreatine: 1 μl (final concentration: 10 mM)
   g. 100 mM ATP: 1 μl (final concentration: 1 mM)
   h. 10 mM GTP: 1 μl (final concentration: 100 μM)
   i. 2 mg/ml Cytochalasin B: 0.75 μl (final concentration: 15 μg/ml)

Gently tap the reaction tube intermittently during these additions to prevent settling of the cells. Preparation of the reprogramming cell extract is described in the next section. As control extracts, we usually use whole cell extracts of the target cells, prepared exactly as the reprogramming extracts. If setting up multiple identical reactions together in bulk, the amounts added of the preceding listed reaction components should be increased accordingly. However, after assembly of the preceding reaction mix in bulk, we find it advisable to aliquot the bulk mix to individual reactions in individual reaction tubes to avoid excessive cell clumping in the following incubation step.

3. To each individual reaction tube, add 10 μl of 0.5 units/μl activated SLO (final SLO concentration: 50 units/ml). The efficiency of SLO-mediated permeabilization varies among cell types. The optimum concentration of SLO should, therefore, be determined empirically for a particular cell type by titration. For these and other optimization experiments, fluorescence-conjugated marker proteins such as rhodamine-labeled dextran (70 kDa) or rhodamine-labeled albumin (68 kDa) are included during the assembly and incubation of the reprogramming reaction (final concentration 10–50 μg/ml). After resealing of the target cell membrane, uptake of the fluorescent proteins is assessed by fluorescence microscopy and is indicative of the efficiency of cell permeabilization, resealing of the membrane and cell survival.

4. Incubate the reactions at 37° for 3 h. To prevent the cells from settling or clumping during this incubation, we use a gentle rocker in a 37° incubator.

Resealing and Recovery of Permeabilized Cells

Materials

- Growth and passaging reagents specific to the target/reprogramming extract cell type.

Protocol

1. After the incubation, gently pipet all the contents of each reaction and dilute in 0.75 ml of cell culture media in one well of a 4-well or 24-well dish. The cell culture media should contain at least 2 mM CaCl$_2$ to initiate resealing of the permeabilized cell membrane. Target cell–specific culture conditions should also be provided: for instance, permeabilized 293T cells need to be seeded on polylysine-coated plates to reattach after permeabilization.

2. Incubate the cells overnight at 37° in standard culture conditions to recover.

3. The next day, aspirate away unattached dead cells and refresh the cell culture media.

4. Examine the cells and/or harvest them for an early time point of assessment of reprogramming. If fluorescently labeled proteins were included in the permeabilization reaction to monitor the process, examine them by fluorescence microscopy over the next few days. Figure 2 depicts uptake and retention of rhodamine-conjugated albumin in a variety of SLO-permeabilized primary cell types. Notably, in all cases, the cells take up the fluorescent protein robustly, recover from the reprogramming reaction to grow to confluence, and seem to retain and partition the input protein through successive doublings— observations that suggest that reprogramming factors from cell extracts could also last long enough in the target cells to exert their influence.

5. Culture the cells as usual until harvested for evaluation of reprogramming, usually over a time course. Cultures that grow to confluence can be passaged to generate subcultures for further time points of evaluation.

Evaluation of Cell Reprogramming

The goal of reprogramming here is to bring about a change in the gene expression profile of the target cell to that of the source of the reprogramming cell extracts. Various assays that examine such a change can be used, including looking directly for the gain of expression of specific marker genes that represent the new cell type at the RNA level by reverse transcriptase-polymerase chain reaction (RT-PCR) analysis or at the protein level by immunofluorescence or immunoblotting. Concomitantly, loss of expression of genes that represent the target cell type is also expected. Initially, RT-PCR analysis is expected to be the most sensitive test. As the reprogramming effect gets more robust, with time or with altered conditions of experimentation, changes at the protein level, in multiple marker genes, in global transcription patterns and, ultimately, in function and morphology are aimed for.

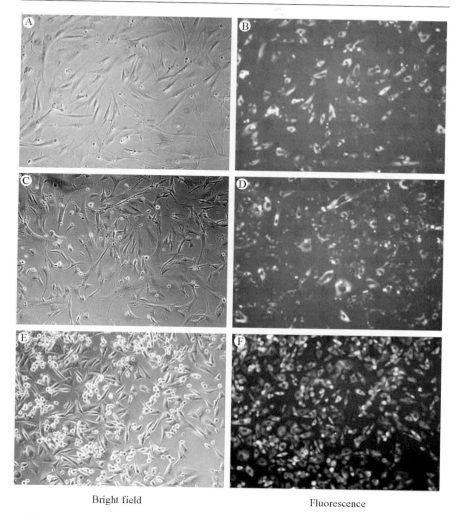

Bright field   Fluorescence

Fig. 2. Streptolysin-O (SLO)-mediated permeabilization and uptake of rhodamine-conjugated albumin in various primary cells. Human primary adult dermal fibroblasts (A and B), human primary neonatal dermal fibroblasts (C and D), and mouse primary fibroblasts (E and F) were permeabilized using SLO in the presence of rhodamine-conjugated albumin. Left panels, bright-field images; right panels, fluorescence views of the same corresponding fields. Original magnification, ×10.

Preparation of Reprogramming Cell Extracts

The quality of the reprogramming cell extracts used in this strategy is critical. Since the identity or levels of the crucial "reprogramming factors" in the extracts is unknown and can, therefore, not be examined directly, it is important that the cells used to prepare extracts be healthy and the extracts be handled carefully at all times, with the aim of preserving all vital components. For instance, if preparing embryonic cell extracts to dedifferentiate target cells, it should be ensured that the starting cultures are primarily undifferentiated themselves. Because the cell extracts will be applied to living cells during the permeabilization and reprogramming reaction, they cannot be prepared using any detergents. Instead, they are generated by a combination of physical disruption by sonication and freezing and thawing. It is important that the genomic DNA of the source cells of these extracts be disrupted as much as possible to avoid any artifacts caused by uptake of this DNA by the permeabilized target cells. Again, because these extracts will be used for cell-based manipulations, all materials and supplies must be maintained in a tissue culture sterile manner.

Materials

- Growth and subculturing reagents specific to the extract cell type (Cell culture media, phosphate-buffered saline (PBS), trypsin-EDTA)
- Phosphate-buffered saline (PBS), without calcium and magnesium (Mediatech, Inc.; Catalog No. 21–040-CV)
- Lysis buffer (20 mM HEPES, pH 8.2, 5 mM MgCl$_2$, 1 mM DTT, 1× protease inhibitors): prepared fresh and kept on ice.

Protocol

1. Begin with healthy, exponentially growing cells. Confluent or overgrown cultures tend to yield extracts that are more toxic to the cells to be permeabilized.

2. Harvest the cells as per their standard protocol, usually with trypsin-EDTA for adherent cells. Rather large quantities of cell extract are required for this strategy, so plan accordingly.

3. Wash the cells in PBS (without calcium and magnesium) two times, sedimenting them in a swinging bucket rotor at 1000 rpm for 5 min at RT. This is important to eliminate any serum proteins or calcium ions that could interfere with the permeabilization/reprogramming reaction. The cell pellet can, after the washes, be snap frozen in liquid nitrogen and stored at −80°. It is often more convenient to collect a few cell pellets and proceed with processing them for cell extracts at the same time. Keep on ice from now on.

4. Estimate the volume of the cell pellet and resuspend well in 1–2 volumes of freshly prepared, ice-cold lysis buffer by pipetting up and down gently. It is preferable to keep the cell suspension as concentrated as possible at this stage; however, overconcentrated suspensions do not lyse well on sonication (see below). In addition, cell suspensions of less than 0.5 ml total volume should be transferred to 1.5-ml microcentrifuge tubes to minimize loss of cells along the walls of larger tubes during sonication.

5. Incubate the cells on ice for 1 h. This incubation of the cells in the hypotonic lysis buffer will cause them to swell, which facilitates their disruption during sonication.

6. Sonicate the cells in short pulses until they are all lysed. We use a Fisher Scientific Sonic Dismembrator, Model 100. Keep the probe of the sonicator as sterile as possible, by cleaning with water and alcohol. Also, wash the probe well if shifting between different cell extracts. The power and time of sonication may vary between cell types. If multiple pulses are required, cool the cells on ice between pulses to avoid heating up and degrading extract components. Complete sonication can be judged by a loss in the viscosity of the lysate. The lysate can also be examined under the microscope for loss of intact cells and nuclei.

7. Transfer the sonicated cell lysate to 1.5-ml microcentrifuge tubes, if not already there.

8. Snap-freeze the lysate in liquid nitrogen. Follow this by a quick thaw in a 37° water bath to fragment any remaining genomic DNA.

9. Centrifuge the lysate for 15–30 min at 4° in a fixed-angle micro-centrifuge at 14,000 rpm.

10. Aliquot the supernatant in 200–500 μl volumes, depending on use, to avoid multiple freezing and thawing cycles. Store at −80°.

11. Determine the protein concentration of the cell extract. Typically, we obtain concentrations of 6–9 mg/ml. For the reprogramming reactions, we have used the cell extracts between 1.5–6 mg/ml. Depending on the specific cell extract, some are very toxic to the permeabilized target cells at higher concentrations. This needs to be determined empirically for each extract and target cell type.

12. It is very important to run some quality control tests on the cell extracts generated: at least initially and, preferably, intermittently thereafter. Examine the cell extracts by resolving the proteins by electrophoresis and inspecting the general protein profile by Coomassie stain to ensure that there is no visible protein degradation. It is also advisable to examine the intactness of a few expected cell type–specific proteins (nuclear and cytoplasmic) in the cell extracts by immunoblotting. In particular, proteins that are known to have critical "master regulatory" roles in a particular cell type could be examined.

The field of reprogramming is clearly in its nascent stages. Several complementary strategies are, however, being explored. Studies that use these strategies as tools to dissect the molecular and biochemical components of the reprogramming phenomenology observed thus far are also emerging. Lessons learned from these studies will prove valuable to our understanding of developmental biology, as well as to therapeutic applications. Lessons learned already (and being learned) from isolating, characterizing, and differentiating embryonic and adult stem cells are being used in developing reprogramming conditions. These studies also have direct application if, for instance, patient-specific cells need to be deprogrammed to an early differentiation stage before desired cell types can be derived from them. Collective efforts of a creative scientific community could very well turn the lofty goal of reprogramming one somatic cell to another into reality.

Acknowledgments

Grateful thanks to Carmin Szynal, Yordanka Ivanova, Katherine Holton, and Jennifer Shepard for experimental help during the course of the development of these methods. This work was performed in part under the support of the U.S. Department of Commerce, National Institutes of Standards and Technology, Advanced Technology Program, Cooperative Agreement Number 70NANB1H3015.

References

Alberio, R., Johnson, A. D., Stick, R., and Campbell, K. H. (2005). Differential nuclear remodeling of mammalian somatic cells by *Xenopus laevis* oocyte and egg cytoplasm. *Exp. Cell Res.* **307,** 131–141.

Andrews, P. W. (2002). From teratocarcinomas to embryonic stem cells. *Philos. Trans. R. Soc. Lond. B Biol. Sci.* **357,** 405–417.

Bhakdi, S., Tranum-Jensen, J., and Sziegoleit, A. (1985). Mechanism of membrane damage by streptolysin-O. *Infect. Immun.* **47,** 52–60.

Blau, H. M., and Baltimore, D. (1991). Differentiation requires continuous regulation. *J. Cell Biol.* **112,** 781–783.

Blau, H. M., and Blakely, B. T. (1999). Plasticity of cell fate: Insights from heterokaryons. *Semin. Cell Dev. Biol.* **10,** 267–272.

Blau, H. M., Chiu, C. P., and Webster, C. (1983). Cytoplasmic activation of human nuclear genes in stable heterokaryons. *Cell* **32,** 1171–1180.

Blau, H. M., Pavlath, G. K., Hardeman, E. C., Chiu, C. P., Silberstein, L., Webster, S. G., Miller, S. C., and Webster, C. (1985). Plasticity of the differentiated state. *Science* **230,** 758–766.

Brockes, J. P., and Kumar, A. (2002). Plasticity and reprogramming of differentiated cells in amphibian regeneration. *Nat. Rev. Mol. Cell. Biol.* **3,** 566–574.

Chiu, C. P., and Blau, H. M. (1984). Reprogramming cell differentiation in the absence of DNA synthesis. *Cell* **37,** 879–887.

Chiu, C. P., and Blau, H. M. (1985). 5-Azacytidine permits gene activation in a previously noninducible cell type. *Cell* **40,** 417–424.

Cibelli, J. B., Stice, S. L., Golueke, P. J., Kane, J. J., Jerry, J., Blackwell, C., Ponce de Leon, F. A., and Robl, J. M. (1998). Transgenic bovine chimeric offspring produced from somatic cell-derived stem-like cells. *Nat. Biotechnol.* **16,** 642–646.

Collas, P., and Hakelien, A. M. (2003). Teaching cells new tricks. *Trends Biotechnol.* **21,** 354–361.

Condorelli, G., Borello, U., De Angelis, L., Latronico, M., Sirabella, D., Coletta, M., Galli, R., Balconi, G., Follenzi, A., Frati, G., Cusella De Angelis, M. G., Gioglio, L., *et al.* (2001). Cardiomyocytes induce endothelial cells to trans-differentiate into cardiac muscle: Implications for myocardium regeneration. *Proc. Natl. Acad. Sci. USA* **98,** 10733–10738.

Cowan, C. A., Atienza, J., Melton, D. A., and Eggan, K. (2005). Nuclear reprogramming of somatic cells after fusion with human embryonic stem cells. *Science* **309,** 1369–1373.

Dabeva, M. D., Hwang, S. G., Vasa, S. R., Hurston, E., Novikoff, P. M., Hixson, D. C., Gupta, S., and Shafritz, D. A. (1997). Differentiation of pancreatic epithelial progenitor cells into hepatocytes following transplantation into rat liver. *Proc. Natl. Acad. Sci. USA* **94,** 7356–7361.

Do, J. T., and Scholer, H. R. (2004). Nuclei of embryonic stem cells reprogram somatic cells. *Stem Cells* **22,** 941–949.

Echeverri, K., and Tanaka, E. M. (2002). Ectoderm to mesoderm lineage switching during axolotl tail regeneration. *Science* **298,** 1993–1996.

Eggan, K., Baldwin, K., Tackett, M., Osborne, J., Gogos, J., Chess, A., Axel, R., and Jaenisch, R. (2004). Mice cloned from olfactory sensory neurons. *Nature* **428,** 44–49.

Eguchi, G., and Kodama, R. (1993). Transdifferentiation. *Curr. Opin. Cell Biol.* **5,** 1023–1028.

Fawcett, J. M., Harrison, S. M., and Orchard, C. H. (1998). A method for reversible permeabilization of isolated rat ventricular myocytes. *Exp. Physiol.* **83,** 293–303.

Ferber, S., Halkin, A., Cohen, H., Ber, I., Einav, Y., Goldberg, I., Barshack, I., Seijffers, R., Kopolovic, J., Kaiser, N., and Karasik, A. (2000). Pancreatic and duodenal homeobox gene 1 induces expression of insulin genes in liver and ameliorates streptozotocin-induced hyperglycemia. *Nat. Med.* **6,** 568–572.

Gaustad, K. G., Boquest, A. C., Anderson, B. E., Gerdes, A. M., and Collas, P. (2004). Differentiation of human adipose tissue stem cells using extracts of rat cardiomyocytes. *Biochem. Biophys. Res. Commun.* **314,** 420–427.

Guan, K., Nayernia, K., Maier, L. S., Wagner, S., Dressel, R., Lee, J. H., Nolte, J., Wolf, F., Li, M., Engel, W., and Hasenfuss, G. (2006). Pluripotency of spermatogonial stem cells from adult mouse testis. *Nature* **440,** 1199–1203.

Gurdon, J. B., and Byrne, J. A. (2003). The first half-century of nuclear transplantation. *Proc. Natl. Acad. Sci. USA* **100,** 8048–8052.

Haggitt, R. C., Tryzelaar, J., Ellis, F. H., and Colcher, H. (1978). Adenocarcinoma complicating columnar epithelium-lined (Barrett's) esophagus. *Am. J. Clin. Pathol.* **70,** 1–5.

Hakelien, A. M., Gaustad, K. G., and Collas, P. (2004). Transient alteration of cell fate using a nuclear and cytoplasmic extract of an insulinoma cell line. *Biochem. Biophys. Res. Commun.* **316,** 834–841.

Hakelien, A. M., Gaustad, K. G., and Collas, P. (2006). Modulation of cell fate using nuclear and cytoplasmic extracts. *Methods Mol. Biol.* **325,** 99–114.

Hakelien, A. M., Gaustad, K. G., Taranger, C. K., Skalhegg, B. S., Kuntziger, T., and Collas, P. (2005). Long-term *in vitro,* cell-type-specific genome-wide reprogramming of gene expression. *Exp. Cell Res.* **309,** 32–47.

Hakelien, A. M., Landsverk, H. B., Robl, J. M., Skalhegg, B. S., and Collas, P. (2002). Reprogramming fibroblasts to express T-cell functions using cell extracts. *Nat. Biotechnol.* **20**, 460–466.

Hansis, C., Barreto, G., Maltry, N., and Niehrs, C. (2004). Nuclear reprogramming of human somatic cells by xenopus egg extract requires BRG1. *Curr. Biol.* **14**, 1475–1480.

Hay, E. D., and Zuk, A. (1995). Transformations between epithelium and mesenchyme: Normal, pathological, and experimentally induced. *Am. J. Kidney Dis.* **26**, 678–690.

Hochedlinger, K., and Jaenisch, R. (2002). Monoclonal mice generated by nuclear transfer from mature B and T donor cells. *Nature* **415**, 1035–1038.

Hochedlinger, K., and Jaenisch, R. (2006). Nuclear reprogramming and pluripotency. *Nature* **441**, 1061–1067.

Hu, E., Tontonoz, P., and Spiegelman, B. M. (1995). Transdifferentiation of myoblasts by the adipogenic transcription factors PPAR gamma and C/EBP alpha. *Proc. Natl. Acad. Sci. USA* **92**, 9856–9860.

Kablar, B., Tajbakhsh, S., and Rudnicki, M. A. (2000). Transdifferentiation of esophageal smooth to skeletal muscle is myogenic bHLH factor-dependent. *Development* **127**, 1627–1639.

Kanatsu-Shinohara, M., Inoue, K., Lee, J., Yoshimoto, M., Ogonuki, N., Miki, H., Baba, S., Kato, T., Kazuki, Y., Toyokuni, S., Toyoshima, M., Niwa, O., *et al.* (2004). Generation of pluripotent stem cells from neonatal mouse testis. *Cell* **119**, 1001–1012.

Lawrence, P. A., and Morata, G. (1983). The elements of the bithorax complex. *Cell* **35**, 595–601.

Li, W. C., Yu, W. Y., Quinlan, J. M., Burke, Z. D., and Tosh, D. (2005). The molecular basis of transdifferentiation. *J. Cell Mol. Med.* **9**, 569–582.

McGann, C. J., Odelberg, S. J., and Keating, M. T. (2001). Mammalian myotube dedifferentiation induced by newt regeneration extract. *Proc. Natl. Acad. Sci. USA* **98**, 13699–13704.

Miller, R. A., and Ruddle, F. H. (1976). Pluripotent teratocarcinoma-thymus somatic cell hybrids. *Cell* **9**, 45–55.

Munsie, M. J., Michalska, A. E., O'Brien, C. M., Trounson, A. O., Pera, M. F., and Mountford, P. S. (2000). Isolation of pluripotent embryonic stem cells from reprogrammed adult mouse somatic cell nuclei. *Curr. Biol.* **10**, 989–992.

Odelberg, S. J., Kollhoff, A., and Keating, M. T. (2000). Dedifferentiation of mammalian myotubes induced by msx1. *Cell* **103**, 1099–1109.

Okada, T. S. (1991). "Transdifferentiation Flexibility in Cell Differentiation." Oxford, Clarendon.

Patapoutian, A., Wold, B. J., and Wagner, R. A. (1995). Evidence for developmentally programmed transdifferentiation in mouse esophageal muscle. *Science* **270**, 1818–1821.

Pomerantz, J., and Blau, H. M. (2004). Nuclear reprogramming: A key to stem cell function in regenerative medicine. *Nat. Cell Biol.* **6**, 810–816.

Poss, K. D., Keating, M. T., and Nechiporuk, A. (2003). Tales of regeneration in zebrafish. *Dev. Dyn.* **226**, 202–210.

Qin, M., Tai, G., Collas, P., Polak, J. M., and Bishop, A. E. (2005). Cell extract-derived differentiation of embryonic stem cells. *Stem Cells* **23**, 712–718.

Raff, M. (2003). Adult stem cell plasticity: Fact or artifact? *Annu. Rev. Cell Dev. Biol.* **19**, 1–22.

Ringertz, N., and Savage, R. E. (1976). "Cell Hybrids." Academic Press, New York.

Shen, C. N., Horb, M. E., Slack, J. M., and Tosh, D. (2003). Transdifferentiation of pancreas to liver. *Mech. Dev.* **120**, 107–116.

Strelchenko, N., Kukharenko, V., Shkumatov, A., Verlinsky, O., Kuliev, A., and Verlinsky, Y. (2006). Reprogramming of human somatic cells by embryonic stem cell cytoplast. *Reprod. Biomed. Online* **12**, 107–111.

Strutz, F., and Muller, G. A. (2000). Transdifferentiation comes of age. *Nephrol. Dial. Transplant.* **15**, 1729–1731.

Surani, M. A. (2005). Nuclear reprogramming by human embryonic stem cells. *Cell* **122**, 653–654.

Tada, M., Morizane, A., Kimura, H., Kawasaki, H., Ainscough, J. F., Sasai, Y., Nakatsuji, N., and Tada, T. (2003). Pluripotency of reprogrammed somatic genomes in embryonic stem hybrid cells. *Dev. Dyn.* **227**, 504–510.

Tada, M., Tada, T., Lefebvre, L., Barton, S. C., and Surani, M. A. (1997). Embryonic germ cells induce epigenetic reprogramming of somatic nucleus in hybrid cells. *EMBO J.* **16**, 6510–6520.

Tada, M., Takahama, Y., Abe, K., Nakatsuji, N., and Tada, T. (2001). Nuclear reprogramming of somatic cells by *in vitro* hybridization with ES cells. *Curr. Biol.* **11**, 1553–1558.

Taranger, C. K., Noer, A., Sorensen, A. L., Hakelien, A. M., Boquest, A. C., and Collas, P. (2005). Induction of dedifferentiation, genomewide transcriptional programming, and epigenetic reprogramming by extracts of carcinoma and embryonic stem cells. *Mol. Biol. Cell* **16**, 5719–5735.

Wakayama, T., Tabar, V., Rodriguez, I., Perry, A. C., Studer, L., and Mombaerts, P. (2001). Differentiation of embryonic stem cell lines generated from adult somatic cells by nuclear transfer. *Science* **292**, 740–743.

Walev, I., Bhakdi, S. C., Hofmann, F., Djonder, N., Valeva, A., Aktories, K., and Bhakdi, S. (2001). Delivery of proteins into living cells by reversible membrane permeabilization with streptolysin-O. *Proc. Natl. Acad. Sci. USA* **98**, 3185–3190.

Wei, G., Schubiger, G., Harder, F., and Muller, A. M. (2000). Stem cell plasticity in mammals and transdetermination in Drosophila: Common themes? *Stem Cells* **18**, 409–414.

Wilmut, I., Schnieke, A. E., McWhir, J., Kind, A. J., and Campbell, K. H. (1997). Viable offspring derived from fetal and adult mammalian cells. *Nature* **385**, 810–813.

Section II

Tissue Engineering and Regenerative Medicine

[13]   Tissue Engineering Using Adult Stem Cells

By DANIEL EBERLI and ANTHONY ATALA

Abstract

Patients with a variety of diseases may be treated with transplanted tissues and organs. However, there is a shortage of donor tissues and organs, which is worsening yearly because of the aging population. Scientists in the field of tissue engineering are applying the principles of cell transplantation, material science, and bioengineering to construct biological substitutes that will restore and maintain normal function in diseased and injured tissues. The stem cell field is also advancing rapidly, opening new options for cellular therapy and tissue engineering. The use of adult stem cells for tissue engineering applications is promising. This chapter discusses applications of these new technologies for the engineering of tissues and organs. The first part provides an overview of regenerative medicine and tissue engineering techniques; the second highlights different adult stem cell populations used for tissue regeneration.

Introduction

Organ damage or loss can occur from congenital disorders, cancer, trauma, infection, inflammation, iatrogenic injuries, or other conditions and often necessitates reconstruction or replacement. Depending on the organ and severity of damage, autologous tissues can be used for reconstruction. However, for most tissues in the body there is not sufficient tissue and there is a degree of morbidity associated with the harvest procedure. For functional replacement, organ transplants are used for damaged tissues. However, there is a severe shortage of donor organs, which is worsening with the aging of the population. Both aforementioned approaches rarely replace the entire function of the original organ. Tissues used for reconstruction can lead to complications because of their inherent different functional parameters. The replacement of deficient tissues with functionally equivalent tissues would improve the outcome for these patients. Therefore, engineered biological substitutes that can restore and maintain normal tissue function would be useful in tissue and organ replacement applications.

Tissue engineering, one of the major components of regenerative medicine, follows the principles of cell transplantation, materials science, and engineering toward the development of biological substitutes that can

METHODS IN ENZYMOLOGY, VOL. 420
0076-6879/06 $35.00
DOI: 10.1016/S0076-6879(06)20013-2

restore and maintain normal function. Tissue engineering strategies generally fall into two categories: the use of acellular matrices, which depend on the body's natural ability to regenerate for proper orientation and direction of new tissue growth, and the use of matrices with cells. Acellular tissue matrices are usually prepared by manufacturing artificial scaffolds or by removing cellular components from tissues by mechanical and chemical manipulation to produce collagen-rich matrices (Chen *et al.*, 1999; Dahms *et al.*, 1998; Piechota *et al.*, 1998; Yoo *et al.*, 1998). These matrices tend to slowly degrade on implantation and are generally replaced by the extracellular matrix (ECM) proteins that are secreted by the ingrowing cells.

When native cells are used for tissue engineering, a small piece of donor tissue is dissociated into individual cells. These cells are expanded in culture, attached to a support matrix, and then reimplanted into the host after expansion. Cells can also be used for therapy through injection, either with carriers such as hydrogels or alone.

The source of donor tissue can be heterologous (different species), allogeneic (same species, different individual), or autologous (same individual). Ideally, both structural and functional tissue replacement will occur with minimal complications. The preferred cells to use are autologous cells, in which a biopsy of tissue is obtained from the host, the cells are dissociated and expanded in culture, and the expanded cells are implanted into the same host (Atala, 2001, 2005; Oberpenning *et al.*, 1999; Schultz *et al.*, 2006; Yoo *et al.*, 1999). The use of autologous cells, although it may cause an inflammatory response, avoids rejection, and thus the deleterious side effects of immunosuppressive medications can be avoided.

Most current strategies for tissue engineering depend on a sample of autologous cells from the diseased organ of the host. However, for many patients with extensive end-stage organ failure, a tissue biopsy may not yield enough normal cells for expansion and transplantation. In other instances, primary autologous human cells cannot be expanded from a particular organ, such as the pancreas. In these situations, embryonic and adult stem cells are an alternative source of cells from which the desired tissue can be derived. Embryonic stem cells can be derived from discarded human embryos or from fetal tissues. Adult stem cells can be harvested from adult tissues, including bone marrow, fat, muscle, and skin. These cells can be differentiated into the desired cell type in culture and then used for bioengineering.

To complete the list of possible cell sources for bioengineering of tissues and organs, therapeutic cloning must be mentioned. Therapeutic cloning, which has also been called *nuclear transplantation* and *nuclear transfer*, involves the introduction of a nucleus from a donor cell into an enucleated oocyte to generate an embryo with a genetic makeup identical to that of the donor. Stem cells can be derived from this source, which may have the potential to be used therapeutically.

The use of native cells and adult stem cells is ethically sound and accepted by all major religions and governments. On the other hand, the use of embryonic stem cells and therapeutical cloning are more controversial because the same methods could theoretically be used to clone human beings.

Major advances have been achieved in engineering of tissues within the past decade. Regenerative medicine may extend the treatment options for various diseases. However, like every new evolving field, regenerative medicine and tissue engineering are expensive. Several of the clinical trials involving bioengineered products have been placed on hold because of costs involved with the specific technology. With a bioengineered product, costs are usually high because of the biological nature of the therapies involved. As with any therapy, the cost that the medical health care system can allow for a specific technology is limited. Therefore, the costs of bioengineered products have to be reduced for them to have an impact clinically. This is currently being addressed for multiple tissue-engineered technologies. As the technologies advance over time and the volume of the application is considered, costs will naturally decrease.

Native Cells and Progenitor Cells

One of the limitations of applying cell-based regenerative medicine techniques to organ replacement has been the inherent difficulty of growing specific cell types in large quantities. By studying the privileged sites for committed precursor cells in specific organs, as well as exploring the conditions that promote differentiation, one may be able to overcome the obstacles that limit cell expansion *in vitro*.

For example, in the past, urothelial cells could be grown in the institution setting, but only with limited expansion. Several protocols were developed over the past two decades that identified the undifferentiated cells and kept them undifferentiated during their growth phase (Cilento *et al.*, 1994; Puthenveettil *et al.*, 1999; Scriven *et al.*, 1997). Using these methods of cell culture, it is now possible to expand a urothelial strain from a single specimen that initially covered a surface area of 1 cm^2 to one covering a surface area of 4202 m^2 (the equivalent of one football field) within 8 weeks (Yoo *et al.*, 1998).

These studies indicated that it should be possible to collect autologous bladder cells from human patients, expand them in culture, and return them to the donor in sufficient quantities for reconstructive purposes (Cilento *et al.*, 1994; Liebert *et al.*, 1997; Nguyen *et al.*, 1999; Puthenveettil *et al.*, 1999; Strem *et al.*, 2005). Major advances have been achieved within the past decade in the possible expansion of a variety of progenitor cells and adult stem cells, with specific techniques that make the use of autologous cells possible for clinical application.

Biomaterials

For cell-based tissue engineering, the expanded cells are seeded onto a scaffold synthesized with the appropriate biomaterial. In tissue engineering, biomaterials replicate the biological and mechanical function of the native ECM found in tissues in the body by serving as an artificial ECM. Biomaterials provide a three-dimensional space for the cells to form into new tissues with appropriate structure and function and also can allow for the delivery of cells and appropriate bioactive factors (e.g., cell adhesion peptides, growth factors) to desired sites in the body (Kim and Mooney, 1998). Because most mammalian cell types are anchorage-dependent and will die if no cell-adhesion substrate is available, biomaterials provide a cell-adhesion substrate that can deliver cells to specific sites in the body with high loading efficiency. Biomaterials can also provide mechanical support against *in vivo* forces such that the predefined three-dimensional structure is maintained during tissue development. Furthermore, bioactive signals, such as cell-adhesion peptides and growth factors, can be loaded along with cells to help regulate cellular function.

The ideal biomaterial should be biodegradable and bioresorbable to support the replacement of normal tissue without inflammation. Incompatible materials are destined for an inflammatory or foreign-body response that eventually leads to rejection and/or necrosis. Degradation products, if produced, should be removed from the body by metabolic pathways at an adequate rate that keeps the concentration of these degradation products in the tissues at a tolerable level. The biomaterial should also provide an environment in which appropriate regulation of cell behavior (adhesion, proliferation, migration, and differentiation) can occur such that functional tissue can form. Cell behavior in the newly formed tissue has been shown to be regulated by multiple interactions of the cells with their microenvironment, including interactions with cell-adhesion ligands and with soluble growth factors (Hynes, 1992).

Because biomaterials provide temporary mechanical support while the cells undergo spatial tissue reorganization, the properly chosen biomaterial should allow the engineered tissue to maintain sufficient mechanical integrity to support itself in early development. In late development, it should have begun degradation such that it does not hinder further tissue growth.

(Kim and Mooney, 1998). Generally, three classes of biomaterials have been used for engineering tissues: naturally derived materials (e.g., collagen and alginate), acellular tissue matrices (e.g., bladder submucosa and small intestinal submucosa), and synthetic polymers such as polyglycolic acid (PGA), polylactic acid (PLA), and poly(lactic-co-glycolic acid) (PLGA). These classes of biomaterials have been tested in respect to their biocompatibility (Pariente *et al.*, 2001, 2002). Naturally derived materials and acellular tissue matrices have the potential advantage of biological recognition. However, synthetic polymers can be produced reproducibly on a large scale with controlled properties of their strength, degradation rate, and microstructure.

Naturally Derived Materials

Collagen is the most abundant and ubiquitous structural protein in the body and may be readily purified from both animal and human tissues with an enzyme treatment and salt/acid extraction. Collagen implants degrade through a sequential attack by lysosomal enzymes. The *in vivo* resorption rate can be regulated by controlling the density of the implant and the extent of intermolecular cross-linking. The lower the density, the greater the interstitial space and generally the larger the pores for cell infiltration, leading to a higher rate of implant degradation. Collagen contains cell adhesion domain sequences (e.g., RGD) that may assist in retaining the phenotype and activity of many types of cells, including fibroblasts (Silver and Pins, 1992) and chondrocytes (Sams and Nixon, 1995).

Alginate, a polysaccharide isolated from seaweed, has been used as an injectable cell delivery vehicle (Smidsrod and Skjak-Braek, 1990) and a cell immobilization matrix (Lim and Sun, 1980) because of its gentle gelling properties in the presence of divalent ions such as calcium. Alginate is relatively biocompatible and approved by the Food and Drug Administration (FDA) for human use as wound-dressing material. Alginate is a family of copolymers of D-mannuronate and L-glucuronate. The physical and mechanical properties of alginate gel are strongly correlated with the proportion and length of polyglcuuronate block in the alginate chains (Smidsrod and Skjak-Braek, 1990).

Acellular Tissue Matrices

Acellular tissue matrices are collagen-rich matrices prepared by removing cellular components from tissues. The matrices are often prepared by mechanical and chemical manipulation of a segment of tissue (Chen *et al.*, 1999; Dahms *et al.*, 1998; Piechota *et al.*, 1998; Strem *et al.*, 2005; Yoo *et al.*, 1998). The matrices slowly degrade on implantation and are replaced and remodeled by ECM proteins synthesized and secreted by transplanted or ingrowing cells.

Synthetic Polymers

Polyesters of naturally occurring α-hydroxy acids, including PGA, PLA, and PLGA, are widely used in tissue engineering. These polymers have gained FDA approval for human use in a variety of applications, including sutures (Gilding, 1981). The ester bonds in these polymers are hydrolytically labile, and these polymers degrade by nonenzymatic hydrolysis. The degradation products of PGA, PLA, and PLGA are nontoxic natural metabolites and are eventually eliminated from the body in the form of carbon dioxide and water (Gilding, 1981). The degradation rate of these polymers can be tailored from several weeks to several years by altering crystallinity, initial molecular weight, and the copolymer ratio of lactic to glycolic acid. Because these polymers are thermoplastics, they can be easily formed into a three-dimensional scaffold with a desired microstructure, gross shape, and dimension by various techniques, including molding, extrusion (Freed *et al.*, 1994), solvent casting (Mikos *et al.*, 1994), phase separation techniques and gas foaming techniques (Harris *et al.*, 1998). Many applications in tissue engineering require a scaffold with high porosity and ratio of surface area to volume. Other biodegradable synthetic polymers, including poly(anhydrides) and poly(ortho-esters), can also be used to fabricate scaffolds for tissue engineering with controlled properties (Peppas and Langer, 1994).

Angiogenic Factors

The engineering of large organs will require a vascular network of arteries, veins, and capillaries to deliver nutrients to each cell. One possible method of vascularization is through the use of gene delivery of angiogenic agents such as vascular endothelial growth factor (VEGF) with the implantation of vascular endothelial cells (ECs) to enhance neovascularization of engineered tissues. Skeletal myoblasts from adult mice were cultured and transfected with an adenovirus encoding VEGF and combined with human vascular ECs (Nomi *et al.*, 2002). The mixtures of cells were injected subcutaneously in nude mice, and the engineered tissues were retrieved up to 8 weeks after implantation. The transfected cells were noted to form muscle with neovascularization by histological and immunohistochemical probing with maintenance of their muscle volume, whereas engineered muscle of nontransfected cells had a significantly smaller mass of cells with loss of muscle volume over time, less neovascularization, and no surviving ECs. These results indicate that a combination of

VEGF and ECs may be useful for inducing neovascularization and volume preservation in engineered tissue.

Adult Stem Cells for Tissue Engineering

Investigators around the world, including our institution, have been working toward the development of several cell types, tissues, and organs for clinical application. The predominant cell type used for tissue engineering applications today is predetermined progenitor cells, which are present in almost every tissue. These cells provide replacement and repair for normal turnover or for injured tissues. Harvested through a biopsy, these cells can be expanded in culture and placed on bio-scaffolds for implantation. Our institute has successfully engineered multiple tissues for organ reconstruction using tissue specific progenitor cells, including urinary bladder (Atala, 2001), uterus (Duel *et al.*, 1996), vagina (De Filippo *et al.*, 2003), and penile tissue (Falke *et al.*, 2003). The first tissue-engineered hollow organ successfully implanted into patients was the urinary bladder, a composite tissue engineered form smooth muscle cells and urothelial cells (Atala *et al.*, 2006).

Because of the limited availability of tissue-specific progenitor cells, there is a growing scientific interest in the potential of adult stem cells. These cells are derived from a large variety of tissues including bone marrow (Pountos and Giannoudis, 2005), fat tissue (Lin *et al.*, 2006), muscle (Sun *et al.*, 2005), amniotic fluid, placenta (Portmann-Lanz *et al.*, 2006), and umbilical cord (Moise, 2005).

When compared with embryonic stem cells, adult stem cells have many similarities: they can differentiate into all three germ layers, they express common markers, and they preserve their telomere length. However, the adult stem cells demonstrate considerable advantages. They easily differentiate into specific cell lineages; they do not form teratomas if injected *in vivo*; they do not need any feeder layers to grow; and they do not require the sacrifice of human embryos for their isolation, thus avoiding the controversies associated with the use of human embryonic stem cells.

Unfortunately, the isolation of adult stem cells at sufficient purity and quality remains challenging. Purification is usually done by preplating techniques and through sorting for surface proteins. Adult stem cells are negative for tissue-specific markers and can be positive for embryonic cell surface antigens (Petersen *et al.*, 1999).

Adult stem cells are unspecialized cells, which show self-renewal and can self-maintain for a long time with the potential to commit to a cell lineage with specialized functions. These cells are able to differentiate into committed cells of other tissues, a feature defined as *plasticity*. This would allow for engineering of composite tissues composed of multiple cell types using one single source of adult stem cells. Therefore, use of adult stem cells opens a new avenue for cellular therapy and for the engineering of tissues and organs.

The most investigated adult stem cells are mesenchymal stem cells (MSCs). This cell type holds significant promise for the engineering of musculoskeletal structures. Bone marrow stroma represents the major source of MSCs. The bone marrow is aspirated from the iliac crest or from long bones and fractionated using a Ficoll density gradient followed by centrifugation. Cells from the low-density fraction are then plated and cultured. A small percentage of these cells grow adherent fibroblastic cells in colonies. These MSCs are characterized by a high proliferation potential and the capability to differentiate into progenitor cells for distinct mesenchymal tissues (Caplan, 1991). MSCs develop into distinct terminal differentiated cells and tissues including bone, cartilage, fat, muscle, tendon, and neural tissue (Ringe *et al.*, 2002). However, even with an increasing number of cell passages, MSCs do not spontaneously differentiate (Pittenger *et al.*, 1999). Taken together MSCs seem to be an optimal cell source for the engineering of bone and cartilage.

Engineering of Bone Tissue

For the bridging of osseous defects, autologous bone is still one of the most effective graft materials. However, there are major disadvantages including donor site morbidity, pain during recovery, and the lack of quality and quantity of bone that can be harvested. A combination of bioactive biomaterial and bone-producing cells could eliminate this problem.

Bone is formed by osteoblasts, which arise from stem cells in a multistep development process (Caplan, 1994). This differentiation is closely guided by bioactive molecules, such as bone morphogenetic proteins and growth and differentiation factors. It involves similar transitional events as those occurring in embryogenesis (Pathi *et al.*, 1999). Although the temporal expression patterns of such molecules are not well understood, they were successfully used to enhance bone engineering. Biodegradable scaffolds impregnated with bone morphogenetic protein, BMP-2, were able to bridge critical bone damage in a rat model (Lane *et al.*, 1999). The authors conclude that the enhanced recruitment of MSCs through the chemoattractant effect of BMP-2 leads to increased bone formation. However, the regenerative capacity of a scaffold with bioactive molecules may be limited because of the decreasing number of MSCs with aging. When compared with a newborn, the number of MSCs decreases fourfold by 50 years of age and up to 20-fold for patients older than 80 (Caplan, 1994). Tissue engineering offers a solution to this problem. Adult stem cells can be isolated and expanded in culture until sufficient cell numbers are achieved. During the same period, the cells can be differentiated into the desired tissues and used for implantation. This approach was successfully applied in rats (Ohgushi *et al.*, 1990). Rat MSCs were expanded *in vitro* with a porous hydroxyapatite under osteogenic conditions. One week after implantation of these constructs, bone formation and maturation was documented. In both control groups—whole rat bone marrow and undifferentiated MSCs—the bone formation was delayed (Ohgushi *et al.*, 1990). This study showed that tissue repair could be enhanced by expanding and differentiating the MSCs before application.

In humans, the treatment with isolated allogeneic MSCs has the potential to enhance the therapeutic effects of conventional bone marrow transplantation in patients with genetic disorders affecting mesenchymal tissues including bone, cartilage, and muscle. In a human trial, allogeneic mesenchymal cells were investigated as a therapy for osteogenesis imperfecta (Horwitz *et al.*, 2002). Each child received two infusions of allogeneic cells. Most children showed engraftment in one or more sites and had an acceleration of growth during the first 6 months after infusion. This improvement ranged from 60–94% of the predicted median values for age-matched and sex-matched unaffected children compared with 0–40% over the 6 months immediately preceding the infusions.

Muscle-derived stem cells might present another cell source for bone regeneration. Although muscle progenitor cells are highly heterogeneous in nature, there seems to be an adult stem cell population that is able to transdifferentiate into other tissues (Sun *et al.*, 2005). Osteogenic differentiation has been shown with cells isolated from skeletal muscle tissue (Bosch *et al.*, 2000). After exposure to BMP-2, *in vitro* cells were injected into the hind limb muscle of immune compromised mice. The injected cells seemed to actively participate in the ectopic bone formation. These results show that muscle may represent an additional source of adult stem cells for bone tissue engineering.

Engineering of Cartilage Tissue

Cartilage tissue is known for its slow turnover and negligible self-healing potential. Only deep osteochondral defects with damage to cartilage and bone show a small fibrous tissue repair. Tissue engineering using adult stem cells would be a promising approach to reconstruct joints after trauma or arthritis.

The reconstruction of cartilage after osteochondral defects was investigated in a rabbit model. MSCs from rabbit bone marrow were embedded in a type I collagen gel and implanted in to a large osteochondral lesion on the distal femur (Wakitani *et al.*, 1994). After 2 weeks the MSCs differentiated into chondrocytes and covered the defect zone. By 24 weeks the subchondral bone was completely repaired, and an articular cartilage layer was formed. However, the neo-cartilage was of low quality, with reduced thickness, minor mechanical properties, and inadequate integration to surrounding tissue. The same research group performed a study in patients with osteoarthritic knees (Wakitani *et al.*, 2002). Autologous mesenchymal cells were expanded in culture and embedded in collagen gel. The collagen–cell mix was placed into the cartilage defect and covered by autologous periosteum. To assess the tissue formation, small biopsy specimens were taken by arthroscopy. By 42 weeks, the defects were covered with soft tissue and formed a hyaline-like cartilage. Although the implantation of the collagen–MSC resulted in an improvement in tissue formation, the clinical outcome was not significantly influenced.

Engineering of Cardiac Tissue

Another area of great clinical and scientific interest is the use of adult stem cells for cardiac tissue engineering. Arteriosclerosis and myocardial infarction is still the number-one cause of mortality in many countries. Unlike skeletal muscle, cardiomyocytes have only limited potential to regenerate heart muscle. Necrotic cardiomyocytes in infracted tissue are replaced with fibroblasts forming a scar, which results in contractile dysfunction (Fukuda, 2001). Studies have shown that fetal rat cardiomyocytes can survive and functionally improve infarcted cardiac muscle. The use of differentiated progenitor cells is valid for a proof-of-principle, but this approach is not favorable for the clinical setting because of difficulties harvesting autologous heart cells. Adult stem cells with cardiomyogenic development potential may represent an alternate approach. MSCs are able to differentiate into skeletal muscle, smooth muscle, and cardiac muscle cells.

The capacity of adult stem cells from bone marrow to regenerate the heart is controversial and currently under intensive debate. Initial studies in mice showed that adult stem cells isolated from bone marrow were able to regenerate new myocardium when injected into the heart of recipient mice after myocardial infarction (Orlic *et al.*, 2001). However, recent studies in rats using the same cell type were not able to show any significant cardiac regeneration (Balsam *et al.*, 2004; Nygren *et al.*, 2004).

A swine myocardial infarct model was used to evaluate the improved cardiac function after implantation of autologous MSCs in a large animal setting (Shake *et al.*, 2002). MSCs were isolated and expanded from bone marrow aspirates. Two weeks after the myocardial infarction, 60 million MSCs were implanted into the infarct zone by direct injection. Robust engraftment of MSCs could be shown in all treated animals, and the degree of contractile dysfunction was significantly attenuated.

A German group (Strauer et al., 2001) reported the first human application of adult stem cells for the treatment of myocardial infarction. After confirmation of an occlusion of the left coronary artery causing an acute myocardial infarction, a 46-year-old man was treated by percutaneous transluminal catheter angioplasty and stent placement. Mononuclear bone marrow cells of the patient were prepared, and 6 days after infraction, 12 million cells were injected in the infarct-related artery. At 10 weeks after the stem cell transplantation, the transmural infarct area had been reduced from 24.6–15.7% of left ventricular circumference, whereas ejection fraction, cardiac index, and stroke volume had increased by 20–30%. These results demonstrate that selective intracoronary transplantation of human autologous adult stem cells is possible under clinical conditions. More research in a randomized setting is needed to evaluate the regeneration of the myocardial scar after stem cell therapy. To summarize, MSCs seem to be powerful candidates for bone, cartilage, and cardiac tissue engineering. The ability to form both bone and cartilage may be useful for the reconstruction of complex tissues such as joints.

Engineering of Neural Tissue

A similar population of adult stem cells derives from fat tissue, termed *adipose tissue–derived stem cells* (ADSCs). These cells share many of the characteristics of their counterparts in bone marrow, including high proliferative capacity and the ability for multilineage differentiation (Zuk et al., 2002). ADSC can be enzymatically digested out of adipose tissue and separated from the adipocytes by centrifugation. Advantages of ADSCs over MSCs include their simple harvest with local anesthesia and the high density of adult stem cells in fat tissue. Although a bone marrow aspiration in healthy adults is generally limited to 40 ml, the harvest of fat tissue can easily exceed 200 ml. Therefore, the number of harvested adult stem cells is approximately 40× higher (Strem et al., 2005), a big advantage if a large number of cells is needed for tissue engineering applications. It has been demonstrated that ADSC can undergo differentiation along classical mesenchymal lineages including fat, cartilage, bone, and muscle (Strem et al., 2005). Nonmesodermal transdifferentiation has also been confirmed into endothelial cells (Planat-Benard et al., 2004) and nerve cells (Safford et al., 2004).

These findings opened up a new avenue for the cellular treatment of brain disorders. ADSC were marked with a reporter gene *(LacZ)* and injected into rat brains after 90 min of middle cerebral artery occlusion (Kang *et al.*, 2003). Marked cells were seen throughout the infarct area 14 days after injection. The protein expression pattern showed signs of neural differentiation, and the ADSC-treated animals showed significant improvement in neurological tests. Similar results were shown when MSCs were injected (Zhao *et al.*, 2002). The implanted cells underwent *in vivo* differentiation with expression of markers consistent with differentiation along astrocytic, oligodendrocytic, and neural lineages. The MSC-treated rats also showed significantly improved performance in a limb placement test.

Fetal Stem Cells

Additional promising cells for tissue engineering applications and cell therapy are fetal stem cells isolated from amniotic fluid and umbilical cord blood.

Fetal stem cells have a higher potential for expansion than cells taken from the adult individual; and for this reason they could represent a better source for therapeutic applications when large numbers of cells are needed. The ability to isolate the progenitor cells during gestation may also be advantageous for babies born with congenital malformations. Furthermore, the progenitor cells can be cryopreserved for future self-use.

Human amniotic fluid stem cells (hAFS cells) are a novel source for tissue engineering of tissues and organs. Human amniotic fluid has been used in prenatal diagnosis for more than 70 years. It has proven to be a safe, reliable, and simple screening tool for a wide variety of developmental and genetic disorders. A subset of cells found in amniotic fluid has been isolated and found to be capable of maintaining prolonged undifferentiated proliferation, as well as differentiating into multiple tissue types encompassing the three germ layers.

hAFS cells are harvested by amniocentesis at about 16 weeks of gestation. The cells are then isolated through positive selection for cells expressing the membrane receptor *c-kit* (Cremer *et al.*, 1981) and can be maintained for >300 population doublings, far exceeding Hayflick's limit. The progenitor cells derived from human amniotic fluid are pluripotent and have been shown to differentiate into osteogenic, adipogenic, myogenic, neurogenic, endothelial, and hepatic phenotypes *in vitro*.

Recently, investigators discovered mesenchymal cells from umbilical cord blood that can be induced in culture to form a variety of tissues, including bone, cartilage, myocardial muscle, and neural tissue (Bieback *et al.*, 2004). Studies in mice were able to show significant advantages for cellular therapy in the treatment of intracranial hemorrhage (Nan *et al.*, 2005), stroke (Xiao *et al.*, 2005), and amyotrophic lateral sclerosis (Ende *et al.*, 2000).

The exact role of each cell type addressed in this chapter will be defined in future studies. The optimal combination of cell source, differentiation state, growth factors, culture conditions, biomaterials, and seeding technique will allow the engineering of tissue and organs for clinical application.

Conclusion

Tissue engineering efforts using adult stem cells experimentally are currently underway for virtually every type of tissue and organ within the human body. As regenerative medicine incorporates the fields of tissue engineering, cell biology, nuclear transfer, and materials science, personnel who have mastered the techniques of cell harvest, culture, expansion, transplantation, and polymer design are essential for the successful application of these technologies. Various tissues are at different stages of development, with some already being used clinically, a few in preclinical trials, and others in the discovery stage. Recent progress suggests that engineered tissues and cell-based therapies using adult stem cells may have an expanded clinical applicability in the future and may represent a viable therapeutic option for those who require tissue replacement or repair.

References

Atala, A., and L.RP.P.I.A.A.L.R.e., A. (2001). "Methods of Tissue Engineering." Academic Press, San Diego.

Atala, A., and M.D.P.I.A.A.ed. (2005). "Tissue Engineering." Birkhauser Press, Boston.

Atala, A. (2001). Bladder regeneration by tissue engineering. *BJU Int.* **88,** 765–770.

Atala, A., Bauer, S. B., Soker, S., Yoo, J. J., and Retik, A. B. (2006). Tissue-engineered autologous bladders for patients needing cystoplasty. *Lancet* **367,** 1241–1246.

Balsam, L. B., Wagers, A. J., Christensen, J. L., Kofidis, T., Weissman, I. L., and Robbins, R. C. (2004). Haematopoietic stem cells adopt mature haematopoietic fates in ischaemic myocardium. *Nature* **428,** 668–673.

Bieback, K., Kern, S., Kluter, H., and Eichler, H. (2004). Critical parameters for the isolation of mesenchymal stem cells from umbilical cord blood. *Stem Cells* **22,** 625–634.

Bosch, P., Musgrave, D. S., Lee, J. Y., Cummins, J., Shuler, T., Ghivizzani, T. C., Evans, T., Robbins, T. D., and Huard, T. D. (2000). Osteoprogenitor cells within skeletal muscle. *J. Orthop. Res.* **18,** 933–944.

Caplan, A. I. (1991). Mesenchymal stem cells. *J. Orthop. Res.* **9,** 641–650.

Caplan, A. I. (1994). The mesengenic process. *Clin. Plast. Surg.* **21,** 429–435.

Chen, F., Yoo, J. J., and Atala, A. (1999). Acellular collagen matrix as a possible "off the shelf" biomaterial for urethral repair. *Urology* **54,** 407–410.

Cilento, B. G., Freeman, M. R., Schneck, F. X., Retik, A. B., and Atala, A. (1994). Phenotypic and cytogenetic characterization of human bladder urothelia expanded *in vitro. J. Urol.* **152,** 665–670.

Cremer, M., Schachner, M., Cremer, T., Schmidt, W., and Voigtlander, T. (1981). Demonstration of astrocytes in cultured amniotic fluid cells of three cases with neural-tube defect. *Hum. Genet.* **56,** 365–370.

Dahms, S. E., Piechota, H. J., Dahiya, R., Lue, T. F., and Tanagho, E. A. (1998). Composition and biomechanical properties of the bladder acellular matrix graft: Comparative analysis in rat, pig and human. *Br. J. Urol.* **82,** 411–419.

De Filippo, R. E., Yoo, J. J., and Atala, A. (2003). Engineering of vaginal tissue *in vivo. Tissue Eng.* **9,** 301–306.

Duel, B. P., Hendren, W. H., Bauer, S. B., Mandell, J., Colodny, A., Peters, C. A., Atala, A., and Retik, A. B. (1996). Reconstructive options in genitourinary rhabdomyosarcoma. *J. Urol.* **156,** 1798–1804.

Ende, N., Weinstein, F., Chen, R., and Ende, M. (2000). Human umbilical cord blood effect on sod mice (amyotrophic lateral sclerosis). *Life Sci.* **67,** 53–59.

Falke, G., Yoo, J. J., Kwon, T. G., Moreland, R., and Atala, A. (2003). Formation of corporal tissue architecture *in vivo* using human cavernosal muscle and endothelial cells seeded on collagen matrices. *Tissue Eng.* **9,** 871–879.

Freed, L. E., Vunjak-Novakovic, G., and Biron, R. J. (1994). "Biodegradable Polymer Scaffolds for Tissue Engineering." Biotechnology, New York.

Fukuda, K. (2001). Development of regenerative cardiomyocytes from mesenchymal stem cells for cardiovascular tissue engineering. *Artif. Organs* **25,** 187–193.

Gilding, D. K. (1981). Biodegradable polymers. *In* "Biocompatibility of Clinical Implant Materials." (D. F. Williams, ed.), CRC Press, Boca Raton, FL.

Harris, L. D., Kim, B. S., and Mooney, D. J. (1998). Open pore biodegradable matrices formed with gas foaming. *J. Biomed. Mater. Res.* **42,** 396–402.

Horwitz, E. M., Gordon, P. L., Koo, W. K., Marx, J. C., Neel, M. D., McNall, R. Y., Muul, L., and Hofmann, T. (2002). Isolated allogeneic bone marrow-derived mesenchymal cells engraft and stimulate growth in children with osteogenesis imperfecta: Implications for cell therapy of bone. *Proc. Natl. Acad. Sci. USA* **99,** 8932–8937.

Hynes, R. O. (1992). Integrins: Versatility, modulation, and signaling in cell adhesion. *Cell* **69,** 11–25.

Kang, S. K., Lee, D. H., Bae, Y. C., Kim, H. K., Baik, S. Y., and Jung, J. S. (2003). Improvement of neurological deficits by intracerebral transplantation of human adipose tissue-derived stromal cells after cerebral ischemia in rats. *Exp. Neurol.* **183,** 355–366.

Kim, B. S., and Mooney, D. J. (1998). Development of biocompatible synthetic extracellular matrices for tissue engineering. *Trends Biotechnol.* **16,** 224–230.

Lane, J. M., Yasko, A. W., Tomin, E., Cole, B. J., Waller, S., Browne, M., Turek, T., and Gross, J. (1999). Bone marrow and recombinant human bone morphogenetic protein-2 in osseous repair. *Clin. Orthop. Relat. Res.* 216–227.

Liebert, M., Hubbel, A., Chung, M., Wedemeyer, G., Lomax, M. I., Hegeman, A., Yuan, T. Y., Brozovich, M., Wheelock, M. J., and Grossman, H. B. (1997). Expression of mal is associated with urothelial differentiation *in vitro*: Identification by differential display reverse-transcriptase polymerase chain reaction. *Differentiation* **61,** 177–185.

Lim, F., and Sun, A. M. (1980). Microencapsulated islets as bioartificial endocrine pancreas. *Science* **210,** 908–910.

Lin, Y., Chen, X., Yan, Z., Liu, L., Tang, W., Zheng, X., Li, Z., Qiao, J., Li, S., and Tian, W. (2006). Multilineage differentiation of adipose-derived stromal cells from GFP transgenic mice. *Mol. Cell Biochem.* **285,** 69–78.

Mikos, A. G., Lyman, M. D., Freed, L. E., and Langer, R. (1994). Wetting of poly(L-lactic acid) and poly(DL-lactic-co-glycolic acid) foams for tissue culture. *Biomaterials* **15,** 55–58.

Moise, K. J., Jr. (2005). Umbilical cord stem cells. *Obstet. Gynecol.* **106,** 1393–1407.

Nan, Z., Grande, A., Sanberg, C. D., Sanberg, P. R., and Low, W. C. (2005). Infusion of human umbilical cord blood ameliorates neurologic deficits in rats with hemorrhagic brain injury. *Ann. N. Y. Acad. Sci.* **1049,** 84–96.

Nguyen, H. T., Park, J. M., Peters, C. A., Adam, R. M., Orsola, A., Atala, A., and Freeman, M. R. (1999). Cell-specific activation of the HB-EGF and ErbB1 genes by stretch in primary human bladder cells. *In vitro Cell Dev. Biol. Anim.* **35**, 371–375.

Nomi, M., Atala, A., Coppi, P. D., and Soker, S. (2002). Principals of neovascularization for tissue engineering. *Mol. Aspects Med.* **23**, 463–483.

Nygren, J. M., Jovinge, S., Breitbach, M., Sawen, P., Roll, W., Hescheler, J., Taneera, J., Fleischmann, B. K., and Jacobsen, S. E. (2004). Bone marrow-derived hematopoietic cells generate cardiomyocytes at a low frequency through cell fusion, but not transdifferentiation. *Nat. Med.* **10**, 494–501.

Oberpenning, F., Meng, J., Yoo, J. J., and Atala, A. (1999). *De novo* reconstitution of a functional mammalian urinary bladder by tissue engineering. *Nat. Biotechnol.* **17**, 149–155.

Ohgushi, H., Okumura, M., Tamai, S., Shors, E. C., and Caplan, A. I. (1990). Marrow cell induced osteogenesis in porous hydroxyapatite and tricalcium phosphate: A comparative histomorphometric study of ectopic bone formation. *J. Biomed. Mater. Res.* **24**, 1563–1570.

Orlic, D., Kajstura, J., Chimenti, S., Jakoniuk, I., Anderson, S. M., Li, B., Pickel, J., McKay, R., Nadal-Ginard, B., Bodine, D. M., Leri, A., and Anversa, P. (2001). Bone marrow cells regenerate infarcted myocardium. *Nature* **410**, 701–705.

Pariente, J. L., Kim, B. S., and Atala, A. (2001). *In vitro* biocompatibility assessment of naturally derived and synthetic biomaterials using normal human urothelial cells. *J. Biomed. Mater. Res.* **55**, 33–39.

Pariente, J. L., Kim, B. S., and Atala, A. (2002). *In vitro* biocompatibility evaluation of naturally derived and synthetic biomaterials using normal human bladder smooth muscle cells. *J. Urol.* **167**, 1867–1871.

Pathi, S., Rutenberg, J. B., Johnson, R. L., and Vortkamp, A. (1999). Interaction of Ihh and BMP/Noggin signaling during cartilage differentiation. *Dev. Biol.* **209**, 239–253.

Peppas, N. A., and Langer, R. (1994). New challenges in biomaterials. *Science* **263**, 1715–1720.

Petersen, B. E., Bowen, W. C., Patrene, K. D., Mars, W. M., Sullivan, A. K., Murase, N., Boggs, S. S., Greenberger, J. S., and Goff, J. P. (1999). Bone marrow as a potential source of hepatic oval cells. *Science* **284**, 1168–1170.

Piechota, H. J., Dahms, S. E., Nunes, L. S., Dahiya, R., Lue, T. F., and Tanagho, E. A. (1998). *In vitro* functional properties of the rat bladder regenerated by the bladder acellular matrix graft. *J. Urol.* **159**, 1717–1724.

Pittenger, M. F., Mackay, A. M., Beck, S. C., Jaiswal, R. K., Douglas, R., Mosca, J. D., Moorman, M. A., Simonetti, D. W., Craig, S., and Marshak, D. R. (1999). Multilineage potential of adult human mesenchymal stem cells. *Science* **284**, 143–147.

Planat-Benard, V., Silvestre, J. S., Cousin, B., Andre, M., Nibbelink, M., Tamarat, R., Clergue, M., Manneville, C., Saillan-Barreau, C., Duriez, M., Tedgui, A., Levy, B., Penicaud, L., and Casteilla, L. (2004). Plasticity of human adipose lineage cells toward endothelial cells: Physiological and therapeutic perspectives. *Circulation* **109**, 656–663.

Portmann-Lanz, C. B., Schoeberlein, A., Huber, A., Sager, R., Malek, A., Holzgreve, W., and Surbek, D. V. (2006). Placental mesenchymal stem cells as potential autologous graft for pre- and perinatal neuroregeneration. *Am. J. Obstet. Gynecol.* **194**, 664–673.

Pountos, I., and Giannoudis, P. V. (2005). Biology of mesenchymal stem cells. *Injury* **36** (Suppl. 3), S8–S12.

Puthenveettil, J. A., Burger, M. S., and Reznikoff, C. A. (1999). Replicative senescence in human uroepithelial cells. *Adv. Exp. Med. Biol.* **462**, 83–91.

Ringe, J., Kaps, C., Burmester, G. R., and Sittinger, M. (2002). Stem cells for regenerative medicine: Advances in the engineering of tissues and organs. *Naturwissenschaften* **89**, 338–351.

Safford, K. M., Safford, S. D., Gimble, J. M., Shetty, A. K., and Rice, H. E. (2004). Characterization of neuronal/glial differentiation of murine adipose-derived adult stromal cells. *Exp. Neurol.* **187,** 319–328.

Sams, A. E., and Nixon, A. J. (1995). Chondrocyte-laden collagen scaffolds for resurfacing extensive articular cartilage defects. *Osteoarthritis Cartilage* **3,** 47–59.

Schultz, S. S., Abraham, S., and Lucas, P. A. (2006). Stem cells isolated from adult rat muscle differentiate across all three dermal lineages. *Wound Repair Regen.* **14,** 224–231.

Scriven, S. D., Booth, C., Thomas, D. F., Trejdosiewicz, L. K., and Southgate, J. (1997). Reconstitution of human urothelium from monolayer cultures. *J. Urol.* **158,** 1147–1152.

Shake, J. G., Gruber, P. J., Baumgartner, W. A., Senechal, G., Meyers, J., Redmond, J. M., Pittenger, M. F., and Martin, B. J. (2002). Mesenchymal stem cell implantation in a swine myocardial infarct model: Engraftment and functional effects. *Ann. Thorac. Surg.* **73,** 1919–1925.

Silver, F. H., and Pins, G. (1992). Cell growth on collagen: A review of tissue engineering using scaffolds containing extracellular matrix. *J. Long Term Eff. Med. Implants* **2,** 67–80.

Smidsrod, O., and Skjak-Braek, G. (1990). Alginate as immobilization matrix for cells. *Trends Biotechnol.* **8,** 71–78.

Strauer, B. E., Brehm, M., Zeus, T., Gattermann, N., Hernandez, A., Sorg, R. V., Kogler, G., and Wernet, P. (2001). Intracoronary, human autologous stem cell transplantation for myocardial regeneration following myocardial infarction. *Dtsch. Med. Wochenschr.* **126,** 932–938.

Strem, B. M., Hicok, K. C., Zhu, M., Wulur, I., Alfonso, Z., Schreiber, R. E., Fraser, J. K., and Hedrick, M. H. (2005). Multipotential differentiation of adipose tissue-derived stem cells. *Keio J. Med.* **54,** 132–141.

Sun, J. S., Wu, S. Y., and Lin, F. H. (2005). The role of muscle-derived stem cells in bone tissue engineering. *Biomaterials* **26,** 3953–3960.

Wakitani, S., Goto, T., Pineda, S. J., Young, R. G., Mansour, J. M., Caplan, A. I., and Goldberg, V. M. (1994). Mesenchymal cell-based repair of large, full-thickness defects of articular cartilage. *J. Bone Joint Surg. Am.* **76,** 579–592.

Wakitani, S., Imoto, K., Yamamoto, T., Saito, M., Murata, N., and Yoneda, M. (2002). Human autologous culture expanded bone marrow mesenchymal cell transplantation for repair of cartilage defects in osteoarthritic knees. *Osteoarthritis Cartilage* **10,** 199–206.

Xiao, J., Nan, Z., Motooka, Y., and Low, W. C. (2005). Transplantation of a novel cell line population of umbilical cord blood stem cells ameliorates neurological deficits associated with ischemic brain injury. *Stem Cells Dev.* **14,** 722–733.

Yoo, J. J., Meng, J., Oberpenning, F., and Atala, A. (1998). Bladder augmentation using allogenic bladder submucosa seeded with cells. *Urology* **51,** 221–225.

Yoo, J. J., Park, H. J., Lee, I., and Atala, A. (1999). Autologous engineered cartilage rods for penile reconstruction. *J. Urol.* **162,** 1119–1121.

Zhao, L. R., Duan, W. M., Reyes, M., Keene, C. D., Verfaillie, C. M., and Low, W. C. (2002). Human bone marrow stem cells exhibit neural phenotypes and ameliorate neurological deficits after grafting into the ischemic brain of rats. *Exp. Neurol.* **174,** 11–20.

Zuk, P. A., Zhu, M., Ashjian, P., De Ugarte, D. A., Huang, J. I., Mizuno, H., Alfonso, Z. C., Fraser, J. K., Benhaim, P., and Hedrick, M. H. (2002). Human adipose tissue is a source of multipotent stem cells. *Mol. Biol. Cell* **13,** 4279–4295.

[14]   Tissue Engineering Using Human Embryonic Stem Cells

By Shahar Cohen, Lucy Leshanski, and Joseph Itskovitz-Eldor

Abstract

The possibility of using stem cells for tissue engineering has greatly encouraged scientists to design new platforms in the field of regenerative and reconstructive medicine. Stem cells have the ability to rejuvenate and repair damaged tissues and can be derived from both embryonic and adult sources. Among cell types suggested as a cell source for tissue engineering (TE), human embryonic stem cells (hESCs) are one of the most promising candidates. Isolated from the inner cell mass of preimplantation stage blastocysts, they possess the ability to differentiate into practically all adult cell types. In addition, their unlimited self-renewal capacity enables the generation of sufficient amount of cells for cell-based TE applications. Yet, several important challenges are to be addressed, such as the isolation of the desired cell type and gaining control over its differentiation and proliferation. Ultimately, combing scaffolding and bioactive stimuli, newly designed bioengineered constructs, could be assembled and applied to various clinical applications. Here we define the culture conditions for the derivation of connective tissue lineage progenitors, design strategies, and highlight the special considerations when using hESCs for TE applications.

Introduction

Tissue engineering (TE) is an evolving interdisciplinary area that combines biological and engineering principles aimed at mimicking the natural processes of tissue formation and providing transplantable substitutes for the field of reconstructive and regenerative medicine (Vacanti and Langer, 1999).

The essentials of TE involve cells, scaffolds, and bioactive factors, such as chemical substances and mechanical stimuli. For cells to be viable for TE, they must be easily isolated, sufficient in number, and have an appropriate defined and controlled phenotype. A number of cell types have already been used for TE applications, including fully matured cells derived from adult tissues and stem cells derived from either embryonic, fetal, or adult tissues (Sharma and Elisseeff, 2004).

Designing the right strategy for engineering tissues using stem cells is especially challenging, because it requires plastic cells to form tissues while

METHODS IN ENZYMOLOGY, VOL. 420   0076-6879/06 $35.00
Copyright 2006, Elsevier Inc. All rights reserved.   DOI: 10.1016/S0076-6879(06)20014-4

differentiating. The formation of stem cell–derived neo-tissues integrates several dynamic processes occurring simultaneously. Primarily, the basic building block, a stem cell, is a very powerful and flexible unit. Its differentiation and proliferation characteristics have an inverse relationship; the more it differentiates, the less it proliferates.

In addition, the surrounding matrix builds and degrades at the same time, enabling cell migration and spatial organization. Thus, the microenvironment is continuously remodeling and, in turn, affects basic cellular processes.

Ultimately, in order for higher-order engineered tissues to be suitable for graftment into patients, it is essential to have a vascular network assimilated, enabling proper nutritional supply and waste disposal. This can be achieved through either stem cell–derived vascular progenitors setting up the infrastructure for functional blood vessels or by promoting host-derived vasculature invading and integrating into the graft. Possibly, stem cell–based tissue engineered grafts, being growing and differentiating biological elements, will continue remodeling once transplanted *in vivo*, adjusting to the specific host requirements.

As for having the ultimate cell source to accomplish these goals, human embryonic stem cells (hESCs) hold great promise to be just that. Ever since they were first isolated (Thomson *et al.*, 1998), they have been shown to possess a developmental potential to differentiate into cells representing all three embryonic germ layers (Itskovitz-Eldor *et al.*, 2000), including neurons (Reubinoff *et al.*, 2001), cardiomyocytes (Kehat *et al.*, 2001), hematopoietic cells (Kaufman *et al.*, 2001), endothelial cells (Levenberg *et al.*, 2002), and more. In addition, their practically unlimited self-renewal capacity can provide a sufficient amount of cells needed for TE applications. Nevertheless, these unique properties raise several critical issues. Because undifferentiated hESCs have the potential to form tumors *in vitro*, it is crucial to study how to direct and control their differentiation and proliferation.

Special Considerations When Using hESCs as the Cell Source for TE

Previous studies have provided protocols for differentiating hESCs along various lineages. Cell phenotype and functionality are usually tested to ensure that genuine differentiation has occurred. The following is an outline of the general principles and special considerations when using hESCs for TE applications.

Growing hESCs in Defined Animal-Free Conditions

Traditionally, hESCs are cocultured with feeder layers made of mouse embryonic fibroblasts (MEFs) and fed with serum-containing media

(Pera *et al.*, 2003); they can, therefore, be considered as xenografts. Although MEF feeders are essential to support the growth of undifferentiated hESCs, the use of animal products is associated with the risk of pathogen transmission, thus major advantages were made in this field. Alternatives include several human-derived feeder layers, feeder-free conditioned medium, and defined medium supplemented with growth factors and matrix proteins (Amit *et al.*, 2003, 2004; Mallon *et al.*, 2006).

Ultimately, new hESC lines should be derived in defined, animal-free culture conditions to be suitable for clinical applications. Guidelines for setting defined, animal-free culture systems are beyond the scope of this chapter and may be found elsewhere (Ludwig *et al.*, 2006).

Obtaining the Desired Cell Population

hESCs are the most potent stem cells available for TE; therefore, controlling their differentiation into the desired cell type is of great challenge. In general, hESCs can be induced to differentiate once removed from the MEF feeders and introduced with bioactive signals. This is done either directly or through the formation of embryoid bodies (EBs). EBs are small clumps of hESC colonies grown in suspension, which form three-dimensional (3-D) spheroid bodies representing a differentiation model with the widest spectrum of cell types that can be achieved *in vitro*. Differentiating cells within the EBs enjoy cell–cell interaction and paracrine effects of the three embryonic germ layers, in a developing 3-D microenvironment that mimics to the closest extent the temporal and spatial processes taking place in the developing embryo (Dvash and Benvenisty, 2004). Although direct differentiation is possible, most differentiation systems rely on EB formation.

Once cells start to differentiate, a variety of bioactive manipulations can be applied to control and direct the differentiation journey. In general, these include:

• Soluble signals, such as growth factors, hormones, and cell-conditioned media
• Genetic modifications, such as overexpression of transcription factors known to derive stem cells into the desired cell type
• Direct or indirect coculturing with other developing or mature somatic cell populations
• Physical stimuli, such as mechanical forces, temperature, and oxygenation changes. Whether differentiation is allowed to occur spontaneously or in a directed manner, the resultant cell population in most known protocols is still heterogeneous, which limits its potential to be used as a cell source for TE.

Thus, the next challenge is the isolation of the desired cell type. Methods for isolating a specific cell type from heterogeneous populations include either positively selecting the desired cells or negatively removing the undesired cells. Both can be done using several approaches, including fluorescence-activated and magnetic-activated cell sorting or genetic modification and selection using antibiotics. Defining the target cell population and its phenotype is crucial when using these strategies and planning the next stages and appropriate time points for seeding cells onto scaffolds and transplanting them into animal models.

Choosing the Right Scaffold

Scaffolds used in TE are designed to provide cells with a solid 3-D framework, allowing cells to attach, migrate, grow, and differentiate, while meeting their nutritional and biological needs (Lavik and Langer, 2004). They could be used as a means of delivering cells to the patient or support cell growth and *ex vivo* tissue formation before transplantation.

Ideally, scaffolds should imitate the chemical and physical properties of the native extracellular matrix and provide the cells with the most "homey" environment. They can be made of either natural materials, such as collagen, hydroxyapatite, alginate, and silica; synthetic materials, such as polyesters; or both. Although natural materials are more biocompatible and recognizable by cells, synthetic materials offer more control over properties such as degradation rate, permeability, specific architecture, and mechanical properties. Their architecture can be processed in various techniques, attaining controlled porous structures, different-scale fibrous matrices, and hydrogels, which are either chemically or physically cross-linked water-soluble polymers that can be mixed with cells and potentially injected in a variety of clinical situations. In addition, the surface properties of a scaffold have a crucial effect on its biocompatibility. A surface can be modified in a range of physical and chemical ways, including applying biological molecules and binding peptides, such as RGD—an ubiquitous peptide found in many extracellular matrix (ECM) proteins (such as fibronectin and laminin), which binds to cells through integrins. In summary, the properties of a scaffold can be specifically tailored and tightly controlled to meet the many biological and physical requirements.

Scaling Up a Regulatable Bioprocess

Large-scale production of functional tissues to be suitable for biomedical applications requires that bioprocesses are scalable, tightly controlled, and easily regulated. Standard, "investigative science"—scale, static culture systems for growing hESCs—offer limited control over the culture conditions.

Although different hESC lines show diversity in growth kinetics, phenotype, and differentiation potential, the variety of culture protocols and laboratory skills result in lack of consistency and different desirable yields. Each step of hESC-based systems should be ultimately scaled up in a regulated and controlled manner. Perhaps the most challenging process to control is the formation and cultivation of EBs. EB remains the preferable approach in many differentiation systems. Made of a small aggregate of hESCs grown in suspension, EBs are independently growing and differentiating units, heterogeneous in size and in spatial arrangement, and may aggregate between themselves to form agglomerates. In addition, cells within the growing EB respond differently and sometimes unpredictably to bioactive stimuli such as growth factors and physical cues. Methods to obtain some control over these processes include encapsulation of EBs in beads made of specific material and in specific size. Ultimately, tissue culture bioreactors, such as spinner flasks and rotating vessels, can be scaled in size to meet specific production needs and offer control over culture conditions such as nutrients and growth factors concentrations, pH, oxygen, and carbon dioxide levels.

hESC-Derived Connective Tissue Progenitors for TE

Defining the desired target cell population derived from hESCs, one could aim to either somatic cell type or earlier committed progenitor cell. The objective of the following protocols developed in our laboratory was to direct hESC progeny along the mesenchymal lineage and to achieve a progenitor cell population that is committed to connective tissue derivatives and meets the basic requirements of being viable for cell-based TE applications. The general principles and special considerations can be applied to other cell types and differentiation assays, with appropriate modifications.

Culture and Maintenance of hESC on MEF Feeders

Preparation of Growth Media

MEF GROWTH MEDIUM

- High-glucose Dulbecco's modified eagle's medium (DMEM), supplemented with:
  - 10% Fetal bovine serum (FBS)

hESC Growth Medium

- Knockout DMEM, supplemented with:
  - 20% Knockout serum replacement
  - 1 mM Glutamine
  - 1% Nonessential amino acids
  - 0.1 mM 2-mercaptoethanol
  - 4 ng/ml basic fibroblast growth factor (bFGF)

EB Growth Medium

- Knockout DMEM, supplemented with:
  - 20% FBS
  - 1 mM glutamine
  - 1% nonessential amino acids

CTP Growth Medium

- Minimum essential medium-alpha (MEM-α), supplemented with:
  - 15% FBS (selected lots)
  - 50 μg/ml ascorbic acid
  - 10 mM beta-glycerophosphate
  - 10–7 M dexamethasone

Use low protein binding, 22-μm pore size filters for sterilizing media components.

Preparation of MEF Feeder Layers

The procedure of deriving MEFs of 13-day-old ICR mouse embryos is described elsewhere (Pera *et al.*, 2003). Once derived, MEFs should be subcultured and used for feeder preparation at passages 3–4. Lower passage use is possible but wasteful.

1. Inactivate MEFs by incubating with 8 μg/ml mitomycin C for 2 h.
2. Wash with Dulbecco's phosphate-buffered saline (PBS).
3. Harvest cells by trypsinization.
4. Plate 40,000 cells/cm^2 on gelatin-pretreated 6-well plates, in MEF growth medium.
   - Overnight incubation is recommended before plating hESCs.
   - The fresher the better; use plates within a week, keep for 2 weeks only.

Starting hESC Culture

1. Make sure MEF feeders are intact and healthy.
2. Change feeders' medium to hESC medium 1 h before plating.

3. Thaw out a frozen hESC vial and resuspend in fresh hESC medium.
4. Gently centrifuge and resuspend pellet in final volume not exceeding 1 ml per feeder well.
5. Plate on feeders, place inside the incubator, and shake plates for evenly distributing hESCs on feeders.
6. Feed cells with fresh medium on a daily basis.

Passaging hESCs

Frequency of Splitting hESC Cultures Changes Between Different Cell Lines

Generally, timing and splitting ratio should be determined according to the following two principles.

Morphology of the Colonies

A high-quality colony is round, has well-defined edges, and shows no signs of differentiation. Cells within the colony are small, with a high nucleus/cytoplasm ratio (Fig. 1).

Poor colonies could be selectively taken out, mechanically, using a sterile needle or pipette tip. Alternately, good colonies could be saved in the same manner.

Density of the Colonies

hESC colonies favor a crowded environment, where they support each other. At the same time, avoid overly crowded cultures. Grow approximately 40–60 medium-size colonies per well (Fig. 2).

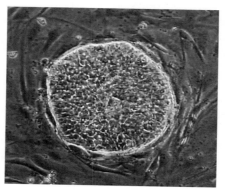

FIG. 1. The appearance of a high-quality human embryonic stem cell (hESC) colony. Note round-shaped, well-defined edges, and high nucleus/cytoplasm ratio of cells within the colony. (See color insert.)

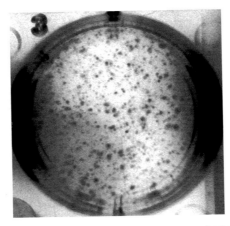

FIG. 2. The optimal density of human embryonic stem cell (hESC) colonies. (See color insert.)

Passaging Protocol

1. Prepare feeders by removing MEF medium and incubating with hESC medium 1 hbefore hESC seeding.
2. Incubate hESCs with type 0.1% type IV collagenase for 20–40 min.
3. Wait for the colonies' edges to lift off the feeders before continuing.
4. Add fresh medium.
5. Use a pipette tip and thoroughly scratch out the colonies.
6. Collect the scratched material into a conical tube.
7. Gently centrifuge and resuspend pellet in final volume not exceeding 1 ml per feeder well.
8. Plate on feeders, place inside the incubator, and shake plates to evenly distribute the hESCs on feeders.
9. Feed cells with fresh hESC medium on a daily basis.

hEB Formation

1. Prepare 60-mm petri dishes (bacterial grade, non-tissue culture treated).
2. Repeat steps 2–5 of passaging protocol.
3. Gently centrifuge and resuspend pellet in fresh human EB medium.
4. Plate into petri dishes.

hEBs are considered to be independently growing units, thus density of culture is of lesser importance. In general, plate one well of a six-well plate content into one 60-mm petri dish.

5. Place inside the incubator.
6. Feed cells with fresh hEB medium every 3–4 days.

Changing hEB Medium

1. Collect the content of the petri dish into a conical tube.
7. Gently centrifuge and resuspend pellet in fresh hEB medium.
2. Plate into new petri dishes

Alternately, the following method can be used:

1. Place the petri dish inside the working hood, topless.
2. Gently swirl the dish until all hEBs are centered.
3. Aspirate off the medium from the edges of the dish.
4. Add fresh hEB medium and place inside the incubator.

Derivation and Propagation of Connective Tissue Progenitors

1. Collect 10-day-old hEBs growing in suspension into a conical tube.
2. Wash with PBS.
3. Trypsinize.
4. Thoroughly pipette up and down, and pass through a 40-μm mesh cell strainer.
5. Resuspend in CTP medium, centrifuge, and resuspend again.
6. Plate 5×10^4 cells per cm^2 on tissue culture-treated flask.
7. On reaching subconfluence, incubate with 0.1% type IV collagenase for 40–60 min.
8. Wash with PBS.
9. Harvest cells by trypsinization.
10. Resuspend in fresh CTP medium, centrifuge and resuspend again.
11. Split 1:3 onto new flasks.

Choosing the Right Scaffold for Connective Tissue Engineering

In contrast to parenchymal organs, which are mainly cellular and function by means of their cells, most of the volume of connective tissues consists of their functional element—the ECM.

Connective tissue ECMs cope with tensile and compressive mechanical stresses. Tension is transmitted and resisted by nanoscaled fibrous proteins such as collagen and elastin, whereas compression is opposed by water-soluble proteoglycans, such as chondroitin sulphate (Scott, 2003). The proteoglycan part forms a highly hydrated, gel-like "ground substance" in which the fibrous proteins are embedded.

So that cells would enjoy the most suitable 3-D surrounding environment resembling the native ECM, we have postulated that nanoscaled fabricated surface topography of a synthetic scaffold would be best one to use. Electrospinning is the most common and practical way to fabricate polymeric nanofiber matrix (reviewed by Ma *et al.* [2005]). We hypothesized that electrospun nanofiber biodegradable polymer scaffolds would support hESC-derived CTPs' organization into complex 3-D tissues, as we show in the following.

Scaffold Fabrication and Cell Seeding

Electrospun nanofiber mash scaffolds were made of a 1:1 blend of polycaprolactone (PCL) and poly(lactic acids) (PLA) by a process described elsewhere (Ma *et al.*, 2005). The average thickness of the prepared scaffold was 500 μm; the fiber diameter ranged between 200–450 nm, with porosity of 85%.

For preparation for cell seeding we recommend the following procedure:

1. Cutting scaffold mat into 0.5×0.5 cm^2 squares, making them fit into 24-well plates.
2. Gas-sterilizing with ethylene oxide.
3. Immersing in 5 M sodium hydroxide and washing in PBS to increase surface hydrophilicity.

CTP Seeding Protocol

1. Incubate subconfluent CTP cultures with 0.1% type IV collagenase for 40–60 min.
2. Rinse with PBS.
3. Harvest cells by trypsinization.
4. Resuspend in fresh CTP medium, centrifuge, and resuspend again.
5. Seeding volume should be minimal: count cells and resuspend to obtain 5×10^5 cells per 10 μl.
6. Seed 10 μl on each scaffold and allow cells to attach for 30 min inside the incubator.
7. Gently add fresh medium and change medium every 3–4 days.

Harvesting Samples for Analyses

Immunofluorescent Staining

To avoid misinterpretation of the staining results, assessing autofluorescence prior to staining is highly recommended.

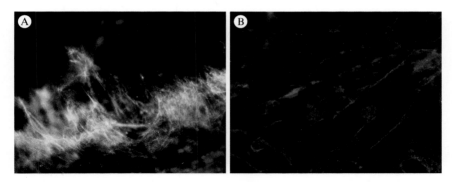

FIG. 3. CTPs stained with antibody against type I collagen (A) and type II collagen (B). DAPI was used for nuclear visualization. Note cells embedded in self-produced extracellular matrix. (See color insert.)

1. Prewash samples with PBS.
2. Soak in 4% paraformaldehyde fixative.
3. Rinse with PBS.
4. Apply primary antibody. Optimal dilution should be calibrated individually.
5. Rinse with PBS.
6. Apply appropriate secondary antibody.
7. Counterstain nuclei with appropriate dye, such as DAPI.
8. Mount cells and view under fluorescent light microscope (Fig. 3A, B).

Electron Microscopy

1. Prewash samples with PBS.
2. Soak in 2.5% glutaraldehyde in 0.1 M sodium cacodylate buffer.
3. Gradually dehydrate in ethanol followed by soaking in hexamethyl-disilazane (HMDS).
4. Coat with carbon and view under scanning electron microscope (Fig. 4A–D).

Histological Analysis

1. Prerinse samples with PBS.
2. Soak in 10% natural buffered formalin fixative.
3. Gradually dehydrate in ethanol and embed in paraffin.
4. Cut sections and stain with hematoxylin-eosin (H&E).
5. View under light microscope (Fig. 5A, B).

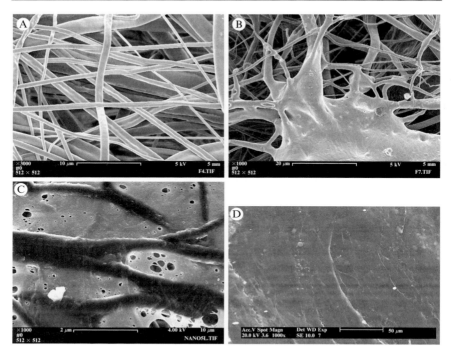

FIG. 4. Scanning electron micrograph of electrospun PCL/PLA nanofiber mash scaffold alone (A), and of seeded CTPs (B), producing extracellular matrix (C) and eventually forming 3-D sheetlike tissue completely covering the scaffold (D).

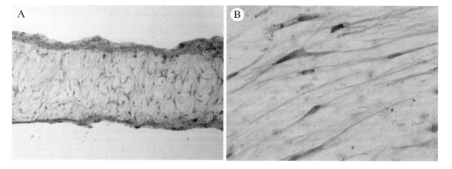

FIG. 5. Hematoxylin-eosin–stained histological images of cross-sectioned CTPs seeded on nanofiber scaffolds at low (A) and high (B) power magnifications. (See color insert.)

References

Amit, M., Margulets, V., Segev, H., Shariki, K., Laevsky, I., Coleman, R., and Itskovitz-Eldor, J. (2003). Human feeder layers for human embryonic stem cells. *Biol. Reprod.* **68,** 2150–2156.

Amit, M., Shariki, C., Margulets, V., and Itskovitz-Eldor, J. (2004). Feeder layer- and serum-free culture of human embryonic stem cells. *Biol. Reprod.* **70,** 837–845.

Dvash, T., and Benvenisty, N. (2004). Human embryonic stem cells as a model for early human development. *Best Pract. Res. Clin. Obstet. Gynaecol.* **18,** 929–490.

Itskovitz-Eldor, J., Schuldiner, M., Karsenti, D., Eden, A., Yanuka, O., Amit, M., Soreq, H., and Benvenisty, N. (2000). Differentiation of human embryonic stem cells into embryoid bodies compromising the three embryonic germ layers. *Mol. Med.* **6,** 88–95.

Kaufman, D. S., Hanson, E. T., Lewis, R. L., Auerbach, R., and Thomson, J. A. (2001). Hematopoietic colony-forming cells derived from human embryonic stem cells. *Proc. Natl. Acad. Sci. USA* **98,** 10716–10721.

Kehat, I., Kenyagin-Karsenti, D., Snir, M., Segev, H., Amit, M., Gepstein, A., Livne, E., Binah, O., Itskovitz-Eldor, J., and Gepstein, L. (2001). Human embryonic stem cells can differentiate into myocytes with structural and functional properties of cardiomyocytes. *J. Clin. Invest.* **108,** 407–414.

Lavik, E., and Langer, R. (2004). Tissue engineering: Current state and perspectives. *Appl. Microbiol. Biotechnol.* **65,** 1–8.

Levenberg, S., Golub, J. S., Amit, M., Itskovitz-Eldor, J., and Langer, R. (2002). Endothelial cells derived from human embryonic stem cells. *Proc. Natl. Acad. Sci. USA* **99,** 4391–4396.

Ludwig, T. E., Levenstein, M. E., Jones, J. M., Berggren, W. T., Mitchen, E. R., Frane, J. L., Crandall, L. J., Daigh, C. A., Conard, K. R., Piekarczyk, M. S., Llanas, R. A., and Thomson, J. A. (2006). Derivation of human embryonic stem cells in defined conditions. *Nat. Biotechnol.* **24,** 185–187.

Ma, Z., Kotaki, M., Inai, R., and Ramakrishna, S. (2005). Potential of nanofiber matrix as tissue-engineering scaffolds. *Tissue Eng.* **11,** 101–109.

Mallon, B. S., Park, K. Y., Chen, K. G., Hamilton, R. S., and McKay, R. D. (2006). Toward xeno-free culture of human embryonic stem cells. *Int. J. Biochem. Cell Biol.* **38,** 1063–1075.

Pera, M. F., Filipczyk, A. A., Hawes, S. M., and Laslett, A. L. (2003). Isolation, characterization, and differentiation of human embryonic stem cells. *Methods Enzymol.* **365,** 429–446.

Reubinoff, B. E., Itsykson, P., Turetsky, T., Pera, M. F., Reinhartz, E., Itzik, A., and Ben-Hur, T. (2001). Neural progenitors from human embryonic stem cells. *Nat. Biotechnol.* **19,** 1134–1140.

Scott, J. E. (2003). Elasticity in extracellular matrix 'shape modules' of tendon, cartilage, etc. A sliding proteoglycan-filament model. *J. Physiol.* **553,** 335–343.

Sharma, B., and Elisseeff, J. H. (2004). Engineering structurally organized cartilage and bone tissues. *Ann. Biomed. Eng.* **32,** 148–159.

Thomson, J. A., Itskovitz-Eldor, J., Shapiro, S. S., Waknitz, M. A., Swiergiel, J. J., Marshall, V. S., and Jones, J. M. (1998). Embryonic stem cell lines derived from human blastocysts. *Science* **282,** 1145–1147.

Vacanti, J. P., and Langer, R. (1999). Tissue engineering: The design and fabrication of living replacement devices for surgical reconstruction and transplantation. *Lancet* **354**(Suppl. 1), SI32–SI34.

[15] Engineering Cardiac Tissue from Embryonic Stem Cells

By Xi-Min Guo, Chang-Yong Wang, X. Cindy Tian, and Xiangzhong Yang

Abstract

Restoration of cardiac function by replacement of diseased myocardium with functional cardiac myocytes may offer a potential cure for cardiac disease and will likely revolutionize treatment methods. During the past 20 years, we have seen the development of tissue engineering; among these types of tissue engineering is cardiac tissue engineering. This type of cardiac tissue engineering includes growing neonatal cardiomyocytes on preformed polymers, liquid collagen, and temperature-responsive surfaces. It also includes the application of neonatal rat or chick cardiomyocytes to skeletal myoblasts, mesenchymal stem cells and embryonic stem cells, static culture, and bioreactor and stretching cultivation. Progress has come step-by-step, but, in recent years, with great technological advances, the progress has been accelerating, moving this area of research from dream to reality. The engineered cardiac tissue not only reproduces *in vitro*, but it can also be shaped so that it will, at some time, be able to form valves or endothelial lining. This chapter describes the currently used protocols for cardiac tissue engineering: liquid collagen–based cardiac tissue engineering and cell sheet–based cardiac tissue engineering, especially cardiac tissue engineering using cardiomyocytes derived from embryonic stem cells.

Introduction

Cardiac tissue engineering is an emerging field that holds great promise for developing revolutionary treatments for heart disease. Heart defects are the most common congenital defect and are the leading cause of death in the first year of life (Hoffman, 1995a,b). Congenital heart defects may occur in as many as 14 of every 1000 live births (Gillum, 1994). Acquired heart diseases also have a profound effect on the population; in 2004, there were 2016 heart transplants in the United States, and slightly more than 3000 patients were on the waiting list for a new heart in 2005 (American Heart Association, 2005). Unfortunately, there are not sufficient numbers of donor hearts for the patients who need them. A large number of patients who are not necessarily candidates for transplant may benefit from smaller structures such as pieces of muscle, valves, or vessels.

METHODS IN ENZYMOLOGY, VOL. 420
0076-6879/06 $35.00
DOI: 10.1016/S0076-6879(06)20015-6

Cardiac tissue engineering may not only provide advanced surgical implant materials for these patients, but the development of tissue equivalents for *in vitro* use could also improve the testing of drugs and potential therapeutic agents and could expand our understanding of cardiac cell biology.

Several tissue-engineering approaches have been explored for cardiac repair. The most common approach has been to seed cardiomyocytes onto porous scaffolds, typically constructed from a biodegradable polymer, such as poly(lactic-co-glycolic acid) or natural polymers, such as collagen. Scaffold seeding has worked well for proliferative, hypoxia-tolerant cells, such as smooth muscle, which expand to fill void spaces after seeding, but it has been more difficult to achieve tissue-like cell densities with nonproliferative rat or mouse cardiomyocytes. Nevertheless, seeded myocardial constructs have been shown to conduct action potentials and beat synchronously (Papadaki *et al.*, 2001), as well as hypertrophy in response to electrical stimulation (Radisic *et al.*, 2004). Li and coworkers (Li *et al.*, 1999, 2000; Sakai *et al.*, 2001) have grown small three-dimensional cardiac grafts and implanted them into host myocardia and the right ventricular outflow tract. Two critical observations from this work were the survival of grafted material and the apparent vascularization of the implants by the host circulation. Highly engineered scaffolds could, in theory, direct the gross conformation of a construct, influence the phenotype of cellular components, or direct particular cells to specific sites within a construct.

Over the past years, Eschenhagen's group developed a principally different technique that does not use preformed scaffolds but rather uses liquid collagen I to reconstitute embryonic chicken or neonatal rat cardiomyocytes onto three-dimensional cardiac grafts (Zimmermann *et al.*, 2000, 2002). The technique, which was further proven by Zhao *et al.* (2005) with minor modification, uses collagen I to support the endogenous capability of immature cardiac cells to form a heart tissue–like structure *in vitro*. Enzymatically disaggregated cardiomyocytes are mixed with freshly neutralized collagen type I from rat tails, extracellular matrix of the Engelbreth–Holm–Swarm tumor, and culture medium. This cell matrix mixture is pipetted into casting molds of the desired size and shape. After 7 days in the casting molds, engineered cardiac tissues (ECTs) were transferred to a stretching device and subjected to phasic stretch by 10% for another 5–7 days. The contractile activity of the constructs was superb, and the method seems to be highly reproducible. By virtue of the method's reproducibility and the characteristics of the constructs described so far, ECTs should represent an excellent source of material for *in vitro* testing. With some modifications to the procedure, ECTs may also provide suitable material for implantation studies. Encouraging success in heart tissue repairs has been achieved as

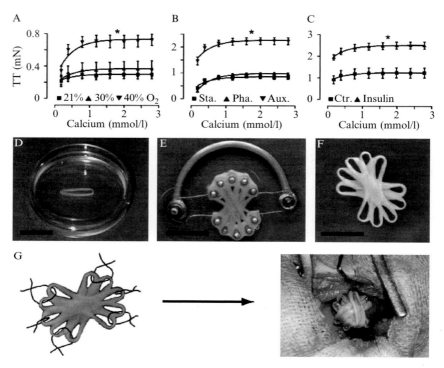

FIG. 1. Construction of optimized EHTs. Effects of oxygen, load, and insulin were analyzed by isometric contraction experiments in EHT rings. TT, twitch tension. Direct comparison of calcium response curves showed that EHTs benefited from oxygen supplementation (O_2, $n = 11$ at 21%; $n = 5$ at 30%; $n = 10$ at 40%; (A) auxotonic (Aux.; $n = 8$) in contrast to static (Sta.; $n = 8$) or phasic (Pha.; $n = 8$) load (B), and addition of insulin (10 $\mu g/ml$; $n = 4$) compared with untreated controls ($n = 3$); (C). Stacking five single EHTs (D) on a custom-made device facilitated EHT fusion and allowed contractions under auxotonic load (E), resulting in synchronously contracting multiloop EHTs (F) ready for *in vivo* engraftment. (G) Six single-knot sutures served to fix multiloop EHTs on the recipients' hearts. *$p < 0.05$ vs. 21% O_2, static load, and culture in the absence of insulin (Ctr.), respectively, by repeated ANOVA. Scale bars, 10 mm (Zimmermann *et al.*, 2006). (See color insert.)

described recently in *Nature Medicine* (Zimmermann *et al.*, 2006). They created large (thickness/diameter, 1–4 mm/15 mm), force-generating engineered heart tissue from neonatal rat heart cells (Fig. 1). Engineered heart tissue formed thick cardiac muscle layers when implanted on myocardial infarcts in immune-suppressed rats. When evaluated 28 days later, engineered heart tissue showed undelayed electrical coupling to the native myocardium without evidence of arrhythmia induction (Figs. 2 and 3).

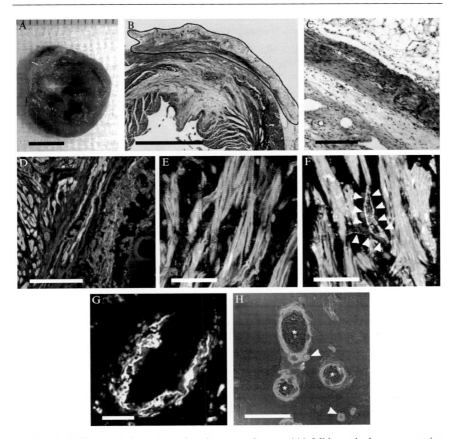

FIG. 2. EHT morphology 4 weeks after engraftment. (A) Midventricular cross-section 28 days after implantation showed that engrafted EHTs remained pale but firmly attached to the infarct scar. (B and C) H&E staining of paraffin sections through the infarcted left ventricular free wall 4 weeks after EHT engraftment showed the formation of thick cardiac muscle on top of the infarct scar (B; EHT circled). High-power magnification of the infarct area showed that engrafted EHTs formed compact and oriented heart muscle (C) spanning the transmural infarct. (D) Engrafted EHTs could be identified by DAPI-labeled nuclei (blue; actin, green; background, red). (E) Laser scanning microscopy showed the highly differentiated sarcomeric organization of engrafted cardiomyocytes (actin, green; nuclei, blue). (F–H) EHT grafts were vascularized *in vivo* (F; actin, green; nuclei, blue; arrows indicate a putative vessel in a reconstituted confocal image). Newly formed vessels contained DAPI$^+$ endothelial (G; lectin, red; nuclei, blue) or smooth muscle cells (H; actin, green; nuclei, blue). Macrophages (ED2, red; highlighted by arrows in H) with blue nuclei were found in close proximity to newly formed vessels. Asterisks indicate erythrocytes visualized by differential interference contrast imaging (H). Scale bar in A,B, 5 mm; in C,D, 500 μm; in E–H, 50 μm (Zimmermann *et al.*, 2006). (See color insert.)

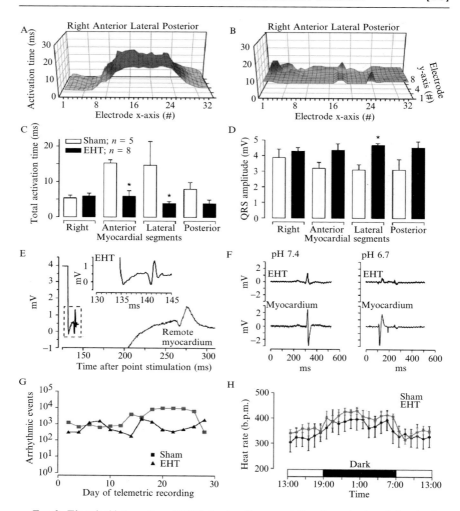

FIG. 3. Electrical integration of EHTs *in vivo*. Representative plots of epicardial activation times in sham-operated (A) and EHT-engrafted (B) hearts. Total activation time (C) and QRS-complex voltage (D) in right, anterior, lateral, and posterior segments of the investigated hearts. (E) Point stimulation of an implanted EHT with simultaneous recording of the propagated potential in the EHT and in remote myocardium showed retrograde coupling. EHT could be uncoupled after acidification of the hearts (F). Telemetric ECG recordings showed a similar frequency of arrhythmias in sham-operated and EHT-grafted groups ($n = 5$ per group; G). (H) Circadian rhythm in sham-operated and EHT groups. *$p < 0.05$ vs. sham-operated rats by ANOVA with Mann–Whitney U test (Zimmermann *et al.*, 2006). (See color insert.)

Moreover, engineered heart tissue prevented further dilation, induced systolic wall thickening of infarcted myocardial segments, and improved fractional area shortening of infarcted hearts compared with controls (sham operation and noncontractile constructs) (Figs. 4 and 5).

On the basis of this method, Guo *et al.* (2006) created cardiac tissue using cardiomyocytes derived from mouse embryonic stem cells (mESCs). In this study, a step-by step strategy was used to derive cardiomyocytes as described in Chapter 1 to produce embryoid bodies in large scale in a bioreactor, induce cardiogenic differentiation of ESCs, and enrich cardiomyocytes from mESCs by Percoll density gradients. The cells were then mixed with liquid collagen to construct cardiac tissue. The engineered cardiac tissue was mechanically stretched *in vitro* and proved both structurally and functionally to resemble neonatal native cardiac muscle (Figs. 6–9).

The basic methods of cell seeding, casting, and culturing ECTs, as well as force measurements, have been described in detail (Eschenhagen *et al.*, 1997, 2002; Zimmermann *et al.*, 2000).

Liquid Collagen–Based Cardiac Tissue Engineering

Cell/Collagen Mix Preparation

1. Mix a 1.33-ml amount of collagen type I (rat tail, 3.6 mg/ml 0.1% acetic acid, Upstate Biotechnology, Lake Placid, NY) with 1.33 ml 2× concentrated culture medium (2× DMEM, 20% horse serum, 4% chick embryo extract, 200 μg/ml streptomycin, 200 U/ml penicillin G).
2. Neutralize the mix with 182 μl 0.1 M NaOH.
3. Add 0.48 ml Matrigel.
4. Mix with 1.48 ml of cell suspension (415 × 10^6 cardiomyocytes).
5. Keep on ice until casting.

Plane (Lattice) System

1. See Fig. 10. Glue the strips of Velcro (thick side) to silicone tubes (A).
2. Assemble 6–8 pairs of Velcro-coated tubes by stainless-steel wire spacers and put in rectangular wells (17 × 10 × 4 mm) cut into a layer of silicone rubber in a 100-mm glass culture dish (B).
3. Autoclave the assembly before use.
4. Pour the cell/collagen/Matrigel mix into each well between the two tubes (C).

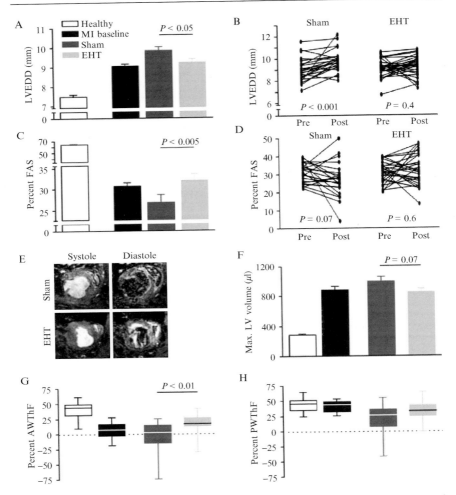

FIG. 4. Changes in left ventricular function after Fig015.4EHT implantation. Left ventricular end-diastolic diameter (LVEDD; A and B) and FAS (C and D) determined by echocardiography. "Healthy" indicates age-matched untreated controls ($n = 29$). "MI baseline" indicates pooled values ($n = 53$) measured 14 days after myocardial infarction in rats that underwent sham ($n = 24$) or EHT ($n = 29$) surgery. These rats were reevaluated after an additional 28 days. Trajectories show the change of LVEDD (B) and FAS (D) for each rat. Pre, values at MI baseline; post, values 28 days after sham or EHT surgery. MRI was performed subsequently (E–H) with five exceptions because of technical reasons. Maximal and minimal volumes of the left ventricle were calculated from 4-D CINE mode MRI images in EHT-grafted ($n = 24$) and sham-operated ($n = 19$) rats (E). Analyses of systolic thickening in anterior (AWThF; G) and posterior (PWThF; H) segments of the ventricular wall served to assess local contractility. MRI data from healthy rats ($n = 29$) and 2 weeks after infarction ($n = 8$) were recorded in an independent series of experiments and are shown for comparison. LV, left ventricular. Statistical evaluations were performed by unpaired (A and B, F–H) and paired (B and D) Student t tests (Zimmermann *et al.*, 2006).

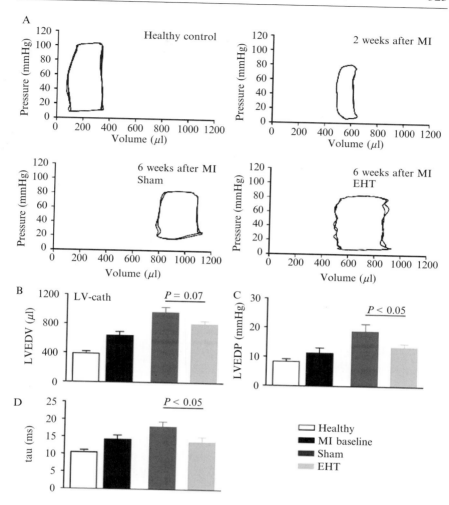

FIG. 5. Influence of EHT grafting on left ventricular hemodynamics. (A) Representative pressure-volume loops and detailed analyses of left ventricular end-diastolic volume (LVEDV) (B) pressure (LVEDP), (C) and relaxation (tau), (D) in EHT-grafted ($n = 7$) and sham-operated rats ($n = 17$). Left ventricular catheterization (LV-cath) data from healthy rats ($n = 6$) and 2 weeks after infarction ($n = 9$) were recorded in an independent series of experiments and are shown for comparison. Statistical evaluations were performed by unpaired Student t tests. MI, myocardial infarction (Zimmermann et $al.$, 2006).

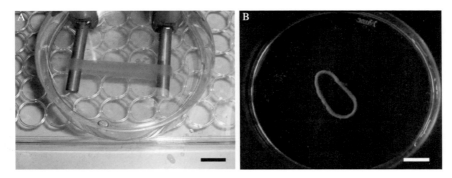

Fig. 6. Macroscopy of ECT. (A) Mechanical stretching of ECTs. The ECTs were fixed between the two rods of the stretching machine and given a unidirectional and cyclic stretch (10%, 2 Hz) in culture medium for 7 days. The medium was changed every day. Scale bar 11 mm. (B) Microscopic view of spontaneously contracting ECT constructed by seeding cardiomyocytes derived from mouse ES cells into liquid type I collagen. Note the vigorous contraction of the ECT in organ bath solution, with a frequency of more than 1 Hz (Guo *et al.*, 2006). (See color insert.)

5. Put the dish into the 37° incubator for about 60 min.
6. Add 20 ml complete culture medium.
7. After 6–10 days of cultivation, the typical biconcave ECTs form, spanning the gap between the two tubes (D).

Ring System

See Fig. 11.

1. Glue silicone tubing (T) to the surface of glass culture dishes.
2. Place either Teflon disks (D) or cylinders (C) over silicone tubing to function as removable spacers during casting mold preparation and ECT culture, respectively.

   NOTE: There will be ECT condensation around the central Teflon cylinder in casting molds between culture days 1 and 4. After condensation, no change of gross morphology was observed.

3. Transfer the ECTs into a stretch apparatus to continue culture under unidirectional and cyclic stretch (10%, 2 Hz).
4. Change medium after overnight incubation and then every other day.

Okano's group (Shimizu *et al.*, 2002b) applied novel cell culture surfaces grafted with a temperature-responsive polymer, poly(*N*-isopropylacrylamide)

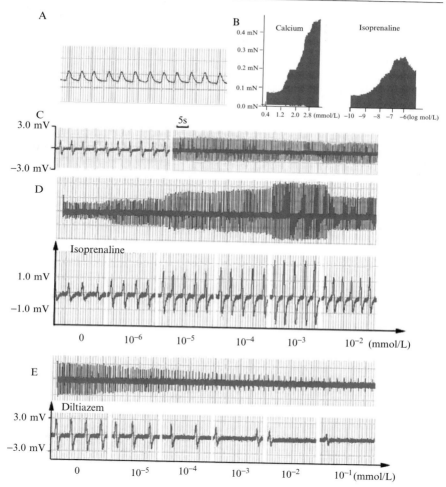

FIG. 7. Contractile properties and electrophysiology of ECTs. Representative contraction of ECTs was recorded as described by Zimmermann *et al.* The spontaneously beating ECTs were immersed in Tyrode's solution supplemented with calcium at 0.4 m*M*/L and stretched to the length of maximal force development. (A) Calcium was lowered to 0.2 m*M*/L and then increased cumulatively to 2.8 m*M*/L. After two washes with 0.2 m*M*/L calcium, isoprenaline was cumulatively added between 0.1–1000 n*M*/L. (B) For electrophysiology, the ECTs beat spontaneously and rhythmically in Tyrode's solution, showing regular ventricular activity. (C) Isoprenaline enhanced the amplitude (D). Addition of diltiazem markedly reduced resting tension to below the baseline (E) (Guo *et al.*, 2006).

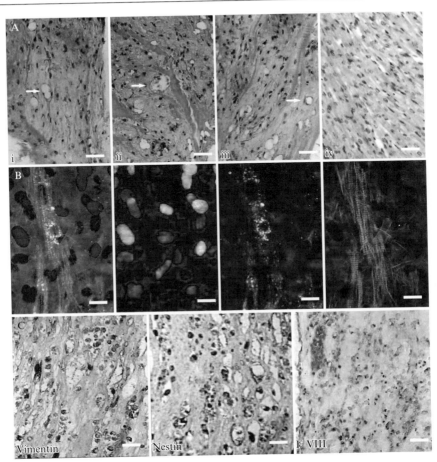

FIG. 8. Histology of and distinct cell types in ECT. Photomicrographs of H&E–stained paraffin sections from ECTs showed formation of complexes of multicellular aggregates and longitudinally oriented cell bundles (A, i–iii). Vascular vessels were notable in the ECTs (arrow). The histological morphology of the ECTs resembles that of immature neonatal cardiac tissue (A, iv). Immunolabeling indicates formation of cardiac cell bundles with significant striations of sarcomeres in the ECT. (Actin appears red; α-sarcomeric actin, green; and nuclear, blue.) (B) Distribution of fibroblasts (vimentin), vascular endothelial cells (F VIII), and neural cell–like cells (nestin) were also observed as indicated by immunolabeling (green) (C). Scale bars, 30 μm (A), 15 μm (B), or 30 μm (C) (Guo et al., 2006). (See color insert.)

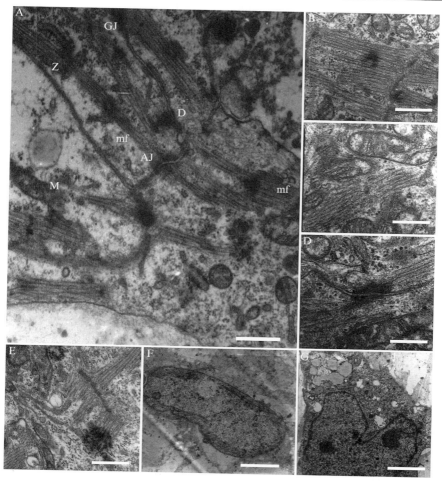

FIG. 9. TEM of ECT. The ECTs displayed sarcomeric structures (A–E), cell–cell junctions (A and D), and rich mitochondria and glycogen granulae (A–E). (A) Myofilament bundles (mf), adherens junctions (AJ), desmosomes (D), Z band (Z), and gap junctions (GJ). Noncardiac cells, such as fibroblasts (F) and macrophages (G), also populate ECT. Scale bars, 500 nm (A–E), 20 μm (F and G) (Guo *et al.*, 2006).

(PIPAAm), from which confluent cells detach as a cell sheet simply by reducing temperature without any enzymatic treatments (Shimizu *et al.*, 2003; Tsuda *et al.*, 2004; Yamato and Okano, 2004; Yang *et al.*, 2005) (Figs. 12 and 13).

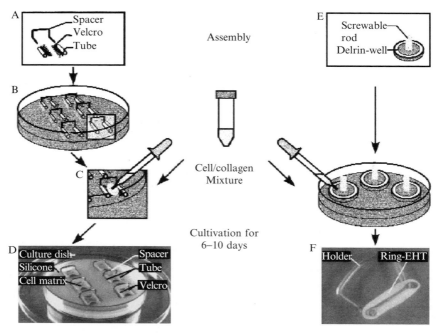

FIG. 10. Mechanism for forming a plane (lattice) system (Zimmermann *et al.*, 2000).

In their innovative study, neonatal rat cardiomyocyte sheets detached from PIPAAm-grafted surfaces were overlaid to construct cardiac grafts. Layered cell sheets began to pulse simultaneously, and morphological communication by means of connexin43 was established between the sheets. When four sheets were layered, engineered constructs were macroscopically observed to pulse spontaneously (Shimizu *et al.*, 2002a,b). *In vivo*, layered cardiomyocyte sheets were transplanted into subcutaneous tissues of nude rats. Three weeks after transplantation, surface electromyograms originating from transplanted grafts were detected and spontaneous beating was macroscopically observed. Histological studies showed characteristic structures of heart tissue and multiple neovascularization within contractile tissues. Constructs transplanted into 3-week-old rats exhibited more cardiomyocyte hypertrophy and less connective tissue than those placed into 8-week-old rats. Long-term survival of pulsatile cardiac grafts was confirmed for up to 12 weeks. In a recent report in *Nature Medicine* from Okano's group, Miyahara *et al.* (2006) cultured adipose tissue–derived mesenchymal stem

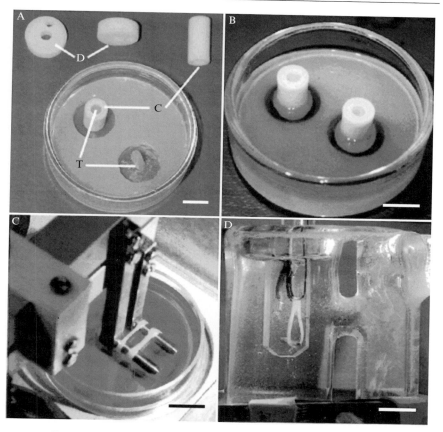

FIG. 11. The ring system (Zimmermann *et al.* 2002). (See color insert.)

cells using the temperature-responsive culture dishes (Fig. 14). Four weeks after coronary ligation, the monolayered mesenchymal stem cells were transplanted onto the scarred myocardium (Fig. 15). After transplantation, the engrafted sheet gradually grew to form a thick stratum that included newly formed vessels, undifferentiated cells, and few cardiomyocytes (Fig. 16). The mesenchymal stem cell sheet also acted through paracrine pathways to trigger angiogenesis. Unlike a fibroblast cell sheet, the monolayered mesenchymal stem cells reversed wall thinning in the scar area and improved cardiac function in rats with myocardial infarction (Figs. 17 and 18). In brief, cell sheet manipulation technology (cell sheet engineering) using

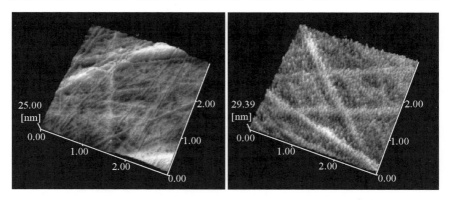

FIG. 12. Atomic force microscope images of temperature-responsive culture dish surfaces. Nongrafted, polystyrene culture dish surfaces (left) and poly(N-isopropylacrylamide)-grafted culture dish surfaces (right) were examined in air. Defects and scratches were observed on both surfaces. Small prickles can be seen on the grafted surface. Image size is 3 μm × 3 μm. Height is 25 nm (left) and 30 nm (right) (Yamato and Okano, 2004). (See color insert.)

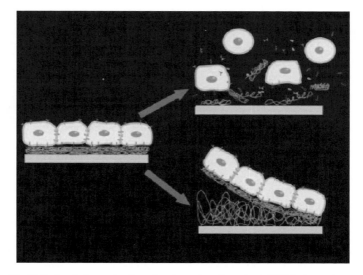

FIG. 13. Cell sheet harvest. Trypsin degrades deposited ECM (green), as well as membrane proteins, so that confluent, monolayer cells are harvested as single cells (upright). The temperature-responsive polymer (orange) covalently immobilized on the dish surface hydrates when the temperature is reduced, decreasing the interaction with deposited ECM. All the cells connected by cell–cell conjunction proteins are harvested as single, contiguous cell sheets without the need for proteolytic enzymes (lower right) (Yamato and Okano, 2004).

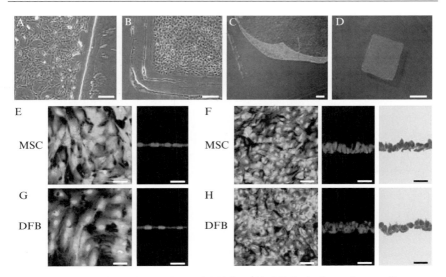

FIG. 14. Preparation of monolayered MSCs. (A) MSCs 2 days after seeding on a temperature-responsive dish. (B) Cultured MSCs expanded to confluence within the square area of the dish by day 3. (C) The monolayered MSCs detached easily from the culture dish at 20°. (D) The completely detached monolayered MSCs were identified as a 12 × 12 mm square sheet. (E–H) Cross-sectional analysis of GFP-expressing monolayered MSCs and DFBs before detachment (E and G, confocal images) and after detachment (F and H, left and center, confocal images; right, Masson trichrome). The thickness of both monolayers was 3.5-fold greater than the thickness before detachment, and constituent cells were compacted. Scale bars in A–C, 100 μm; in D, 5 mm; in E–H, 20 μm (Miyahara *et al.*, 2006). (See color insert.)

temperature-responsive cell culture surfaces has been shown to be very useful for fabricating electrically communicative, pulsatile cardiac grafts both *in vitro* and *in vivo*. This technology should have enormous potential for constructing *in vitro* 3-D heart tissue models and improving viable functional cardiac graft materials for clinical tissue repair.

This chapter mainly describes the protocols for creation of cardiac tissue on the basis of cell sheets.

Cell Sheet

Preparation of Square-Designed PIPAAm-grafted Polystyrene Cell Culture Dishes

1. Prepare poly(*N*-isopropylacrylamide) (PIPAAm) monomer in 2-propanol solution.

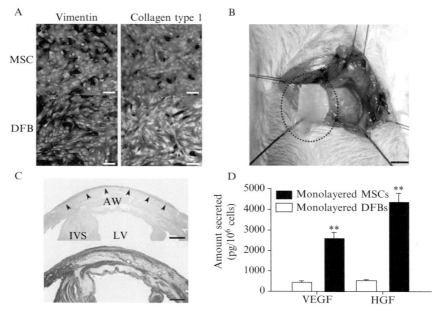

FIG. 15. Characteristics of monolayered MSCs. (A) Properties of constituent cells in the monolayered grafts. Compared with DFBs (green), MSCs (green) are positive for vimentin (red) and slightly positive for collagen type 1 (red). (B) Monolayered MSCs (in the dotted circle) transferred to the infarcted heart. (C) Extent of monolayered MSCs 48 h after transplantation (arrows). AW, anterior wall; LV, left ventricle; RV right ventricle; IVS, interventricular septum. (D) Comparison of secretion of growth factors between monolayered MSCs and DFBs. **$p < 0.01$ vs. DFBs. Scale bar in A, 20 μm; in B, 5 mm; in C, 100 μm (Miyahara et al., 2006). (See color insert.)

2. Spread the PIPAAm solution onto tissue culture polystyrene (TCPS) dishes (Falcon 3002, Becton Dickinson, Franklin Lakes, NJ).

3. Subject the dishes to irradiation (0.25 MGy electron beam dose) using an Area Beam Electron Processing System (Nisshin High Voltage, Kyoto, Japan) to generate polymerization and covalent bonding of PIPAAm to the dish surface.

4. Rinse PIPAAm-grafted dishes with cold distilled water to remove ungrafted PIPAAm.

5. Dry in nitrogen gas.

6. Mask PIPAAm-grafted surface with a square glass coverslip (24 × 24 mm, Matsunami, Osaka, Japan).

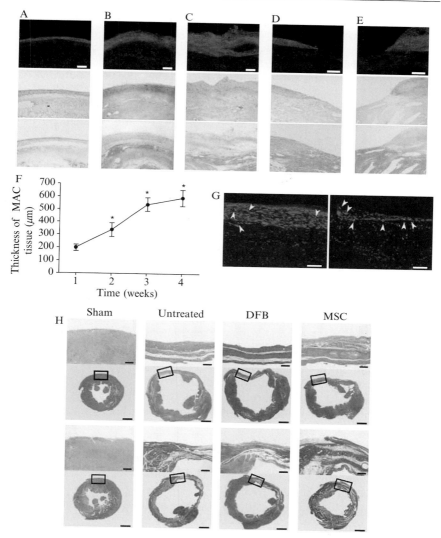

FIG. 16. Engraftment, survival, and growth of monolayered MSCs. To identify the transplanted cells within myocardial sections, we used GFP-expressing cells derived from GFP-transgenic Sprague-Dawley rats. (A–C) MSC tissue above the anterior scar at day 2 (A), day 14 (B), and day 28 (C). GFP-expressing monolayered MSCs were grafted to the native myocardium and grew gradually *in situ*, resulting in increased wall thickness. (D and E) MSC tissue above the surrounding area of the scar at day 2 (D) and day 28 (E). In A–E, upper row shows immunofluorescent staining of MSC tissue (green); nuclei are stained with DAPI (blue). Middle row shows identical sections stained with antibody to GFP and DAB by

7. Spread acrylamide (AAm) monomer solution in 2-propanol onto the masked dish surface.
8. Irradiate the dish surface with the electron beam.
9. Wash with PBS three times.
10. As a result, the center, square area of each dish will be PIPAAm-grafted (temperature-responsive) and the surrounding border will be poly-AAm–grafted (non–cell adhesive).
11. Gas sterilize square-geometry PIPAAm-grafted dishes by using ethylene oxide before use in culture.

Manipulation of Cardiomyocyte Sheets into Layered Constructs

1. Culture cardiomyocytes for 4 days at 37° on thermoresponsive cell culture surfaces.
2. Incubate culture dishes in another CO_2 incubator set at 20° to release confluent cells as a cell sheet. Cardiomyocyte sheets will detach spontaneously within 1 h and float into the aqueous media.
3. Gently aspirate the entire cell sheet with media into the tip of a 10-ml pipette and transfer onto appropriate culture surfaces.
4. Once placed, drop the media onto the center of the sheet to spread folded parts of the transferred cardiomyocyte sheets.
5. After sheet spreading, aspirate the media to adhere the cell sheet to the culture surface.
6. Add new media for further culture when the transferred sheet is reattached. This generally happens within 30 min.
7. To layer cell sheets, transfer another cardiomyocyte sheet detached from a PIPAAm-grafted dish into the first dish in the same way.
8. Position the second sheet above the first sheet and place it onto the original sheet by slow aspiration of media (30 min is sufficient for adhesion of layered sheets).
9. Repeat identical procedures to layer additional sheets.

---

bright-field microscopy. Lower row shows hematoxylin and eosin–stained sections. (F) Time course of growth of MSCs expressing GFP. $*p < 0.05$ vs. thickness of GFP$^+$ MSC tissue at 1 week. (G) TUNEL staining of transplanted MSCs (green, left) and DFBs (green, right) 48 h after transplantation. Nuclei are stained with DAPI (blue). Arrows indicate TUNEL-positive nuclei (red). (H) Photomicrographs show two cases of representative myocardial sections stained with Masson trichrome in the individual groups. Left ventricle enlargement was attenuated by the transplantation of monolayered MSC. Scale bars in A–E and upper panels of H, 100 μm; in g, 20 μm; in lower panels of H, 1 mm (Miyahara *et al.*, 2006). (See color insert.)

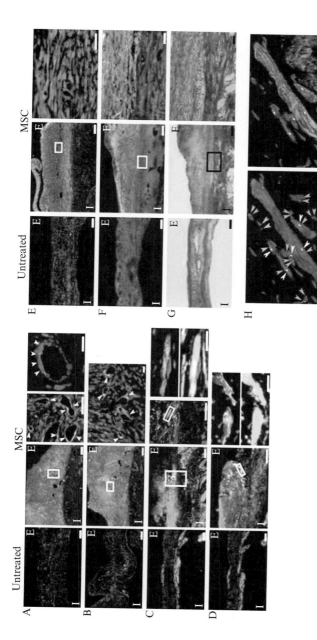

FIG. 17. Differentiation of MSC tissue within the MSC tissue after growth *in situ*. (A and B) GFP-expressing MSCs (green) were identified as a thick stratum at the epicardial side of the myocardium. The MSC tissue contained a number of blood vessel formation were only rarely positive for vascular structures positive for vWF (red, A) and αSMA (red, B). MSCs that did not participate in blood vessel formation were only rarely positive for αSMA, a marker for myofibroblasts. Arrows indicate transplanted MSCs positive for vWF or αSMA. (C and D) Some MSCs within the MSC tissue were positive for cardiac markers cardiac troponin T (red, C) and desmin (red, D). (E) Most of the MSC tissue was positive for vimentin (red). (F) The MSC tissue modestly stained for collagen type 1 (red). (G) Collagen deposition was also detected by picrosirius red staining. (H) FISH analysis. Newly formed cardiomyocytes (desmin, red) that were positive for GFP (green) had only one set of X (purple) and Y chromosomes (white), whereas two X chromosomes were detected exclusively in GFP⁻ host-derived cells. Nuclei are stained with DAPI (blue, A–F and H). Scale bars in left three panels of A and C and in two left panels of B and D–G, 100 μm; in H and far right panels of A–G, 20 μm. E, epicardial side; I, intimal side (Miyahara *et al.*, 2006). (See color insert.)

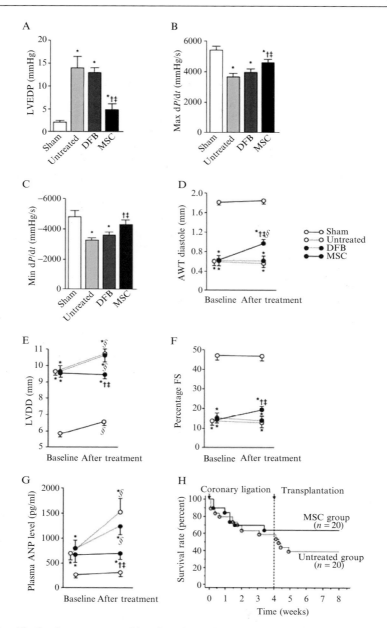

FIG. 18. Cardiac structure and function after transplantation of monolayered MSCs. (A–C) Hemodynamic parameters obtained by catheterization. LVEDP, left ventricle end-diastolic pressure. (D–F) Echocardiographic findings. AWT, anterior wall thickness; LVDD, left

10. To construct pulsatile grafts *in vitro*, prepare collagen membranes (20-mm square, Cellgen, Koken, Tokyo, Japan) with the center 5-mm square part cut out to create an open frame.
11. Overlay cardiomyocyte sheets on the collagen frame with center regions unsupported.

Conclusions

With the recent significant progress, liquid collagen and cell sheet–based cardiac tissue engineering has been proven so far to be the best strategy for engineering cardiac tissue. This method points to a realistic therapeutic perspective. However, significantly more work is necessary to optimize the protocols so as to increase, most importantly, the thickness of the engineered cardiac muscle.

---

ventricle end-diastolic dimension; FS, fractional shortening. (G) Plasma atrial natriuretic peptide (ANP) level. Baseline represents measurements 4 weeks after coronary ligation; "after treatment" represents measurements taken 4 weeks after transplantation (8 weeks after coronary ligation). Data are mean ±S.E.M. *$p < 0.05$ vs. sham group; $^{\dagger}p < 0.05$ vs. untreated group; $^{\ddagger}p < 0.05$ vs. DFB group; $^{\S}p < 0.05$ vs. baseline. (H) Survival of rats with chronic heart failure with or without monolayered MSC transplantation. The Kaplan–Meier survival curve demonstrates an 8-week survival rate of 65% for the MSC group vs. 45% for the untreated group. Survival rate after transplantation was significantly higher in the MSC group than in the untreated group (100% vs. 71% 4-week survival rate after transplantation, log rank test, $p < 0.05$) (Miyahara *et al.*, 2006).

References

American Heart Association. (2005). "Heart Disease and Stroke Statistics—2006 Update." Dallas, Texas: American Heart Association.

Eschenhagen, T., Didie, M., Munzel, F., Shubert, P., Schneiderbanger, K., and Zimmerman, W. H. (2002). 3D engineered heart tissue for replacement therapy. Basic Research in Cardiology, **97**(Suppl. 1), I145–152.

Eschenhagen, T., Fink, C., Remmers, U., Scholz, H., Wattchow, J., Weil, J., and Elson, E. L. (1997). Three dimensional reconstitution of embryonic cardiomycytes in collagen matrix: A new heart muscle model system. *FASEB J.* **11**, 683–694.

Gillum, R. F. (1994). Epidemiology of congenital heart disease in the United States. *Am. Heart J.* **127**, 919–927.

Guo, X.-M., Zhao, Y.-S., Wang, C.-Y., E, L.-L., Chang, H.-X., Zhang, X.-A., Duan, C.-M., Dong, L.-Z., Jiang, H., Li, J., Song, Y., and Yang, X. (2006). Creation of engineered cardiac tissue *in vitro* from mouse embryonic stem cells. *Circulation* **113**, 2229–2237.

Hoffman, J. I. (1995a). Incidence of congenital heart disease: I, Postnatal incidence. *Pediatr. Cardiol.* **16**, 103–113.

Hoffman, J. I. (1995b). Incidence of congenital heart disease: II, Prenatal incidence. *Pediatr. Cardiol.* **16**, 155–165.

Li, R. K., Yau, T. M., Weisel, R. D., Mickle, D. A., Sakai, T., Choi, A., and Jia, Z. Q. (2000). Construction of a bioengineered cardiac graft. *J. Thorac. Cardiovasc. Surg.* **119**, 368–375.

Li, R. K., Jia, Z. Q., Weisel, R. D., Mickle, D. A., Choi, A., and Yau, T. M. (1999). Survival and function of bioengineered cardiac grafts. *Circulation* **100**(Suppl.), II63–II69.

Miyahara, Y., Nagaya, N., Kataoka, M., Yanagawa, B., Tanaka, K., Hao, H., Ishino, K., Ishida, H., Shimizu, T., Kangawa, K., Sano, S., Okano, T., Kitamura, S., and Mori, H. (2006). Monolayered mesenchymal stem cells repair scarred myocardium after myocardial infarction. *Nat. Med.* **12**, 459–465.

Papadaki, M., Bursac, N., Langer, R., Merok, J., Vunjak-Novakovic, G., and Freed, L. E. (2001). Tissue engineering of functional cardiac muscle: Molecular, structural, and electrophysiological studies. *Am. J. Physiol. Heart Circ. Physiol.* **280**, H168–H178.

Radisic, M., Park, H., Shing, H., Consi, T., Schoen, F. J., Langer, R., Freed, L. E., and Vunjak-Novakovic, G. (2004). Functional assembly of engineered myocardium by electrical stimulation of cardiac myocytes cultured on scaffolds. *Proc. Natl. Acad. Sci. USA* **101**, 18129–18134.

Sakai, T., Li, R. K., Weisel, R. D., Mickle, D. A., Kim, E. T., Jia, Z. Q., and Yau, T. M. (2001). The fate of a tissue-engineered cardiac graft in the right ventricular outflow tract of the rat. *J. Thorac. Cardiovasc. Surg.* **121**, 932–942.

Shimizu, T., Yamato, M., Akutsu, T., Shibata, T., Isoi, Y., Kikuchi, A., Umezu, M., and Okano, T. (2002a). Electrically communicating three-dimensional cardiac tissue mimic fabricated by layered cultured cardiomyocyte sheets. *J. Biomed. Mater. Res.* **60**, 110–117.

Shimizu, T., Yamato, M., Isoi, Y., Akutsu, T., Setomaru, T., Abe, K., Kikuchi, A., Umezu, M., and Okano, T. (2002b). Fabrication of pulsatile cardiac tissue grafts using a novel 3-dimensional cell sheet manipulation technique and temperature-responsive cell culture surfaces. *Circ. Res.* **90**, e40.

Shimizu, T., Yamato, M., Kikuchi, A., and Okano, T. (2003). Cell sheet engineering for myocardial tissue reconstruction. *Biomaterials* **24**, 2309–2316.

Tsuda, Y., Kikuchi, A., Yamato, M., Sakurai, Y., Umezu, M., and Okano, T. (2004). Control of cell adhesion and detachment using temperature and thermoresponsive copolymer grafted culture surfaces. *J. Biomed. Mater. Res.* Part A, **69**, 70–78.

Yamato, M., and Okano, T. (2004). Cell sheet engineering. *Materials Today* **7**, 42–47.

Yang, J., Yamato, M., Kohno, C., Nishimoto, A., Sekine, H., Fukai, F., and Okano, T. (2005). Cell sheet engineering: Recreating tissues without biodegradable scaffolds. *Biomaterials* **26**, 6415–6422.

Zhao, Y. S., Wang, C. Y., Li, D. X., Zhang, X. Z., Qiao, Y., Guo, X. M., Wang, X. L., Duan, C. M., Dong, L. Z., and Song, Y. (2005). Construction of a unidirectionally beating 3-dimensional cardiac muscle construct. *J. Heart Lung Transpl.* **24**, 1091–1097.

Zimmermann, W. H., Fink, C., Kralisch, D., Remmers, U., Weil, J., and Eschenhagen, T. (2000). Three-dimensional engineered heart tissue from neonatal rat cardiac myocytes. *Biotechnol. Bioeng.* **68**, 106–114.

Zimmermann, W. H., Schneiderbanger, K., Schubert, P., Didié, M., Münzel, F., Heubach, J. F., Kostin, S., Neuhuber, W. L., and Eschenhagen, T. (2002). Tissue engineering of a differentiated cardiac muscle construct. *Circ. Res.* **90**, 223–230.

Zimmermann, W. H., Melnychenko, I., Wasmeier, G., Didie, M., Naito, H., Nixdorff, U., Hess, A., Budinsky, L., Brune, K., Michaelis, B., Dhein, S., Schwoerer, A., Ehmke, H., and Eschenhagen, T. (2006). Engineered heart tissue grafts improve systolic and diastolic function in infarcted rat hearts. *Nat. Med.* **12**, 452–458.

[16] Mesenchymal Stem Cells and Tissue Engineering

By Nicholas W. Marion and Jeremy J. Mao

Abstract

Mesenchymal stem cells (MSCs) have become one of the most studied stem cells, especially toward the healing of diseased and damaged tissues and organs. MSCs can be readily isolated from a number of adult tissues by means of minimally invasive approaches. MSCs are capable of self-replication to many passages and, therefore, can potentially be expanded to sufficient numbers for tissue and organ regeneration. MSCs are able to differentiate into multiple cell lineages that resemble osteoblasts, chondrocytes, myoblasts, adipocytes, and fibroblasts and express some of the key markers typical of endothelial cells, neuron-like cells, and cardiomyocytes. MSCs have been used alone for cell delivery or seeded in biomaterial scaffolds toward the healing of tissue and organ defects. After an increasing number of the "proof of concept" studies, the remaining tasks are many, such as to determine MSC interactions with host cells and signaling molecules, to investigate the interplay between MSCs and biological scaffold materials, and to apply MSC-based therapies toward clinically relevant defect models. The ultimate goal of MSC-based therapies has valid biological rationale in that clusters of MSCs differentiate to form virtually all connective tissue during development. MSC-based therapies can only be realized our improved understanding of not only their fundamental properties such as population doubling and differentiation pathways but also translational studies that use MSCs in the *de novo* formation and/or regeneration of diseased or damaged tissues and organs.

MSCs: Definition and Therapeutic Promise

"Mesenchymal stem cells" (MSCs) are named out of compromise. During embryonic development, mesenchyme or the embryonic mesoderm contains stem cells that differentiate into virtually all connective tissue phenotypes such as bone, cartilage, bone marrow stroma, interstitial fibrous tissue, skeletal muscle, dense fibrous tissues such as tendons and ligaments, as well as adipose tissue. In vertebrates, mesenchyme is usually abundant and contains unconnected cells in contrast to rows of tightly connected epithelial cells that derive from the ectoderm (Alberts *et al.*, 2002). Mesenchymal–epithelial interactions are critical for both appendicular skeletogenesis and craniofacial morphogenesis (Gilbert, 2000; Mao *et al.*, 2006). On the

METHODS IN ENZYMOLOGY, VOL. 420
0076-6879/06 $35.00
DOI: 10.1016/S0076-6879(06)20016-8

completion of prenatal morphogenesis, clusters of mesenchymal cells likely continue to reside in various tissues and are the logical sources of adult mesenchymal stem cells.

In the adult, the definition of a common progenitor for all connective tissues inevitably elicits controversy. Strictly speaking, mesenchyme defined as embryonic mesenchyme should not exist in the adult. Despite this textbook dilemma, it is without doubt that adult connective tissues contain progenitor cells that maintain physiologically necessary tissue turnover and, on trauma or pathological conditions, are responsible for tissue regeneration. Whereas amicable and dispassionate debate continues regarding the appropriateness of the term *mesenchymal stem cells* (MSCs), or sibling terms such as *mesenchymal progenitor cells* (MPCs), *bone marrow progenitor cells* (*BMPCs*), or *bone marrow stromal cells (BMSCs)*, the scientific community and health care industry demand a workable term for communication. The editors' choice of "Mesenchymal Stem Cells" as the chapter's title is yet another indication of this need.

What we now know as mesenchymal stem cells were first identified as colony-forming unit fibroblast-like cells in the 1970s (Friedenstein *et al.*, 1970, 1976). Numerous reports since have demonstrated that bone marrow, adipose tissue, tooth pulp, etc., contain a subset of cells that not only are capable of self-replication for many passages but also can differentiate into multiple end-stage cell lineages that resemble osteoblasts, adipocytes, chondrocytes, myoblasts, etc. (Alhadlaq and Mao, 2004). Recently, bone marrow–derived cells have been shown to differentiate into nonmesenchymal lineages such as hepatic, renal, cardiac, and neural cells (Alhadlaq and Mao, 2004). MSCs have been identified in an increasing number of vertebrate species including humans (Alhadlaq and Mao, 2004).

Our understanding of MSCs has advanced tremendously because of their demonstrated and perceived therapeutic capacity (Alhadlaq and Mao, 2004; Aubin, 1998; Bianco *et al.*, 2001; Krebsbach *et al.*, 1999; Kuo and Tuan, 2003; Mao *et al.*, 2006; Pittenger *et al.*, 1999; Tuli *et al.*, 2003). Why are MSCs perceived superior to autologous tissue grafts in the regeneration of human tissue and organs? Autologous tissue grafts often represent the current clinical "gold standard" for the reconstruction of defects resulting from trauma, chronic diseases, congenital anomalies, and tumor resection. However, autologous tissue grafting is based on the concept that a diseased or damaged tissue must be replaced by like tissue that is healthy. Thus, the key drawback of autologous tissue grafting is donor site trauma and morbidity. For example, healthy cartilage must be surgically isolated to repair arthritic cartilage. A patient who receives a bone graft harvested from his or her illiac crest for facial bone reconstruction is hospitalized for an extended stay because of donor site trauma and morbidity of the illiac crest, instead of facial surgery.

Also, spare healthy tissue is scarce because of biological design during evolution. In contrast, MSC-based therapeutic approaches may circumvent the key deficiencies associated with autologous grafting procedures. First, a teaspoonful of MSC-containing aspirates can be obtained from bone marrow, or other sources, and expanded to sufficient numbers for healing large, clinically relevant defects. Second, MSCs can differentiate into multiple cell lineages, thus providing the possibility that a common cell source can heal many tissues, as opposed to the principle of harvesting healthy tissue to heal like tissue in association with autologous tissue grafting. Finally, MSCs or MSC-derived cells can be seeded in biocompatible scaffolds, which can be shaped into the anatomical structure that is to be replaced by MSCs. The construct is then surgically implanted to heal the defect.

MSC-based therapies can be autologous (from self) and thus eliminate the issues of immunorejection and pathogen transmission or allogenic for potentially off-the-shelf availability. Autologous MSC-based therapies are also expected to be superior to other surgical approaches such as allogenic grafts, xenogenic grafts, or synthetic materials such as total joint replacement prosthesis. Besides the issues associated with immunorejection, pathogen transmission, wear and tear, and allergic metal reactions, the key drawback allogenic tissue grafts, xenogenic tissue grafts, or synthetic materials is a general deficiency of physiologically necessary remodeling that must take place over years of postsurgical ageing (Barry, 2003; Mao, 2005). For example, the general life span of a surgically successful total joint replacement is 8–10 years, far too short for arthritic patients in their 40s, 50s, or even 60s. Recently, we and others have reported the tissue engineering of an entire articular condyle with both cartilage and bone layers from a single population of MSCs (Mao, 2005). The biological rationale for MSC-based total joint replacement is that clusters of MSCs initiate joint morphogenesis during embryonic development (Archer et al., 2003; Dowthwaite et al., 2003).

Isolation and Expansion of MSCs

When bone marrow content was isolated and cultured, a subset of fibroblast-like cells were observed to differentiate into osteoblasts (Friedenstein, 1995; Friedenstein et al., 1970, 1976). Numerous reports since then have shown that these fibroblast-like cells that adhere to tissue culture polystyrene are capable of not only population doubling but also differentiating into multiple cell lineages in addition to osteoblasts, such as chondrocytes, myoblasts, and adipocytes (Alhadlaq and Mao, 2004). The protocol by centrifugation in a density gradient to separate bone marrow–derived mononucleated cells from plasma and red blood cells is still widely used. The mononucleated cells can then be plated on tissue culture polystyrene with frequent changes of culture medium. Nonadherent cells such as hematopoietic cells are discarded on medium change. Some of the adherent cells are MSCs (Aubin, 1998; Caplan, 1991).

The isolation of MSCs has been recently reviewed (Alhadlaq and Mao, 2004). Bone marrow extracts contain heterogeneous cell populations. MSCs represent a small fraction of total mononucleated cells within bone marrow (Barry, 2003). Further enrichment techniques have been explored such as positive selection using cell surface markers including STRO-1, CD133 (prominin, AC133), p75LNGFR (p75, low-affinity nerve growth factor receptor), CD29, CD44, CD90, CD105, c-kit, SH2 (CD105), SH3, SH4 (CD73), CD71, CD106, CD120a, CD124, and HLA-DR (Alhadlaq and Mao, 2004; Lee et al., 2004; Pittenger et al., 1999). Flow cytometry is another helpful enrichment tool based on an array of cell surface markers. Negative selection is also helpful by the use of antibody cocktails that label bone marrow–derived cells that are not MSCs (Alhadlaq and Mao, 2004; Marion et al., 2005). For example, CD34 can be used as a specific marker for hematopoietic cells. Once the enriched bone marrow sample is placed atop the Percoll or Ficoll gradient and centrifuged, the dense cells and cell–antibody units are drawn to the bottom, leaving the desired cells atop the gradient (Marion et al., 2005). The enriched layer likely will contain a high concentration of MSCs that can be plated and expanded. An example of culture-expanded human MSCs is provided in Fig. 1A.

MSCs can undergo population doubling to a substantial number of passages, but perhaps not unlimited, although unlimited implies a process that cannot be experimentally tested. Human MSCs (hMSCs) may demonstrate an initial lag phase during expansion, but this is followed by rapid proliferation with an average population doubling time of 12–24 h, and with some anticipated variation among donors and with aging (Spees et al., 2004). The estimated number of hMSCs in a 2 ml bone marrow aspirate is between 12.5 and 35.5 billion (Spees et al., 2004). The multipotency of hMSCs is retained up to 23 population doublings (Banfi et al., 2000), whereas no visible change in morphology of MSCs takes place until after 38 population doublings (Bruder et al., 1997). Interestingly, osteogenic differentiation of hMSCs seems to be preserved despite apparent cell senescence and slowdown in proliferation rate (Banfi et al., 2000; Bruder et al., 1997). Numerous studies have attempted to improve the culture conditions and to increase the expandability of primary MSCs. For example, fibroblast growth factor-2 (FGF2) enhances the proliferation rate of primary MSCs without substantial reduction in their differentiation potential (Banfi et al., 2000; Bruder et al., 1997; Tsutsumi et al., 2001). Similar to other somatic cells, MSCs undergo telomere shortening with each cell division, which eventually results in a cessation in

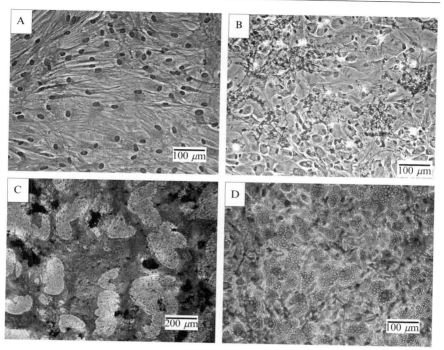

Fig. 1. (A) Human mesenchymal stem cells (MSCs) isolated from anonymous adult human bone marrow donor after culture expansion (H&E staining). Further enrichment of MSCs can be accomplished by positive selection using cell surface markers including STRO-1, CD133 (prominin, AC133), p75LNGFR (p75, low-affinity nerve growth factor receptor), CD29, CD44, CD90, CD105, c-kit, SH2 (CD105), SH3, SH4 (CD73), CD71, CD106, CD120a, CD124, and HLA-DR or negative selection (Alhadlaq and Mao, 2004; Lee et al., 2004; Pittenger et al., 1999). (B) Chondrocytes derived from human mesenchymal stem cells showing positive staining to Alcian blue. Additional molecular and genetic markers can be used to further characterize MSC-derived chondrocytes (Alhadlaq and Mao, 2004; Lee et al., 2004; Pittenger et al., 1999). (C) Osteoblasts derived from human mesenchymal stem cells showing positive von Kossa staining for calcium deposition (black) and active alkaline phosphatase enzyme (red). Additional molecular and genetic markers can be used to further characterize MSC-derived chondrocytes (Alhadlaq and Mao, 2004; Lee et al., 2004; Pittenger et al., 1999). (D) Adipocytes derived from human mesenchymal stem cells showing positive Oil Red–O staining of intracellular lipids. Additional molecular and genetic markers can be used to further characterize MSC-derived chondrocytes (Alhadlaq and Mao, 2004; Lee et al., 2004; Pittenger et al., 1999).

cell proliferation. FGF-2 delays, but does not eliminate, cell senescence (Derubeis and Cancedda, 2004; Martin et al., 1997). Although telomere shortening usually leads to the cessation of cell proliferation, telomerase can repair telomeres after each cell division, thus increasing the cell's lifespan

(Derubeis and Cancedda, 2004). Immortalized MSC cell lines have been developed such as the HMPC32F (Osyczka *et al.*, 2002). HMPC32F has been shown to possess multilineage differentiation potential toward osteogenic, chondrogenic, and adipogenic lineages, while exceeding the lifespan of normal adult human mesenchymal stem cells (Osyczka *et al.*, 2002). This MSC cell line was created by infecting primary MSCs with the human papilloma virus Type16 with E6/E7genes within a viral vector. Immortalization was determined after multilineage differentiation for up to a year in culture and up to approximately 20 passages. Cell lines are valuable experimental tools but are not intended for clinical translation.

Isolation Protocol

Human Bone Marrow–Derived MSCs

- Ficoll-Paque—room temperature (e.g., StemCells, Inc., Vancouver, BC, Canada).
- Bone marrow sample—room temperature (e.g., AllCells, LLC, Berkeley, CA).
- 10 ml marrow + 5 ml DPBS + 125 U/ml heparin (total volume, 15 ml).
- Basal culture media (89% DMEM-low glucose, 10% fetal bovine serum [FBS], 1% antibiotics).
- RosetteSep MSC enrichment cocktail (StemCells, Inc.).
- 100 ml PBS with 2% FBS and 1 mM EDTA.
- Transfer the bone marrow sample to a 50-ml conical tube. Add 750 μl RosetteSep (50 μl/1 ml of bone marrow, 50 μl × 15 ml = 750 μl).
- Incubate for 20 min at room temperature.
- Add 15 ml of PBS 2% FBS 1 mM EDTA solution to bone marrow. Total volume is 30 ml.
- Add 15 ml Ficoll-Paque to two new 50-ml conical tubes.
- Layer bone marrow solution gently on top of the Ficoll-Paque in each tube. Do not allow marrow to mix with the Ficoll-Paque.
- Centrifuge for 25 min at 300g with brake off at room temperature.
- Remove enriched cells from Ficoll-Paque interface.
- Wash enriched cells with PBS-FBS-EDTA solution in 50-ml tube and centrifuge at 1000 rpm for 10 min, brake off.
- Plate cells approximately 0.5–1 million total per petri dish with basal culture media. (Now referred to *as primary cultures* or *passage 0* [P0]).
- Change medium every 2 days. Remove nonadherent cells during medium changes. Some of the adherent colonies are of mesenchymal lineage.

Multilineage Differentiation of MSCS

MSCs are clearly capable of multilineage differentiation into osteoblasts, chondrocytes, myoblasts, adipocytes, etc. in *ex vivo* culture (Alhadlaq and Mao, 2004; Barry, 2003; Caplan, 1991; Caplan and Bruder, 2001; Derubeis and Cancedda, 2004; Gao and Caplan, 2003; Gregory *et al.*, 2005a,b; Indrawattana *et al.*, 2004; Pittenger *et al.*, 1999; Sekiya *et al.*, 2002). The differentiation of MSCs toward osteogenic, chondrogenic, and adipogenic lineages is reviewed later. For myogenic differentiation, the reader is referred to several comprehensive reviews (Bhagavati and Xu [2004]; Gang *et al.* [2004]; Xu *et al.* [2004]).

Chondrogenic Differentiation

Chondrogenic differentiation of MSCs has tremendous significance in cartilage regeneration. Cartilage has poor capacity for self-regeneration because of the scarcity of resident chondroprogenitor cells in the adult (Alberts *et al.*, 2002; Mao, 2005). Most of the sparse cells in adult articular cartilage are mature chondrocytes engaged in matrix maintenance instead of active chondroprogenitor cells capable of proliferation and differentiation into chondrocytes (Hunziker, 2002). Recent work demonstrates that articular cartilage contains a small population of cells that possess some of the same properties as progenitor cells (Dowthwaite *et al.*, 2003). However, the full capacity of these progenitor-like cells is yet to be explored. The clinical observation that injuries to articular cartilage beyond certain degrees fail to self-repair still serves as the rationale for exploring the healing capacity of MSCs in cartilage regeneration (Mao, 2005).

Chondrogenic Stimulants

Transforming growth factors including TGF-β1, TGF-β2, or TGF-β3 have been repeatedly demonstrated to stimulate chondrogenesis of MSCs (Barry, 2003). A combination of TGF-β3 and bone morphogenetic protein-6 (BMP-6) increases cartilage matrix deposition (Sekiya *et al.*, 2001). Cyclical exposure to TGF-β induces a significant increase in matrix deposition compared with continuous exposure of TGF-β3 alone, BMP-6 alone, or in combination (Sekiya *et al.*, 2001, 2002).

Although MSCs can differentiate into chondrocyte-like cells in a 2D culture system, there is a tendency for 2D differentiated chondrocytes to dedifferentiate and/or transdifferentiate into fibroblast-like cells. Even mature chondrocytes isolated from articular cartilage have a tendency to dedifferentiate and/or transdifferentiate on prolonged culture in 2D (Haudenschild *et al.*, 2001; Jakob *et al.*, 2001). Alternatives to 2D culture of chondrocytes include approaches such as micromass culture or pellet culture, differentiating MSCs toward chondrocytes in 3D biomaterials, or self-assembly of MSCs into 3D chondrogenic structures. By centrifuging a known quantity of MSCs in the bottom of a conical tube, for example, 250,000–1.5 million cells, and using a variety of serum-free medium solutions combined with growth factor administration, hMSCs will differentiate toward the chondrogenic lineage. Chondrogenic differentiation medium is frequently high-glucose DMEM as opposed to the medium for hMSC expansion. Fetal bovine serum does not seem to be necessary for chondrogenic differentiation of MSCs. In some formulations, selected bioactive factors are added such as L-proline at 40 μg/ml, ITS (insulin, transferring, and sodium selenite) at $1\times$ solution, and sodium pyruvate at 100 μg/ml. Dexamethasone at 100 nM and L-ascorbic acid 2-phosphate (AsAP) at 50 μg/ml has also been incorporated (Johnstone et al., 1998; Sekiya et al., 2001, 2002; Yoo et al., 1998).

MSCs can be differentiated into chondrocytes in 3D biocompatible scaffolds, partially to circumvent the possibility of dedifferentiation and/or transdifferentiation in extended 2D culture system. Polymeric scaffolds such as alginate, agarose, chitosan, and poly (ethylene glycol) diacrylate (PEGDA) hydrogels have been used to provide 3D environments for chondrogenic differentiation of MSCs (Alhadlaq et al., 2004; Anseth et al., 2002; Hung et al., 2003; Kim et al., 2003; Williams et al., 2003; Woodfield et al., 2006). The feasibility to polymerize biomaterials into complex anatomical structures makes several hydrogels well suited for cartilage tissue engineering. MSCs can be exposed to chondrogenic-supplemented medium, such as TGF-β family, while encapsulated in hydrogels (Alhadlaq et al., 2004; Anseth et al., 2002; Kim et al., 2003; Williams et al., 2003). The advantage of 3D hydrogel encapsulation is that of minimizing the need to disrupt 2D monolayer culture or pellet culture before seeding cells in 3D.

Several reports have demonstrated that chondrocytes can elaborate 3D matrices and self-assemble into cartilage-like structures, sometimes when seeded on top of a biomaterial instead of within it (Klein et al., 2003; Masuda et al., 2003). Isolated chondrocytes are initially cultured on top of agarose or alginate gels to produce the cell-associated matrix, rather than encapsulated within gels, followed by additional 2D culture until cell–matrix structures reach a certain size. This represents a convenient variation of the 3D culture approach and may have therapeutic relevance in cartilage tissue engineering.

Chondrogenic Differentiation Protocol: Rat MSCs

- Rat chondrogenic medium: 89% DMEM-low glucose, 10% FBS, 1% antibiotic solution, supplemented with 10 ng/ml recombinant rat TGF-β1.

- Plate rat MSCs in monolayer culture with basal medium until 80% confluent.
- Remove basal medium and continue monolayer culture with rat chondrogenic medium (previously) for an additional 2 weeks, and change medium biweekly.
- Monolayer cultures may be fixed for histological analysis or for quantification of biochemical markers using 1% Triton-X100.

Chondrogenic Differentiation Protocol: Human MSCs

- Human chondrogenic media: 95% DMEM–high glucose, 1% 1× ITS + 1 solution, 1% antibiotic, 100 μg/ml sodium pyruvate, 50 μg/ml L-ascorbic acid 2-phosphate (AsAP), 40 μg/ml L-proline, 0.1 μM dexamethasone, and 10 ng/ml recombinant human TGF-β3.
- Centrifuge approximately 2.5×10^5 hMSCs in a 15-ml conical tube at 500g for 5 min at 4°.
- Culture with human chondrogenic medium for at least 14 days and change medium biweekly.
- Pellets may be removed from tube by inverting and gently tapping for quantitative and histological analyses.
    a. 1% Triton-X100 may be used to disrupt cell pellets for quantitative biochemical assays such as DNA, collagen, and proteoglycans.
    b. Samples may be dehydrated and embedded in paraffin before sectioning and staining for histological analysis.

Chondrogenic Differentiation Markers

A number of histological dyes provide the most convenient indication of chondrogenic differentiation of MSCs. Histological dyes are reagents sensitive to the presence of proteoglycans or sulfated glycosaminoglycans. Stains for glycosaminoglycans and proteoglycans include Safranin–O/fast green and Alcian blue. These histological dyes have been conventionally used in labeling native articular cartilage and growth plate cartilage and, therefore, are reliable markers of chondrogenic differentiation.

Chondrogenic differentiation is driven by a number of transcription factors such as the SOX family (Lefebvre *et al.*, 2001; Ylostalo *et al.*, 2006). *SOX9* is expressed in differentiating chondrocytes; deletions of SOX9 elicit abnormal endochondral bone formation and hypoplasia of the developing bone (Lefebvre *et al.*, 2001). *SOX5* and *SOX6* are expressed during chondrogenic differentiation. Biosynthesis of type II collagen and aggrecan are regulated by the expression of *SOX9* and *SOX5* through their activation of *COL2A1* and *aggrecan* genes (Lefebvre *et al.*, 2001; Ng *et al.*, 1997; Ylostalo *et al.*, 2006). Furthermore, collagen genes such as *COL9A1*, *COL9A2*, *COL9A3*, and *COL11A2* are expressed in response to the expression of *SOX9* (Ylostalo *et al.*, 2006). RT-PCR, Western blotting, *in situ* hybridization, and immunohistochemistry are effective approaches to identify the presence of type II collagen, type X collagen, various proteoglycans such as aggrecan, decorin, and biglycan in engineered cartilage tissue. Quantitatively, collagen and sulfated GAG contents can be measured using commercially available reagent and ELISA kits or biochemical assays. Genetic analysis such as RT-PCR aims to identify the expression of chondrogenic mRNAs such as collagen II, collagen IX, *SOX 9*, *SOX5*, *SOX6*, *COL9A1*, *COL9A2*, *COL9A3*, and *COL11* because of their presence during early chondral development. Gene arrays can provide a comprehensive portrait of not only cartilage-related genes but also other genes that may be important in chondrogenesis. An example of chondrogenic differentiation of rat MSCs in monolayer is provided in Fig. 1B.

Structural analysis is necessary to determine whether tissue-engineered cartilage has microstructural and ultrastructural characteristics as native cartilage. For instance, native chondrocyte matrix is characterized with pericellular matrix and interterritorial matrix (Allen and Mao, 2004; Guilak, 2000; Guilak and Mow, 2000; Poole *et al.*, 1988, 1991). Although tissue-engineered cartilage apparently has structures similar to pericellular matrix and interterritorial matrix in a number of reports, more attention has yet to be paid to structural analysis of tissue-engineered cartilage. The reader is referred to several excellent reviews of structural properties of native and engineered cartilage (Cohen *et al.* [1998]; Grodzinsky *et al.* [2000]; Hunziker [2002]; Kerin *et al.* [2002]; Nesic *et al.* [2006]; Woodfield *et al.* [2002]).

Mechanical testing is necessary to ascertain that tissue-engineered cartilage has the proper mechanical properties in addition to the "right ingredients" such as type II collagen and glycosaminoglycans, as well as having the "right" structural characteristics. The reader is referred to a number of excellent reviews on the mechanical properties of native and tissue-engineered cartilage (Hung *et al.*, 2004; Hunziker, 2002; Mow *et al.*, 1984, 1999; Troken *et al.*, 2005).

Osteogenic Differentiation

Osteogenic differentiation was the first identified end-stage lineage of MSC differentiation (Friedenstein, 1995; Friedenstein *et al.*, 1970, 1976). Given that bone marrow is a rich source for MSCs, it should come as no surprise that MSCs can be readily differentiated into osteoblasts. An array of genetic and matrix markers have been used to verify the osteogenic differentiation of MSCs.

Osteogenic Stimulants

Several well-explored cocktails have been shown to induce MSCs to differentiate into osteoblasts. MSCs have been shown to express alkaline phosphatase after 7–14 days of exposure to 100 nM dexamethasone, 50 μg/ml L-ascorbic acid 2-phosphate (AsAP), and 100 mM β-glycerophosphate (Alhadlaq and Mao, 2003, 2005; Alhadlaq et al., 2004; Marion et al., 2005). Long-term exposure of MSCs to the formula of dexamethasone, AsAP, and β-glycerophosphate results in calcium matrix deposition and the expression of late osteogenesis markers such as bone sialoprotein, osteocalcin, and osteonectin. Dexamethasone is a glucocorticoid steroid capable of either stimulating or inhibiting osteogenic differentiation of MSCs depending on dosage (Bruder et al., 1997). High dexamethasone dose stimulates adipogenic differentiation of MSCs, whereas lower doses stimulate osteogenic differentiation (Bruder et al., 1997). The addition of AsAP further facilities osteogenic differentiation, including collagen biosynthesis, in addition to its stimulatory effects on cell proliferation (Graves, 1994a,b; Jaiswal et al., 1997). A number of studies have used ascorbic acid, the bioactive component of AsAP as an osteogenic supplement. However, ascorbic acid is somewhat unstable at 37° and neutral pH, a problem not associated with AsAP (Jaiswal et al., 1997). High doses of ascorbic acid can also be toxic to cells (Jaiswal et al., 1997). Last, β-glycerophosphate is critical to stimulate calcified matrix formation in combination with the effects of dexamethasone and AsAP (Jaiswal et al., 1997). Without β-glycerophosphate, MSC-derived osteoblasts are slow to mediate a calcium phosphate matrix (Jaiswal et al., 1997).

Several members of bone morphogenetic proteins (BMPs) have also been shown to induce the osteogenic differentiation of MSCs, including BMP-2, BMP-6, and BMP-9 (Dayoub et al., 2003; Friedman et al., 2006; Katagiri et al., 1994; Li et al., 2006; Long et al., 1995; Rickard et al., 1994; Wang et al., 1990; Wozney, 1992). BMPs are usually supplemented in combination with dexamethasone to stimulate the osteogenic differentiation of MSCs (Rickard et al., 1994). Osteogenic differentiation of MSCs using BMP-2 is dose dependent, with measurable effects between 25–100 ng/mL (Fernando-Lecanda, 1997; Rickard et al., 1994).

Osteogenic Differentiation Protocol

- Osteogenic-supplemented medium: 89% DMEM–low glucose, 10% fetal bovine serum, 1% antibiotics, 50 μg/ml AsAP, 0.1 μM dexamethasone, 100 mM β-glycerophosphate.
- Plate cells approximately 10,000 cells/cm^2 in monolayer.
- Culture 14–28 days and change medium biweekly.

- Monolayer cultures can be fixed for histological analysis or quantitative biochemical assays after 1% Triton-X100 is used to disrupt cells.
- Alkaline phosphatase activity may be detected within 2 weeks, whereas other bone markers may be detected later (Alhadlaq and Mao, 2003, 2005; Alhadlaq *et al.*, 2004; Aubin, 1998; Frank *et al.*, 2002; Malaval *et al.*, 1999; Marion *et al.*, 2005; Rodan and Noda, 1991).

Osteogenic Differentiation Markers

The osteogenic differentiation of MSCs is verified by several osteogenic matrix molecules, accumulation of mineral crystals and nodules, and ultimately the regeneration of bone *in vivo* both ectopically, such as the dorsum of immunodeficient mice, and orthotopically, such as calvarial, axial (e.g., spinal fusion) or appendicular (e.g., segmental) defects.

Up-regulation of alkaline phosphatase activity is an early indicator for the osteogenic differentiation of MSCs and can be detected quantitatively using a commercially available kinetic kit and/or histologically using a naphthol-based chemical stain (Aubin, 1998; Frank *et al.*, 2002; Malaval *et al.*, 1999; Rodan and Noda, 1991). Furthermore, calcium matrix synthesis is histologically verified using either von Kossa (silver nitrate) or alizarin red stains, by means of selective binding with calcium-phosphate matrix components (Aubin, 1998; Frank *et al.*, 2002; Malaval *et al.*, 1999; Rodan and Noda, 1991). Immunohistochemical staining for type I collagen is helpful but nonspecific. Bone sialoprotein, osteocalcin, osteopontin, and osteonectin are late osteogenic differentiation markers and can be measured genetically using RT-PCR or proteomically using ELISA (Aubin, 1998; Malaval *et al.*, 1999; Rodan and Noda, 1991). Immunohistochemistry with antibodies will localize matrix markers in relation to cells. An example of osteogenic differentiation of hMSCs is provided in Fig. 1C.

Tissue-engineered bone must have the appropriate structural characteristics that approximate native bone. Bone is one of the highly hierarchical structures in the body. The structure of cortical bone differs substantially from that of cancellous bone. A number of biomaterials have been used to simulate cortical bone and cancellous bone structures in cell-based or non–cell-based approaches (Lin *et al.*, 2004; Taboas *et al.*, 2003). However, given the extent of bone modeling and remodeling, whether complete maturation of tissue-engineered bone is necessary before *in vivo* is in question. The reader is referred to several excellent reviews of structural properties of native and engineered bone (El-Ghannam, 2005; Mauney *et al.*, 2005; Mistry and Mikos, 2005; Wan and Longaker, 2006). Mechanical testing of tissue-engineered bone is of paramount importance because bone is designed to withstand mechanical stresses as its primary function. The reader is referred to a number of excellent reviews on the mechanical properties of native and tissue-engineered bone (El-Ghannam, 2005; Mauney et al., 2005; Mistry and Mikos, 2005; Wan and Longaker, 2006).

Adipogenic Differentiation

Adipogenic differentiation of MSCs has a number of perhaps underappreciated areas of significance. First, MSC differentiation into osteoblasts and adipocytes is delicately regulated and balanced (Gregory et al., 2005). Second, our knowledge of obesity is likely improved by understanding the genetic regulation of adipogenic differentiation of MSCs. Third, adipose tissue is a key structure to restore in reconstructive and augmentative surgeries such as facial cancer reconstruction and breast cancer reconstruction. Current approaches for soft tissue reconstruction and/or augmentation suffer from shortcomings such as donor site trauma and morbidity, suboptimal volume retention, donor site morbidity, and poor biocompatibility. One of the central issues of poor healing of adipose tissue grafts is a shortage and/or premature apoptosis of adipogenic cells. MSCs self-replenish, and as demonstrated later, can readily differentiate into adipogenic cells in 2D and 3D (Pittenger et al., 1999; Stosich and Mao, 2005, 2006).

Adipogenic Stimulants

With the addition of dexamethasone (0.5 μM), 1-methyl-3-isobutylxanathine (IBMX) (0.5 μM–0.5 mM), and indomethacin (50–100μM), MSCs in monolayer culture will undergo adipogenic differentiation (Alhadlaq and Mao, 2004; Alhadlaq et al., 2005; Gregory et al., 2005; Janderova et al., 2003; Lee et al., 2006; Nakamura et al., 2003; Pittenger et al., 1999; Rosen and Spiegelman, 2000; Stosich and Mao, 2005, 2006; Ylostalo et al., 2006). Insulin is another key ingredient, for example, in adipogenic differentiating medium (dexamethasone, IBMX, indomethacin) for 2–5 days, and then to a maintenance supplement of insulin (Janderova et al., 2003; Nakamura et al., 2003). In most reports of adipogenic differentiation of MSCs, dexamethasone dose is 0.5 μM or five times higher than for osteogenic differentiation of MSCs. Adipogenic differentiation is believed to take place on cell confluence, cell-to-cell contacts, a serum-free culture, or a suspension culture in methylcellulose (Rosen and Spiegelman, 2000). The growth arrest of MSC-derived chondrocytes is crucial for the subsequent activation of adipogenic differentiation processes. IBMX is a phosphodiesterase inhibitor that blocks the conversion of cAMP to 5′AMP (Gregory et al., 2005). This causes an up-regulation of protein kinase A, which results in decreased cell proliferation and upregulation of hormone sensitive lipase (HSL).

HSL has been shown to convert triacylglycerides to glycerol and free fatty acids, a known adipogenic process (Gregory *et al.*, 2005). The activation of CCAAT/enhancer binding proteins (C/EBP) coincides with the expression of peroxisome proliferator-activated receptor γ (PPARγ), which occurs in the presence of indomethacin, a known ligand for PPARγ (Rosen and Spiegelman, 2000). This early transcription factor is essential for adipogenesis because it suppresses the canonical wingless (Wnt) signaling, suggesting the regulation of osteogenesis and adipogenesis by PPARγ expression in MSCs (Gregory *et al.*, 2005). Positive Wnt signaling inhibits osteogenic differentiation but is required for adipogenic differentiation (Gregory *et al.*, 2005). Therefore, a delicate balance exists in the regulation of adipogenic and osteogenic differentiation, because PPARγ has been reported to inhibit osteogenic differentiation of progenitor cells (Cheng *et al.*, 2003; Khan and Abu-Amer, 2003). Furthermore, loss of function for PPARγ or C/EBP (C/EBPα, C/EBPβ, or C/EBPγ) results in detrimental effects for adipogenesis and reduced adipocyte proliferation, as well as reduced lipid vacuole deposition (Rosen and Spiegelman, 2000).

Adipogenic Differentiation Protocol

- Human adipogenic media: 89% DMEM–low glucose, 10% FBS, 1% antibiotic, 0.5 μM dexamethasone, 0.5 μM 1-methyl-3-isobutylxanathine (IBMX), 50 μM indomethacin.
- Plate cells at approximately 20,000 cells/cm^2 or 80% confluence in monolayer.
- Continue culture in human adipogenic media for up to 28 days.
- Lipids may be visible as early as 7 days and can be viewed under phase-contrast microscope.
- Monolayer cultures can be processed for histological examination after fixation or for quantitative biochemical analysis after 1% Triton-X100 is used to disrupt cells.

Adipogenic Differentiation Markers

One of the key transcriptional factors of adipogenic differentiation of MSCs is peroxisome proliferator–activated receptor γ 2 (PPARγ2), which can be detected by RT-PCR or gene arrays. Oil Red–O staining is a convenient and commonly performed histological stain. On fixing the cultures with 10% formalin, lipid vacuoles synthesized intracellularly by MSC-derived adipogenic cells bind to Oil Red-O and stain red. Hematoxylin counterstaining may be used to visualize cell nuclei in blue. Free glycerol may be quantified by lysing the cells with 1% Triton X-100 and quantitatively analyzed with a glycerol kit. Glycerol-3-phosphate dehydrogenase (G-3-PDH) can be measured as one of the key enzymes in triglyceride synthesis (Pairault and Green, 1979). RT-PCR can be used to amplify and detect additional adipogenic gene products such as lipoprotein lipase (LPL) and the polyclonal antibody a-P2 (Pittenger et al., 1999). An example of adipogenic differentiation of hMSCs is provided in Fig. 1D.

Structural analysis is necessary to determine whether engineered adipose tissue has the appropriate microstructural characteristics as native adipose tissue. Adipose tissue is unique in the sense that lipid vacuoles are accumulated intracellularly. The extracellular matrix of adipose tissue consists of primarily interstitial fibrous tissue, nerve supplies, and vascular and lymphatic network.

Mechanical testing is necessary to ascertain that tissue-engineered adipose tissue has the proper mechanical properties in addition to the "right ingredients" such as adipocytes, intracellular lipid vacuoles, and vascular and lymphatic supplies. The reader is referred to a number of excellent reviews on the mechanical properties of native and tissue-engineered adipose tissue, as well as biomaterials that have been used as scaffolds for adipose tissue regeneration (Beahm et al., 2003; McKnight et al., 2002; Patel et al., 2005; Patrick, 2004; Stosich and Mao, 2006).

Clinical Translation of MSC-Based Therapies

MSC-based therapies are being translated toward clinical practice to heal defects resulting from trauma, chronic diseases, congenital anomalies, and tumor resection. Because of space limitation, it is impossible to outline all the ongoing effort on the clinical translation of MSC-based therapeutic approaches. Several examples are briefly introduced in the following.

Recent reports suggest the roles of MSCs in the repair of myocardial infarctions in rats and pigs on intracardiac injection (Shake et al., 2002). The precise mechanisms are unclear, although it has been suggested that MSCs may induce the homing of cardiomyocytes to the infarct site (Saito et al., 2003). Also proposed is MSC differentiation into cardiomyocytes and/or paracrine effects on intravenous MSC injection. Labeled MSCs are found in bone marrow and the site of myocardial infarction (Saito et al., 2003). Several clinical trials are ongoing at universities and biotechnology companies to explore the healing effects of MSCs on myocardial infarctions (Laflamme and Murry, 2005; Pittenger and Martin, 2004).

Several experiments have demonstrated that an entire articular condyle in the same shape and dimensions of a human temporomandibular joint can be grown in vivo with both cartilage and bone layers from a single population of MSCs (Mao, 2005; Mao et al., 2006). A visionary diagram of MSC-based therapies for total joint replacement is shown in Fig. 2, based

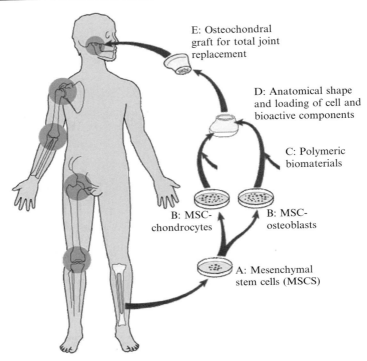

Fig. 2. Schematic diagram of autologous, MSC-based tissue-engineering therapy for total joint replacement. MSC, mesenchymal stem cells. Progenitor cells such as MSCs are isolated from the bone marrow or other connective sources such as adipose tissue, culture-expanded, and/or differentiated *ex vivo* toward chondrocytes and osteoblasts. Cells are seeded in biocompatible materials shaped into the anatomical structures of the synovial joint condyle and implanted *in vivo*. Preliminary proof of concept studies have been reported (Alhadlaq and Mao, 2003, 2005; Alhadlaq *et al.*, 2004; Mao, 2005).

on the work by ourselves and others (Alhadlaq and Mao, 2003, 2005; Alhadlaq *et al.*, 2004). Although bone marrow is the most characterized source of MSCs at this time (Fig. 2), it is probable that MSCs needed for total joint replacement can also be isolated from adipose tissue by aspiration or lipectomy, fresh or banked human umbilical cord blood, placental tissue, or human teeth (Mao, 2005). Total joint replacement is one of the many examples of MSC-based therapies whose proof of concept has been demonstrated in recent years (Rahaman and Mao, 2005).

An emerging concept is that MSCs have trophic effects by secreting a variety of cytokines that function by both paracrine and autocrine pathways (Caplan and Dennis, 2006). The interactions between exogenously delivered growth factors and intrinsic cytokines synthesized by MSCs are one of the most complex and meritorious approaches in cell-based therapies. Our understanding of these fundamental paracrine and autocrine pathways will undoubtedly advance the more practical approaches in MSC-based tissue engineering. The trophic effects, as proposed by Caplan and Denis (2006), include local immune suppression, fibrosis inhibition, and angiogenesis enhancement. A number of translational and clinical studies in the areas of cardiac infarct, synovial joint regeneration, and stroke regeneration models may provide initial data to test the proposed trophic effects of MSCs.

Conclusions

MSCs are somatic stem cells that can be readily isolated from several tissues in the adult and in multiple species. MSCs are capable of undergoing self-replication, up to the number of passages that are meaningful for potential healing of diseased tissues. Recently, we have obtained anecdotal data that that human MSCs isolated from the bone marrow of single donors can be expanded to sufficient numbers for encapsulating in osteochondral constructs as large as synovial joint condyles for *in vivo* implantation. MSCs are able to differentiate into multiple cell lineages that resemble osteoblasts, chondrocytes, myoblasts, adipocytes, and fibroblasts and express some of the key markers typical of endothelial cells, neuron-like cells, and cardiomyocytes. Whether a population of presumably MSCs used in a given study are truly MSCs is a biologically relevant question and can be tested by arrays of cell surface and/or genetic markers. On the other hand, once a functional biological tissue is engineered, it matters little whether the original population of tissue-forming cells are truly MSCs, as long as they can be readily isolated from the patient. Most native tissues, and certainly all organs, are formed by heterogeneous cell populations. It seems that both stem cell biology and tissue engineering approaches are necessary to advance our understanding of how MSCs can be used to heal diseased and damaged tissues and organs. For example, parallel experiments can explore the healing of tissue defects from purified or cloned MSCs, as well as MSCs among heterogeneous cell populations. Despite their first discovery in the mid 1970s, investigations of MSCs have only intensified in recent years. We submit that the true healing power of MSCs is yet to be realized.

Acknowledgments

We thank our colleagues whose work has been cited, and those whose work cannot be cited because of space limitation, for their highly meritorious work that has energized the process of composing this review. We are grateful to the remaining members of Tissue

Engineering Laboratory for their dedication and hard work, in particular. Eduardo Moioli in our laboratory is gratefully acknowledged for his contribution of Fig. 1B, which demonstrates chondrogenic differentiation of rat MSCs in monolayer. We thank Janina Acloque, Maryann Wanner, and Richard Abbott for administrative support. Generous support from the National Institutes of Health is gratefully acknowledged, through NIH grants DE15391 and EB02332 to J. J. M., for the effort spent on composing this manuscript along with some of the experimental data presented in this manuscript from our laboratory.

References

Alberts, B., Johnson, A., Lewis, J., Raff, M., Roberts, K., and Walter, P. (2002). "Molecular Biology of the Cell." Garland Science, New York, NY.

Alhadlaq, A., Elisseeff, J. H., Hong, L., Williams, C. G., Caplan, A. I., Sharma, B., Kopher, R. A., Tomkoria, S., Lennon, D. P., Lopez, A., and Mao, J. J. (2004). Adult stem cell driven genesis of human-shaped articular condyle. *Ann. Biomed. Eng.* **32,** 911–923.

Alhadlaq, A., and Mao, J. J. (2003). Tissue-engineered neogenesis of human-shaped mandibular condyle from rat mesenchymal stem cells. *J. Dent. Res.* **82,** 951–956.

Alhadlaq, A., and Mao, J. J. (2004). Mesenchymal stem cells: Isolation and therapeutics. *Stem Cells Dev.* **13,** 436–448.

Alhadlaq, A., and Mao, J. J. (2005). Tissue-engineered osteochondral constructs in the shape of an articular condyle. *J. Bone Joint Surg. Am.* **87,** 936–944.

Alhadlaq, A., Tang, M., and Mao, J. J. (2005). Engineered adipose tissue from human mesenchymal stem cells maintains predefined shape and dimension: Implications in soft tissue augmentation and reconstruction. *Tissue Eng.* **11,** 556–566.

Allen, D. M., and Mao, J. J. (2004). Heterogeneous nanostructural and nanoelastic properties of pericellular and interterritorial matrices of chondrocytes by atomic force microscopy. *J. Struct. Biol.* **145,** 196–204.

Anseth, K. S., Metters, A. T., Bryant, S. J., Martens, P. J., Elisseeff, J. H., and Bowman, C. N. (2002). *In situ* forming degradable networks and their application in tissue engineering and drug delivery. *J. Control Release* **78,** 199–209.

Archer, C. W., Dowthwaite, G. P., and Francis-West, P. (2003). Development of synovial joints. *Birth Defects Res. C. Embryo Today* **69,** 144–155.

Aubin, J. E. (1998). Bone stem cells. *J. Cell Biochem. Suppl.* **30–31,** 73–82.

Banfi, A., Muraglia, A., Dozin, B., Mastrogiacomo, M., Cancedda, R., and Quarto, R. (2000). Proliferation kinetics and differentiation potential of *ex vivo* expanded human bone marrow stromal cells: Implications for their use in cell therapy. *Exp. Hematol.* **28,** 707–715.

Barry, F. P. (2003). Biology and clinical applications of mesenchymal stem cells. *Birth Defects Res. C. Embryo Today* **69,** 250–256.

Beahm, E. K., Walton, R. L., and Patrick, C. W., Jr. (2003). Progress in adipose tissue construct development. *Clin. Plast. Surg.* **30,** 547–558viii.

Bhagavati, S., and Xu, W. (2004). Isolation and enrichment of skeletal muscle progenitor cells from mouse bone marrow. *Biochem. Biophys. Res. Commun.* **318,** 119–124.

Bianco, P., Riminucci, M., Gronthos, S., and Robey, P. G. (2001). Bone marrow stromal stem cells: Nature, biology, and potential applications. *Stem Cells* **19,** 180–192.

Bruder, S. P., Jaiswal, N., and Haynesworth, S. E. (1997). Growth kinetics, self-renewal, and the osteogenic potential of purified human mesenchymal stem cells during extensive subcultivation and following cryopreservation. *J. Cell Biochem.* **64,** 278–294.

Caplan, A. I. (1991). Mesenchymal stem cells. *J. Orthop. Res.* **9,** 641–650.

Caplan, A. I., and Bruder, S. P. (2001). Mesenchymal stem cells: Building blocks for molecular medicine in the 21st century. *Trends Mol. Med.* **7**(6), 259–264.

Caplan, A. I., and Dennis, J. E. (2006). Mesenchymal stem cells as trophic mediators. *J. Cell Biochem.*

Cheng, S. L., Shao, J. S., Charlton-Kachigian, N., Loewy, A. P., and Towler, D. A. (2003). MSX2 promotes osteogenesis and suppresses adipogenic differentiation of multipotent mesenchymal progenitors. *J. Biol. Chem.* **278,** 45969–45977.

Cohen, N. P., Foster, R. J., and Mow, V. C. (1998). Composition and dynamics of articular cartilage: Structure, function, and maintaining healthy state. *J. Orthop. Sports Phys. Ther.* **28,** 203–215.

Dayoub, H., Dumont, R. J., Li, J. Z., Dumont, A. S., Hankins, G. R., Kallmes, D. F., and Helm, G. A. (2003). Human mesenchymal stem cells transduced with recombinant bone morphogenetic protein-9 adenovirus promote osteogenesis in rodents. *Tissue Eng.* **9,** 347–356.

Derubeis, A. R., and Cancedda, R. (2004). Bone marrow stromal cells (BMSCs) in bone engineering: Limitations and recent advances. *Ann. Biomed. Eng.* **32,** 160–165.

Dowthwaite, G. P., Flannery, C. R., Flannelly, J., Lewthwaite, J. C., Archer, C. W., and Pitsillides, A. A. (2003). A mechanism underlying the movement requirement for synovial joint cavitation. *Matrix Biol.* **22,** 311–322.

El-Ghannam, A. (2005). Bone reconstruction: From bioceramics to tissue engineering. *Exp. Rev. Med. Dev.* **2,** 87–101.

Frank, O., Heim, M., Jakob, M., Barbero, A., Schafer, D., Bendik, I., Dick, W., Heberer, M., and Martin, I. (2002). Real-time quantitative RT-PCR analysis of human bone marrow stromal cells during osteogenic differentiation *in vitro. J. Cell Biochem.* **85,** 737–746.

Friedenstein, A. J. (1995). Marrow stromal fibroblasts. *Calcif. Tissue Int.* **56**(Suppl. 1), S17.

Friedenstein, A. J., Chailakhjan, R. K., and Lalykina, K. S. (1970). The development of fibroblast colonies in monolayer cultures of guinea-pig bone marrow and spleen cells. *Cell Tissue Kinet.* **3,** 393–403.

Friedenstein, A. J., Gorskaja, J. F., and Kulagina, N. N. (1976). Fibroblast precursors in normal and irradiated mouse hematopoietic organs. *Exp. Hematol.* **4,** 267–274.

Friedman, M. S., Long, M. W., and Hankenson, K. D. (2006). Osteogenic differentiation of human mesenchymal stem cells is regulated by bone morphogenetic protein-6. *J. Cell. Biochem.* **98,** 538–554.

Gang, E. J., Jeong, J. A., Hong, S. H., Hwang, S. H., Kim, S. W., Yang, I. H., Ahn, C., Han, H., and Kim, H. (2004). Skeletal myogenic differentiation of mesenchymal stem cells isolated from human umbilical cord blood. *Stem Cells* **22,** 617–624.

Gao, J., and Caplan, A. I. (2003). Mescenchymal stem cells and tissue engineering for orthopaedic surgery. *Chir. Organi. Mov.* **3,** 305–316.

Gilbert, S. F. (2000). "Developmental Biology." Sinauer Associates, Inc., Sunderland, MA.

Graves, S. E., Francis, M. J. O., Gundle, R., and Beresoford, J. N. (1994a). Primary culture of human trabecular bone: Effects of L-ascorate-2-phosphate. *Bone* **15,** 132–133.

Graves, S. E., Gundle, R., Francis, M. J. O., and Beresoford, J. N. (1994b). Ascorbate increases collagen synthesis and promote differentiation in human bone derived cell cultures. *Bone* **15,** 133.

Gregory, C. A., Gunn, W. G., Reyes, E., Smolarz, A. J., Munoz, J., Spees, J. L., and Prockop, D. J. (2005a). How wnt signaling affects bone repair by mesenchymal stem cells from the bone marrow. *Ann. N. Y. Acad. Sci.* **1049,** 97–106.

Gregory, C. A., Prockop, D. J., and Spees, J. L. (2005b). Non-hematopoietic bone marrow stem cells: Molecular control of expansion and differentiation. *Exp. Cell Res.* **306,** 330–335.

Grodzinsky, A. J., Levenston, M. E., Jin, M., and Frank, E. H. (2000). Cartilage tissue remodeling in response to mechanical forces. *Annu. Rev. Biomed. Eng.* **2,** 691–713.

Guilak, F. (2000). The deformation behavior and viscoelastic properties of chondrocytes in articular cartilage. *Biorheology* **37,** 27–44.

Guilak, F., and Mow, V. C. (2000). The mechanical environment of the chondrocyte: A biphasic finite element model of cell-matrix interactions in articular cartilage. *J. Biomech.* **33,** 1663–1673.

Haudenschild, D. R., McPherson, J. M., Tubo, R., and Binette, F. (2001). Differential expression of multiple genes during articular chondrocyte redifferentiation. *Anat. Rec.* **263,** 91–98.

Hung, C. T., Lima, E. G., Mauck, R. L., Takai, E., LeRoux, M. A., Lu, H. H., Stark, R. G., Guo, X. E., and Ateshian, G. A. (2003). Anatomically shaped osteochondral constructs for articular cartilage repair. *J. Biomech.* **36,** 1853–1864.

Hung, C. T., Mauck, R. L., Wang, C. C., Lima, E. G., and Ateshian, G. A. (2004). A paradigm for functional tissue engineering of articular cartilage via applied physiologic deformational loading. *Ann. Biomed. Eng.* **32,** 35–49.

Hunziker, E. B. (2002). Articular cartilage repair: Basic science and clinical progress. A review of the current status and prospects. *Osteoarthritis Cartilage* **10,** 432–463.

Indrawattana, N., Chen, G., Tadokoro, M., Shann, L. H., Ohgushi, H., Tateishi, T., Tanaka, J., and Bunyaratvej, A. (2004). Growth factor combination for chondrogenic induction from human mesenchymal stell cell. *Biochem. Biophys. Res. Commun.* **320**(3), 914–919.

Jaiswal, N., Haynesworth, S. E., Caplan, A. I., and Bruder, S. P. (1997). Osteogenic differentiation of purified, culture-expanded human mesenchymal stem cells *in vitro.* *J. Cell. Biochem.* **64,** 295–312.

Jakob, M., Démarteau, O., Schäfer, D., Hintermann, B., Dick, W., Heberer, M., and Martin, I. (2001). Specific growth factors during the expansion and redifferentiation of adult human articular chondrocytes enhance chondrogenesis and cartilaginous tissue formation *in vitro.* *J. Cell. Biochem.* **81,** 368–377.

Janderova, L., McNeil, M., Murrell, A. N., Mynatt, R. L., and Smith, S. R. (2003). Human mesenchymal stem cells as an *in vitro* model for human adipogenesis. *Obes. Res.* **11,** 65–74.

Johnstone, B., Hering, T. M., Caplan, A. I., Goldberg, V. M., and Yoo, J. U. (1998). *In vitro* chondrogenesis of bone marrow-derived mesenchymal progenitor cells. *Exp. Cell. Res.* **238,** 265–272.

Katagiri, T., Yamaguchi, A., Komaki, M., Abe, E., Takahashi, N., Ikeda, T., Rosen, V., Wozney, J. M., Fujisawa-Sehara, A., and Suda, T. (1994). Bone morphogenetic protein-2 converts the differentiation pathway of C2C12 myoblasts into the osteoblast lineage. *J. Cell. Biol.* **127,** 1755–1766.

Kerin, A., Patwari, P., Kuettner, K., Cole, A., and Grodzinsky, A. (2002). Molecular basis of osteoarthritis: Biomechanical aspects. *Cell Mol. Life Sci.* **59,** 27–35.

Khan, E., and Abu-Amer, Y. (2003). Activation of peroxisome proliferator-activated receptor-gamma inhibits differentiation of preosteoblasts. *J. Lab. Clin. Med.* **142,** 29–34.

Kim, T. K., Sharma, B., Williams, C. G., Ruffner, M. A., Malik, A., McFarland, E. G., and Elisseeff, J. H. (2003). Experimental model for cartilage tissue engineering to regenerate the zonal organization of articular cartilage. *Osteoarthritis Cartilage* **11,** 653–664.

Klein, T. J., Schumacher, B. L., Schmidt, T. A., Li, K. W., Voegtline, M. S., Masuda, K., Thonar, E. J., and Sah, R. L. (2003). Tissue engineering of stratified articular cartilage from chondrocyte subpopulations. *Osteoarthritis Cartilage* **11,** 595–602.

Krebsbach, P. H., Kuznetsov, S. A., Bianco, P., and Robey, P. G. (1999). Bone marrow stromal cells: Characterization and clinical application. *Crit. Rev. Oral Biol. Med.* **10,** 165–1681.

Kuo, C. K., and Tuan, R. S. (2003). Tissue engineering with mesenchymal stem cells. *IEEE Eng. Med. Biol. Mag.* **22,** 51–56.

Laflamme, M. A., and Murry, C. E. (2005). Regenerating the heart. *Nat. Biotechnol.* **23,** 845–856.

Lee, R. H., Kim, B., Choi, I., Kim, H., Choi, H. S., Suh, K., Bae, Y. C., and Jung, J. S. (2004). Characterization and expression analysis of mesenchymal stem cells from human bone marrow and adipose tissue. *Cell Physiol. Biochem.* **14,** 311–324.

Lefebvre, V., Behringer, R. R., and de Crombrugghe, B. (2001). L-Sox5, Sox6 and Sox9 control essential steps of the chondrocyte differentiation pathway. *Osteoarthritis Cartilage* **9**(Suppl. A), S69–S75.

Li, C., Vepari, C., Jin, H. J., Kim, H. J., and Kaplan, D. L. (2006). Electrospun silk-BMP-2 scaffolds for bone tissue engineering. *Biomaterials* **27**, 3115–3124.

Lin, C. Y., Kikuchi, N., and Hollister, S. J. (2004). A novel method for biomaterial scaffold internal architecture design to match bone elastic properties with desired porosity. *J. Biomech.* **37**, 623–636.

Long, M. W., Robinson, J. A., Ashcraft, E. A., and Mann, K. G. (1995). Regulation of human bone marrow-derived osteoprogenitor cells by osteogenic growth factors. *J. Clin. Invest.* **95**, 881–887.

Malaval, L., Liu, F., Roche, P., and Aubin, J. E. (1999). Kinetics of osteoprogenitor proliferation and osteoblast differentiation *in vitro*. *J. Cell Biochem.* **74**, 616–627.

Mao, J. J. (2005). Stem-cell-driven regeneration of synovial joints. *Biol. Cell* **97**, 289–301.

Mao, J. J., Giannoble, W. V., Helms, J. A., Hollister, S. J., Krebsbach, P. H., Longaker, M. T., and Shi, S. (2006). Craniofacial tissue engineering. *J. Dent. Res.* In Press.

Marion, N. W., Liang, W., Reilly, G., Day, D. E., Rahaman, M. N., and Mao, J. J. (2005). Borate glass supports the *in vitro* osteogenic differentiation of human mesenchymal stem cells. *Mech. Adv. Mater. Struct.* **3**, 239–246.

Martin, I., Muraglia, A., Campanile, G., Cancedda, R., and Quarto, R. (1997). Fibroblast growth factor-2 supports *ex vivo* expansion and maintenance of osteogenic precursors from human bone marrow. *Endocrinology* **138**, 4456–4462.

Masuda, K., Sah, R. L., Hejna, M. J., and Thonar, E. J. (2003). A novel two-step method for the formation of tissue-engineered cartilage by mature bovine chondrocytes: The alginate-recovered-chondrocyte (ARC) method. *J. Orthop. Res.* **21**, 139–148.

Mauney, J. R., Volloch, V., and Kaplan, D. L. (2005). Role of adult mesenchymal stem cells in bone tissue engineering applications: Current status and future prospects. *Tissue Eng.* **11**, 787–802.

McKnight, A. L., Kugel, J. L., Rossman, P. J., Manduca, A., Hartmann, L. C., and Ehman, R. L. (2002). MR elastography of breast cancer: Preliminary results. *AJR Am. J. Roentgenol.* **178**, 1411–1417.

Mistry, A. S., and Mikos, A. G. (2005). Tissue engineering strategies for bone regeneration. *Adv. Biochem. Eng. Biotechnol.* **94**, 1–22.

Mow, V. C., Holmes, M. H., and Lai, W. M. (1984). Fluid transport and mechanical properties of articular cartilage: A review. *J. Biomech.* **17**, 377–394.

Mow, V. C., Wang, C. C., and Hung, C. T. (1999). The extracellular matrix, interstitial fluid and ions as a mechanical signal transducer in articular cartilage. *Osteoarthritis Cartilage* **7**, 41–58.

Nakamura, T., Shiojima, S., Hirai, Y., Iwama, T., Tsuruzoe, N., Hirasawa, A., Katsuma, S., and Tsujimoto, G. (2003). Temporal gene expression changes during adipogenesis in human mesenchymal stem cells. *Biochem. Biophys. Res. Commun.* **303**, 306–312.

Nesic, D., Whiteside, R., Brittberg, M., Wendt, D., Martin, I., and Mainil-Varlet, P. (2006). Cartilage tissue engineering for degenerative joint disease. *Adv. Drug Deliv. Rev.* **58**, 300–322.

Ng, L. J., Wheatley, S., Muscat, G. E., Conway-Campbell, J., Bowles, J., Wright, E., Bell, D. M., Tam, P. P., Cheah, K. S., and Koopman, P. (1997). SOX9 binds DNA, activates transcription, and coexpresses with type II collagen during chondrogenesis in the mouse. *Dev. Biol.* **183**, 108–121.

Osyczka, A. M., Noth, U., O'Connor, J., Caterson, E. J., Yoon, K., Danielson, K. G., and Tuan, R. S. (2002). Multilineage differentiation of adult human bone marrow progenitor cells transduced with human papilloma virus type 16 E6/E7 genes. *Calcif. Tissue Int.* **71,** 447–458.

Pairault, J., and Green, H. (1979). A study of the adipose conversion of suspended 3T3 cells by using glycerophosphate dehydrogenase as differentiation marker. *Proc. Natl. Acad. Sci. USA* **76,** 5138–5142.

Patel, P. N., Gobin, A. S., West, J. L., and Patrick, C. W., Jr. (2005). Poly(ethylene glycol) hydrogel system supports preadipocyte viability, adhesion, and proliferation. *Tissue Eng.* **11,** 1498–1505.

Patrick, C. W. (2004). Breast tissue engineering. *Annu. Rev. Biomed. Eng.* **6,** 109–130.

Pittenger, M. F., Mackay, A. M., Beck, S. C., Jaiswal, R. K., Douglas, R., Mosca, J. D., Moorman, M. A., Simonetti, D. W., Craig, S., and Marshak, D. R. (1999). Multilineage potential of adult human mesenchymal stem cells. *Science* **284,** 143–147.

Pittenger, M. F., and Martin, B. J. (2004). Mesenchymal stem cells and their potential as cardiac therapeutics. *Circ. Res.* **95,** 9–20.

Poole, C. A., Flint, M. H., and Beaumont, B. W. (1988). Chondrons extracted from canine tibial cartilage: Preliminary report on their isolation and structure. *J. Orthop. Res.* **6,** 408–419.

Poole, C. A., Glant, T. T., and Schofield, J. R. (1991). Chondrons from articular cartilage. (IV). Immunolocalization of proteoglycan epitopes in isolated canine tibial chondrons. *J. Histochem. Cytochem.* **39,** 1175–1187.

Rahaman, M. N., and Mao, J. J. (2005). Stem cell-based composite tissue constructs for regenerative medicine. *Biotechnol. Bioeng.* **91,** 261–284.

Rickard, D. J., Sullivan, T. A., Shenker, B. J., Leboy, P. S., and Kazhdan, I. (1994). Induction of rapid osteoblast differentiation in rat bone marrow stromal cell cultures by dexamethasone and BMP-2. *Dev. Biol.* **161,** 218–228.

Rodan, G. A., and Noda, M. (1991). Gene expression in osteoblastic cells. *Crit. Rev. Eukaryot. Gene Expr.* **1,** 85–98.

Rosen, E. D., and Spiegelman, B. M. (2000). Molecular regulation of adipogenesis. *Annu. Rev. Cell Dev. Biol.* **16,** 145–171.

Saito, T., Kuang, J. Q., Lin, C. C., and Chiu, R. C. (2003). Transcoronary implantation of bone marrow stromal cells ameliorates cardiac function after myocardial infarction. *J. Thorac. Cardiovasc. Surg.* **126,** 114–123.

Sekiya, I., Colter, D. C., and Prockop, D. J. (2001). BMP-6 enhances chondrogenesis in a subpopulation of human marrow stromal cells. *Biochem. Biophys. Res. Commun.* **284,** 411–418.

Sekiya, I., Vuoristo, J. T., Larson, B. L., and Prockop, D. J. (2002). *In vitro* cartilage formation by human adult stem cells from bone marrow stroma defines the sequence of cellular and molecular events during chondrogenesis. *Proc. Natl. Acad. Sci. USA* **99,** 4397–4402.

Shake, J. G., Gruber, P. J., Baumgartner, W. A., Senechal, G., Meyers, J., Redmond, J. M., Pittenger, M. F., and Martin, B. J. (2002). Mesenchymal stem cell implantation in a swine myocardial infarct model: Engraftment and functional effects. *Ann. Thorac. Surg.* **73,** 1919–1925; discussion 1926.

Spees, J. L., Gregory, C. A., Singh, H., Tucker, H. A., Peister, A., Lynch, P. J., Hsu, S. C., Smith, J., and Prockop, D. J. (2004). Internalized antigens must be removed to prepare hypoimmunogenic mesenchymal stem cells for cell and gene therapy. *Mol. Ther.* **9,** 747–756.

Stosich, M. S., and Mao, J. J. (2005). Stem cell-based soft tissue grafts for plastic and reconstructive surgeries. *Semin. Plast. Surg.* **19,** 251–260.

Stosich, M. S., and Mao, J. J. (2006). Adipose tissue engineering from human mesenchymal stem cells: Clinical implication in plastic and soft tissue reconstructive surgeries. *Plast. Reconstr. Surg.* In Press.

Taboas, J. M., Maddox, R. D., Krebsbach, P. H., and Hollister, S. J. (2003). Indirect solid free form fabrication of local and global porous, biomimetic and composite 3D polymer-ceramic scaffolds. *Biomaterials* **24,** 181–194.

Troken, A. J., Wan, L. Q., Marion, N. W., Mao, J. J., and Mow, V. C. (2005). Properties of cartilage and meniscus. *In* "The Wiley Encyclopedia of Medical Devices and Instrumentation" (J. G. Webster, ed.).

Tsutsumi, S., Shimazu, A., Miyazaki, K., Pan, H., Koike, C., Yoshida, E., Takagishi, K., and Kato, Y. (2001). Retention of multilineage differentiation potential of mesenchymal cells during proliferation in response to FGF. *Biochem. Biophys. Res. Commun.* **288,** 413–419.

Tuli, R., Seghatoleslami, M. R., Tuli, S., Wang, M. L., Hozack, W. J., Manner, P. A., Danielson, K. G., and Tuan, R. S. (2003). A simple, high-yield method for obtaining multipotential mesenchymal progenitor cells from trabecular bone. *Mol. Biotechnol.* **23,** 37–49.

Wan, N., and Longaker, M. T. (2006). Craniofacial bone tissue engineering. *Dent. Clin. North Am.* **50,** 175–190.

Wang, E. A., Rosen, V., D'Alessandro, J. S., Bauduy, M., Cordes, P., Harada, T., Israel, D. I., Hewick, R. M., Kerns, K. M., and LaPan, P. (1990). Recombinant human bone morphogenetic protein induces bone formation. *Proc. Natl. Acad. Sci. USA* **87,** 2220–2224.

Williams, C. G., Kim, T. K., Taboas, A., Malik, A., Manson, P., and Elisseeff, J. (2003). *In vitro* chondrogenesis of bone marrow-derived mesenchymal stem cells in a photopolymerizing hydrogel. *Tissue Eng.* **9,** 679–688.

Woodfield, T. B., Bezemer, J. M., Pieper, J. S., van Blitterswijk, C. A., and Riesle, J. (2002). Scaffolds for tissue engineering of cartilage. *Crit. Rev. Eukaryot. Gene Expr.* **12,** 209–236.

Wozney, J. M. (1992). The bone morphogenetic protein family and osteogenesis. *Mol. Reprod. Dev.* **32,** 160–167.

Xu, W., Zhang, X., Qian, H., Zhu, W., Sun, X., Hu, J., Zhou, H., and Chen, Y. (2004). Mesenchymal stem cells from adult human bone marrow differentiate into a cardiomyocyte phenotype *in vitro. Exp. Biol. Med. (Maywood)* **229,** 623–631.

Ylostalo, J., Smith, J. R., Pochampally, R. R., Matz, R., Sekiya, I., Larson, B. L., Vuoristo, J. T., and Prockop, D. J. (2006). Use of differentiating adult stem cells (MSCs) to identify new downstream target genes for transcription factors. *Stem Cells.*

Yoo, J. U., Barthel, T. S., Nishimura, K., Solchaga, L., Caplan, A. I., Goldberg, V. M., and Johnstone, B. (1998). The chondrogenic potential of human bone-marrow-derived mesenchymal progenitor cells. *J. Bone Joint Surg. Am.* **80,** 1745–1757.

[17] Bone Reconstruction with Bone Marrow Stromal Cells

By WEI LIU, LEI CUI, and YILIN CAO

Abstract

Bone marrow stromal/stem cells (BMSCs) are multipotent adult stem cells and have become the important cell source for cell therapy and engineered tissue repair. Their osteogenic differentiation potential has been well characterized in many *in vitro* studies. In addition, small animal model–based studies also reveal their capability of bone formation *in vivo* when implanted with biodegradable scaffold, indicating the great potential for therapeutic application. Bone defect is a common clinical problem that deserves an optimal therapy. Unlike traditional surgical repair that needs to sacrifice donor site tissue, the tissue-engineering approach can achieve the goal of bone regeneration and repair without the necessity of donor site morbidity. To safely translate experimental study into a clinical trial of engineered bone repair, *in vivo* study using large animal models has become the key issue. Our *in vivo* study in this aspect and the published results indicate that bone regeneration and repair by BMSCs and biodegradable scaffold is a realistic goal that can be achieved.

Introduction

Bone tissue repair is an important task for plastic and orthopedic surgeons. One of the disadvantages of the traditional surgical repair procedure is the need to harvest autologous tissues from a donor site of the human body for the repair of a defect on the other site, thus leaving a secondary tissue defect. The advantage of tissue engineering offers an approach for tissue repair and regeneration without the necessity of donor site morbidity. The basic principle of tissue engineering is to apply seed cells and biodegradable material to the generation of bone or other tissues *in vivo* and thus to achieve the goal of tissue defect repair. In this process, seed cells play a key role in bone regeneration and repair. Thus, the proper choice of seed cells is essential for the success in engineered bone repair. Although many types of stem cells have been discovered and well characterized, bone marrow stem cells (also named *bone marrow stromal cells*, BMSCs) are obviously an optimal cell source for bone engineering because of their strong potential for osteogenic differentiation on chemical

METHODS IN ENZYMOLOGY, VOL. 420   0076-6879/06 $35.00
Copyright 2006, Elsevier Inc. All rights reserved.   DOI: 10.1016/S0076-6879(06)20017-X

induction as revealed in numerous *in vitro* studies. More importantly, many *in vivo* studies have reported the success in bone formation when osteo-genically induced BMSCs were transplanted along with biodegradable polymer. However, for practical application, a series of experiments should be performed to prove the concept and practical feasibility. In the initial phase, immunodeficient animal models are usually used to screen all potential components of the proposed construct, such as matrix, cells, and signaling substances. In the second phase, an appropriate tissue defect model in small animals is used to prove the principle of engineered tissue repair. In the preclinical phase, clinically relevant models are established in large animals to further study the tissue formation process and the out-comes of engineered tissue repair to safely translate animal studies into human clinical trials. Regarding bone engineering, a large number of studies have been performed in the initial and the second phases according to published literature. On the basis of the published and our own results of early phase studies, we have focused on tissue engineering and repair in large animal models in the past few years and have further conducted clinical trials of bone repair in patients on a small scale. This chapter will review the related literature and introduce our experience in bone reconstruction and repair by using BMSCs as the cell source.

Cell Source for Bone Engineering

In the early phase, the non-stem–cell approach was usually used to prove the concept of bone regeneration. For example, Vacanti *et al.* reported that bone tissue could be generated in the subcutaneous tissue of nude mice after implantation of degradable polymer seeded with osteo-blasts isolated from periosteum (Vacanti *et al.*, 1993; Vacanti and Upton, 1994), which clearly demonstrated that the tissue-engineering approach can regenerate bone tissue *in vivo*.

However, harvest of periosteum for seed cell isolation will cause pa-tients' suffering and donor site morbidity. Fortunately, the discovery of adult mesenchymal stem cells provides an optimal solution. As early as 1968, Friedenstein found there were osteogenic precursor cells located in the bone marrow in a population of fibroblastic cells that could form a cell colony, named colony-forming units–fibroblastic, CFU-Fs (Friedenstein *et al.*, 1968). This type of cell was further defined to have the potential for osteogenic, chondrogenic, and adipogenic differentiation in later studies (Owen, 1988; Prockop, 1997), indicating they are mesenchymal stem cells. They are thus named *marrow stromal cells* or *marrow stem cells* (MSC, Prockop, 1997) or *mesenchymal stem cell* (MSC, Caplan, 1994). Because these cells were originally isolated from bone marrow, BMSCs has become a common term to name mesenchymal stem cells isolated from bone marrow.

Regarding osteogenic differentiation of BMSCs, chemical induction is the most commonly used method and has proved to be very effective. Jaiswal et al. reported osteogenic induction by culturing human BMSCs in an induction medium containing dexamethasone, L-ascorbic acid, and beta-glycerophosphate. After 16 days of culture, induced cells exhibited an osteogenic phenotype by alkaline phosphatase expression, reactivity with anti-osteogenic cell surface monoclonal antibodies, modulation of osteocalcin mRNA production, and the formation of a mineralized extracellular matrix containing hydroxyapatite (Jaiswal et al., 1997). The chemically inductive effect can be further enhanced by adding vitamin D_3 (Jorgensen et al., 2004; Rickard, et al., 1994). Similar inductive effect can also be achieved by using growth factor, such as bone morphogenetic protein (BMP)-2 (Jorgensen et al., 2004; Rickard et al., 1994), and BMP-7 (Yeh et al., 2002). Recently, gene transfection of osteogenesis-related transcription factors such as Osterix (Tu et al., 2006) and Runx2 (Byers et al., 2004) has been shown to effectively induce an osteogenic phenotype of BMSCs.

Adipose-derived stem cells (ADSCs) are another type of adult stem cells that have been shown to have potential for osteogenic, adipogenic, chondrogenic, and other lineage differentiation (Gimble, 2003; Zuk et al., 2001, 2002). Importantly, a study showed that ADSCs have the same ability as BMSCs to regenerate bone and repair bone defect in vivo (Cowan et al., 2004). Recently, adult MSCs have also been isolated from muscles (Deasy et al., 2001), peripheral blood (Kuznetsov et al., 2001), cord blood (Erices et al., 2000), and placenta (Fukuchi et al., 2004), etc. These new types of MSCs could become the new cell source for bone engineering. Among all adult MSCs, BMSCs remain the most commonly used cell source for bone regeneration and repair in the studies using different animal models.

Animal Models for BMSC-Mediated Bone Engineering

Calvarial bone defect is a commonly used model to test the feasibility of bone engineering and repair in different animal studies and to define the role of seed cells or scaffold material in bone repair process. Although relatively small, the mouse model is still being used for bone-engineering studies. Kaplan's group has recently used silk as a scaffold material for bone engineering (Meinel et al., 2005). In their study, human mesenchymal stem cells (hMSCs) were first isolated and seeded on a porous silk fibroin scaffold, in vitro engineered for 5 weeks in a bioreactor, and then transplanted to repair the calvarial bone defects with a size of 4 mm in diameter created in nude mice. Their results showed that hMSC could undergo osteogenic differentiation on this novel scaffold, and *in vitro* engineered bone could achieve better reparative results than the cell–scaffold complex without *in vitro* engineering.

Compared with the mouse model, rabbit calvarial repair seems to be a more often used model. In an *in vivo* study, Chang *et al.* (2004) also demonstrated that BMP-2 gene-transfected BMSCs could repair the calvarial bone defect better than nontransfected stem cells when applied with biomaterial to the bone defect site. In several other studies, the rabbit calvarial model was used to test scaffold materials for bone formation. For example, Schantz's study (2003) showed that customized, three-dimensional polycaprolactone could be used as a scaffold for repairing a rabbit calvarial defect when implanted with BMSCs.

The bone-engineering studies in mouse and rabbit calvarial models provide convincing data that critical-sized defects of flat bone in small animals can be completely healed with a tissue-engineering approach. However, these results may not necessarily represent the bone formation and repairing process in human beings, because low-level mammals usually have a stronger ability than human beings for tissue regeneration. In contrast, large mammals such as sheep, dogs, and pigs may better reflect the actual bone formation process in human beings than small animals, which will provide a guide to clinical application. Therefore, our center has focused on engineered bone formation studies in large mammals in the past few years. For example, in a sheep cranial bone defect repairing study (Shang *et al.*, 2001), expanded and osteogenically induced BMSCs were mixed with calcium alginate for *in vivo* implantation. In created bilateral cranial defects (20 mm in diameter), the experimental side was repaired with a bone graft constituted with *in vitro*–induced autologous BMSCs and calcium alginate. Histological examination demonstrated new bone formation 6 weeks after repair, which became more mature by 18 weeks (Fig. 1). Three-dimensional computed tomography (3D-CT) scanning confirmed that the bone defects were almost completely repaired by engineered bone at 18 weeks. In contrast, the control defect that was implanted with calcium alginate alone remained unrepaired (Fig. 2). Furthermore, chemical analysis showed that the engineered bone tissues contained a high level of calcium (71.6% of normal bone tissue), suggesting that engineered bone can achieve good mineralization.

As a gel form scaffold, calcium alginate might be more suitable for engineering injectable bone than for flat bone. In addition, tight contact between host bone and implanted bone construct might be important for better regeneration of engineered bone *in vivo*; therefore, a relatively solid scaffold material should be a preferred choice. Furthermore, a scaffold with natural tissue structure and components should be more suitable

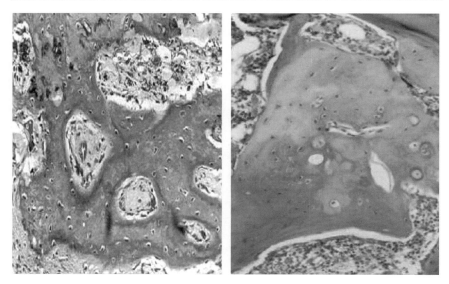

FIG. 1. Histology of tissue-engineered cranial bone at 6 weeks (left) and 18 weeks (right). (Reprinted by permission of *Journal of Craniofacial Surgery*, Shang *et al.*, 2001).

for clinical trials. Considering these, we have performed a similar study in a canine model by use of demineralized bone matrix (DBM) and BMSCs (manuscript in preparation). First, bilateral bone defects with a size of 2 cm × 2 cm were created, then a BMSC-DMB construct that had been preincubated in osteogenic medium for 7 days was implanted on the experimental side. A similarly treated scaffold construct without cell loading was implanted in the other side defect as a control. As shown in Fig. 3, bone formation was observed on the experimental side and maintained stability when examined by x-ray and 3D-CT scanning 12 months after implantation, and the defect was well repaired by the engineered bone. Histological examination also verified the bone formation on the experimental side, but not on the control side. Of note, the engineered bone formed cancellous bone structure instead of lamellar structure of natural calvarial bone (Fig. 4). As expected, the control side remained unhealed when evaluated by x-ray and 3D-CT scanning examination at 12 months. Only fibrotic tissue was observed in its histological examination (Figs. 3 and 4). This work demonstrated that DBM could serve as a suitable scaffold material for bone engineering in large animals and it might be an appropriate material for a clinical trial. Recently, Mauney *et al.* (2005) also demonstrated *de novo* bone formation after *in vivo* implantation of DBM seeded

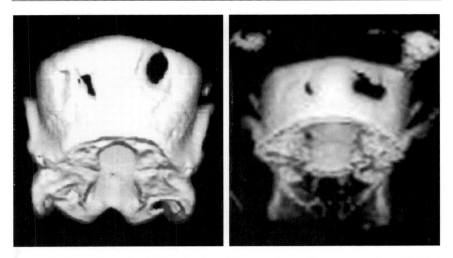

FIG. 2. Three-dimensional CT evaluation of tissue-engineered bone repair of cranial defect at 12 weeks (left panel) and 18 weeks (right panel). Left side, Experimental group; right side, control group. (Reprinted by permission of *Journal of Craniofacial Surgery*, Shang *et al.*, 2001).

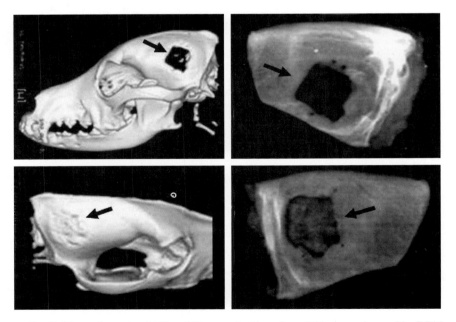

FIG. 3. Three-dimensional CT and X-ray evaluation of cranial bone engineered by DBM and BMSCs at 12 months. Left panels, CT scanning; right panels, X-ray; top panels, control group; bottom panels, experimental group. Arrow indicates the location of created defect.

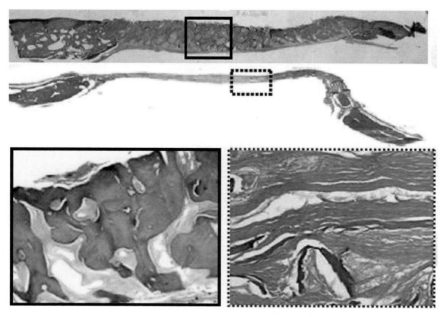

Fig. 4. Histological evaluation of cranial bone engineered by DBM and BMSCs at 12 months. Top panel, Histology of experimental repaired structure including interface and central areas (merged picture); middle panel, histology of control repaired structure including interface and central areas (merged picture); bottom panels, cancellous bone structure of experimental group at central area (solid lined picture, left) and fibrotic tissue structure of control group at central area (dotted lined picture, right).

with human BMSCs. In addition, they found that the level of mineralization of DBM also has influence on the osteogenic differentiation of seeded BMSCs.

Of interest is that engineered flat bone did not form a typical lamellar structure as natural flat bone has; instead, a cancerous bone structure was observed in the engineered cranial bone. This phenomenon is probably due to the lack of proper mechanical loading during engineered bone formation *in vivo*. Unlike the bone engineering process, during the development and growth, a natural calvarial bone may sustain a continuous and long-term pressure force by growing brain tissue and eventually forms a lamellar structure.

Therefore, an *in vivo* model that allows for bone remodeling by mechanical loading is particularly important for generating a bone that has the structure and mechanical strength similar to those of the natural bone counterpart. Different from flat bone, weight-bearing long bones usually sustain mechanical loading in their physiological activities during one's lifetime. This kind of bone, including the femur, tibia, and metatarsus, might be fit for such a model for engineering weight-bearing bone. In 2000, Petite *et al.* succeeded in engineering a metatarsus in a sheep model using coral and BMSCs and showed the feasibility of generating a weight-bearing bone in large animals (Petite *et al.*, 2002).

Femur is the largest weight-bearing bone in animals and human beings. In a recently published study (Zhu *et al.*, 2006), we tested the possibility of engineering the femoral bone in a goat model by using BMSCs and coral scaffold. Expanded and osteogenically induced BMSCs were seeded onto a natural coral scaffold and *in vitro* cultured for 1 week before *in vivo* implantation. In the surgical procedure, adult goats were anesthetized and a 25-mm (20% of the femur's total length) segmental osteoperiosteal defect was created in each of the animals; the defects were then treated either with cell-loaded scaffold (experimental group), scaffold alone (control group), or left untreated (blank control). Animals were sacrificed at either 4 months or 8 months, respectively, for gross observation and histological and biomechanical analyses. To enhance tissue remolding, interlocking nails were removed at 6 months in animals that would be sacrificed at 8 months to give the newly formed bone a mechanical loading.

As shown in Fig. 5, radiographic examination demonstrated new bone formation 1 month after implantation at the site where BMSCs were implanted with coral. At 6 months, bone union was achieved at the defect site by engineered bone tissue, and thus the interlocking nails were removed. After 2 months of mechanical loading, the engineered femur was further remodeled to become a mature bone. As observed radiologically, cortex bone was formed 8 months after implantation. Interestingly, marrow cavity formation inside the engineered bone was also observed at this time. Grossly, the engineered bone also exhibited an appearance similar to that of natural femoral bone (Fig. 6). Histological examination demonstrated the formation of trabecular and woven bone at 4 months. At 8 months, the engineered bone became obviously more mature. Although still being an irregular pattern, the formed Haversian system became observable, indicating that mechanical loading plays an important role in the remodeling of engineered bone (Fig. 7). In contrast, implantation of scaffold alone without cell seeding could not generate femoral bone tissue sufficiently to achieve a bone union both grossly and histologically (Figs. 5–7).

In addition to structural restoration by engineered bone, functional recovery is another important requirement for engineered bone repair. In this study, a three-point bending test demonstrated that engineered femoral bones at 8 months were much stronger than those at 4 months. Besides, no significant difference was found in respect to bending load strength and

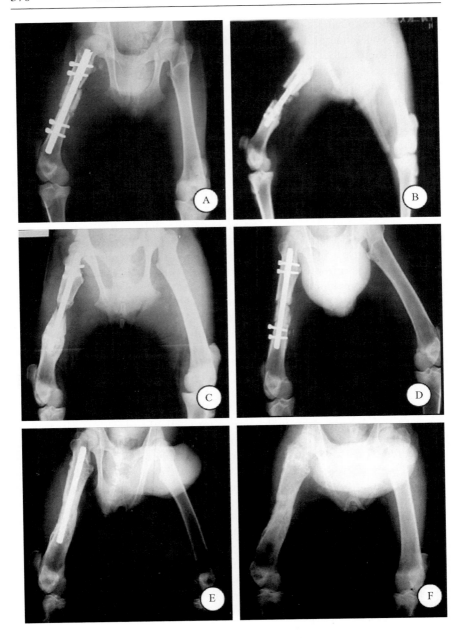

bend rigidity between the 8-month engineered bones and natural counter-part bones. However, the engineered bones were still inferior to natural counterpart bones in regard to bend intention and bend displacement (Zhu et al., 2006).

Clinical Application of Engineered Bone

Vacanti et al. (2001) performed the first clinical trial of engineered bone in thumb reconstruction using degradable polymer and autologous osteo-genic precursor cells isolated from periosteum, and it initially seemed to have succeeded; however, long-term follow-up was not reported. Recently, Warnke et al. (2004) reported successful clinical treatment of mandibular bone defect in a male patient with tissue-engineered bone. A titanium mesh cage with the mandibular shape of the patient was first filled with bone mineral blocks infiltrated with recombinant human BMP-7 and bone marrow mixture and then implanted into the patient's latissimus dorsi muscle for 7 weeks to form a vascularized bone graft. The combined engineered bone graft was then transplanted to functionally repair the mandibular defect, and the bone remodeling and mineralization were also observed by scintigraphy examination.

Our center initiated a small-scale clinical trial of engineered bone approximately 5 years ago, mainly focused on the repair of human cranio-maxillofacial bone defects using autologous BMSCs and demineralized bone matrix (Chai et al., 2003). As a typical case, shown in Fig. 8, we started the clinical trial on a small-size cranial defect. Bone marrow was harvested from the patient to isolate BMSCs; after in vitro expansion and osteogenic induction, cells were seeded on DBM scaffold and in vitro cultured for 7 days and then implanted to repair the patient's defect. As illustrated by 3D-CT scanning, bone formation was observed 3 months after implantation and maintained stable when followed up at 12 months

---

Fig. 5. Radiographs taken of the treated goat's femur at different time frames. (A–C) Femur defects treated with coral alone. (D–F) Femur defects treated with coral loaded with culture-expanded and osteo-inducted BMSCs. (A) Femur defect treated with coral alone at day 1 after implantation. The cylinder with a density less than that of cortex can be found. (B) Coral density mostly disappeared 1 month after implantation. (C) At 8 months after implantation, minimal bone formation at the bone cut ends without bridging defect. (D) Femur defect treated with coral loaded with culture-expanded and osteo-inducted BMSCs 1 month after implantation. The shape of the implant was maintained with callus formation at the interface to the bone cut ends. (E) At 6 months after implantation, newly formed bone can afford weight bearing after removing interlocking nails. (F) At 8 months after implantation, the density of newly formed bone is equal to that of cortex. (Reprinted by permission of Tissue Engineering, Zhu et al., 2006).

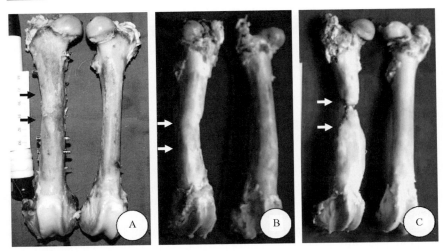

FIG. 6. Gross view of repaired defects in experimental and control groups. (A) Femur defect implanted with coral loaded with culture-expanded and osteo-inducted BMSCs at 4 months. Newly formed cancellous bone with red color. (B) Femur defect implanted with coral loaded with culture-expanded and osteo-inducted BMSCs at 8 months. White-colored, remodeled cortex formed. (C) Femur defect implanted with coral alone at 8 months. Nonunion formed. (A–C) Left, experimental bone defects; right, normal bone serving as a positive control. (Reprinted by permission of *Tissue Engineering*, Zhu *et al.*, 2006).

and 5 years after operation. During a secondary revision operation, a bone biopsy was taken 18 months after implantation, and the histological examination showed the typical structure of cancellous bone. Therefore, we proved that engineered bone can form and maintain stable for the long-term in human beings. On the basis of the success in small-size bone repair, we further challenged ourselves to repair a craniofacial bone defect with larger size and more complicated 3D. Figure 9 demonstrates another typical case. The patient had a craniofacial bone defect involving both frontal and orbital roof bones. To proceed the repair, the patient's 3D-CT scanning data were first obtained and then used to 3D-print a mold that was exactly fitted into the defect site. According to the 3D shape of the mold, DBM materials were trimmed and assembled to form a 3D-shape scaffold. After cell seeding and *in vitro* culture for 7 days, the cell–scaffold construct was implanted to repair the defect. The patient has been followed up for up to 3 years with 3D-CT scanning, which demonstrated that the engineered bone not only satisfactorily repaired the defect with a complicated 3D structure but also maintained stable without absorption even after 3 years. Our clinical trial results

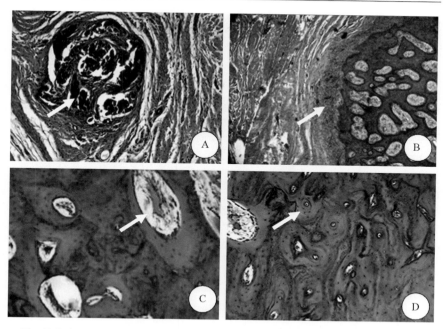

FIG. 7. H&E staining of repaired bone tissues. (A) Femur defect treated with coral alone 4 months after implantation. Residual coral particle remained, surrounded by fibrous tissue (arrow, ×100). (B) Femur defect treated with coral alone 8 months after implantation. Coral particle disappeared completely, and a certain level of bone formed at bone cut end (arrow, ×100). (C) Femur defect implanted with coral loaded with culture-expanded and osteo-inducted BMSCs at 4 months. Coral completely disappeared, and woven bone was formed. White regions indicated by the arrow are newly formed medullary canal (×100). (D) Femur defect implanted with coral loaded with culture-expanded and osteo-inducted BMSCs at 8 months. Mature bone structure was formed, and Haversian system became observable (arrow, ×100). (Reprinted by permission of *Tissue Engineering*, Zhu *et al.*, 2006).

indicate that tissue engineering will become a novel approach for bone regeneration and repair.

Protocol for Dog Cranial Bone Engineering

1. Isolation and osteogenic induction of BMSCs (Weng *et al.*, 2006): After animals were anesthetized, bone marrow (2 ml) was harvested from the proximal end of a canine femoral bone. The mononuclear cells in bone marrow were separated by Percoll gradient centrifugation and cultured in medium. To induce osteogenic differentiation, BMSCs were cultured in DMEM containing 10% FBS, dexamethasone (10^{-8} M), L-glutamine

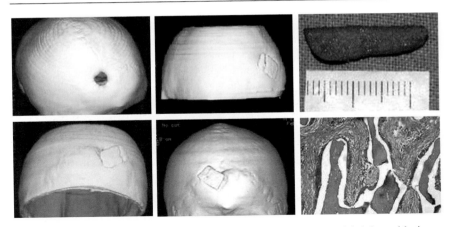

FIG. 8. 3D CT and histological evaluation of clinical repair of cranial defect with tissue-engineered bone. Top left, before operation; top middle, 3 months after repair; bottom left, 12 months after repair; bottom middle, 5 years after repair; top right, bone biopsy; bottom right, biopsy shows cancellous bone structure of engineered bone 18 months after repair (HE).

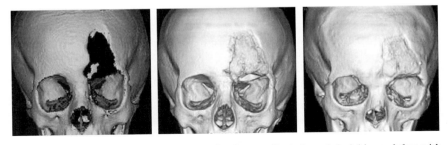

FIG. 9. 3D CT evaluation of clinical repair of a complicated craniofacial bone defect with tissue-engineered bone. Left, before operation; middle, 1 year after repair; right, 3 years after repair.

(0.3 g/L), β-phosphoglycerol (10 mM), and ascorbic acid (50 μg/l) at 37° in humidified atmosphere containing 95% air and 5% CO_2.

2. Characterization of osteogenically induced BMSCs (Weng *et al.*, 2006): Cells at passage 3 were prepared for immunocytochemical staining to determine the expression of core binding factor α 1, osteopontin, bone sialoprotein, osteocalcin, and type I collagen in the induced cells. In addition, cells of passage 3 were also examined for alkaline phosphatase expression and further subjected to a Von Kossa staining.

3. Preparation of cell–scaffold constructs: Pig's caput femoris was harvested and sliced. After washing, the tissue was decellulized by Triton-X treatment and then degreased with methyl chloride/methanol mixture followed by decalcification with diluted hydrochloric acid. The sample was thoroughly washed, dried, and sterilized with radiation to generate DBM scaffold (for animal study). To prepare cell–scaffold constructs, *in vitro* expanded and induced BMSCs were evenly seeded on the DBM at a concentration of 1×10^7/ml. The cell–coral constructs were then placed in an incubator for 4 h at 37° in 95% air and 5% CO_2, allowing complete adhesion of cells to DBM. Subsequently, induced medium was added, and the constructs were *in vitro* cultured for 7 days before *in vivo* implantation.

4. Surgical procedure: Under anesthesia, bilateral defects with a size of 2×2 cm^2 were created in the dogs' parietal bones, and the periosteum surrounding the defects was completely removed. On the experimental side, a cell–scaffold was implanted. On the other side, DBM alone was implanted as a control. The bone formation was monitored with 3D-CT scanning at the time points of months 6, 9, and 12 after implantation. All animals were sacrificed at 12 months, and the calvarial bone tissues were harvested for x-ray and histological examination.

Protocol for Goat Femoral Bone Engineering (Zhu *et al.*, 2006)

1. Isolation and osteogenic induction of BMSCs: After anesthetization, autologous bone marrow (5 ml in total volume) was harvested by iliac aspiration from each adult goat and transferred to a sterile tube containing 20 ml of serum-free DMEM and 1000 U/ml heparin. After centrifugation at 200g for 5 min and removal of the fat layer and the supernatant, cells were rinsed with PBS and then resuspended in osteogenic induction DMEM medium plus 10% FBS, 10^{-8} M dexamethasone, 0.3 g/Lμ L-glutamine, 10 mM β-phosphoglycerol, and 50 μg/L ascorbic acid. The isolated cells were plated on 100-mm culture dishes at a density of 5×10^6 cells per dish for primary culture at 37° in 95% air and 5% CO_2. BMSCs were cultured for a minimum of 5 days without medium change to facilitate cell attachment to the culture dish. The nonadherent cells were then removed from the cultures by medium change. Subsequent medium changes were performed every 3 days and cells were subcultured at a density of 5×10^5 per 100-mm dish in osteogenic induction medium.

2. Characterization of osteogenically induced BMSCs: Performed similarly as previously described (Weng *et al.*, 2006).

3. Preparation of coral scaffold: On the basis of the anatomical data of goat femora, a cylinder shape of coral construct was generated with the

height of 25 mm, outer diameter of 16 mm, and inner diameter of 10 mm (Fig. 10).

4. Design of femur fixation device: To provide a fixation way that allows for mechanical loading to remodel the engineered bone, a special internal fixation device was developed on the basis of the anatomical data of goat femora. This device contains an internal fixation rod with a diameter a littler smaller than that of marrow cavity and two sets of interlocking nails for fixing the rod at two ends (Fig. 11B). After bone formation, the interlocking nails can be removed, leaving the rod in the marrow cavity and thus allowing for mechanical loading by the body weight.

5. Surgical procedure (Fig. 11): Twenty-two adult goats, 12–14 months of age and weighing from 16.5–23 kg (an average of 19.6 kg), were included in this study and randomly divided into experimental group (implanted with cell-scaffold construct, $n = 10$), scaffold control group (implanted with scaffold alone, $n = 10$), and a blank control (without implantation, $n = 2$). After anesthesia, the aspect of the right femoral shaft was exposed and a 25-mm-long (20% of the femur's total length) osteoperiosteal segmental defect was created with proper fixation by using the device. The defects were then treated either with cell-loaded scaffold, scaffold alone, or left untreated. Animals were sacrificed at either 4 months or 8 months, respectively, for gross observation and histological and biomechanical analyses. To enhance tissue remolding, interlocking nails were removed at 6 months in those animals that would be sacrificed at 8 months to give the newly formed bone a mechanical loading.

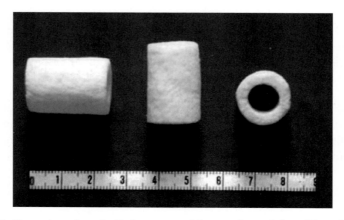

FIG. 10. Gross view of coral cylinders prepared for goat femur defects. The cylinders are 25 mm high, 16 mm in outer diameter, and 10 mm in inner diameter. (Reprinted by permission of *Tissue Engineering*, Zhu *et al.*, 2006).

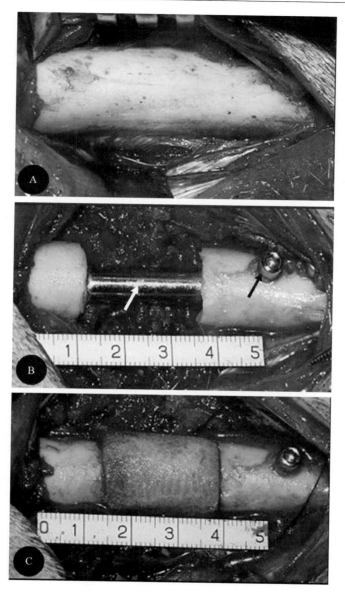

FIG. 11. Surgical procedure: (A) Goat femur is exposed and periosteum is removed; (B) a segmental bone defect is created followed by fixation with a special device (white arrow, fixation rod; black arrow, interlocking nail at one end); (C) cell-loaded coral was implanted to repair the defect.

6. Radiographic and gray-density analyses: Radiographs of both sides of the femurs were obtained under general anesthesia on the first day and postoperatively at 1–8 months. One stepped aluminum wedge with graduated thickness was included in the field of each radiograph, acting as a standard for density correction of radiographic technique. Radiographs were evaluated for evidence of new bone formation within the defect and for development of bone union. Through the use of a computer program, the area of newly formed bone in the defect was digitized, and an average density of each radiograph taken on day 1 and 1–4 months were obtained, according to the standard gray density generated from the same stepped aluminum wedge. The gray density representing newly formed bone (average density × area) within the defect was also quantitatively analyzed.

7. Biomechanical analysis: A three-point bending test was applied to measure the biomechanical property of engineered femoral bone. The femurs harvested from both side legs of the experimental group animals at 4 ($n = 4$) and 8 months ($n = 4$) were immediately frozen and stored at $-80°$ for mechanical testing. All the femurs were thawed for 24 h in a refrigerator before the test. Because of the non-union bone in the control group, only experimental femurs were subjected to the mechanical test, and their contralateral normal femurs served as a positive control. Each femur was placed in a three-point bending system, providing an unsupported length of 8 cm. Both ends of the tested femurs were not fixed. The condyles were directed upward, so that the anterior surface of the femur was placed in tension under the test. Load was applied in the posterior-to-anterior direction to the midpoint of the unsupported length, approximately in the middle of the repaired defect. The same approach was applied to the same point on the left femurs as a positive control. Testing was conducted in a hydraulic materials testing machine (Shimadzu AG-20kNH, Kyoto, Japan) and stopped after bone fracture. Deformation was measured using the strain gauge at a loading rate of 1.4 mm/min. Data from the strain gauge and the displacement of deformation were all recorded in 50 newton increments. Then, on the basis of the results, the bend intention and bend stiffness were determined.

Acknowledgment

The authors thank Drs. Lei Cui, Yulai Weng, Ming Wang, Zhuo Wang, and Lian Zhu for the contribution in bone engineering and Dr. Gang Chai for clinical trial of engineered bone. The research projects are supported by National "973" (2005CB522700) and "863" Project Foundation, Shanghai Science and Technology Development Foundation, and Key Laboratory Foundation of Shanghai Education Committee.

References

Byers, B. A., Guldberg, R. E., and Garcia, A. J. (2004). Synergy between genetic and tissue engineering: Runx2 overexpression and *in vitro* construct development enhance *in vivo* mineralization. *Tissue Eng.* **10,** 1757–1766.

Caplan, A. I. (1994). The mesengenic process. *Clin. Plast. Surg.* **21,** 429–435.

Chai, G., Zhang, Y., Liu, W., Cui, L., and Cao, Y. L. (2003). Clinical application of tissue engineered bone repair of human craniomaxillofacial bone defects. *Zhonghua Yi Xue Za Zhi.,* **83,** 1676–1681.

Chang, S. C., Chuang, H., Chen, Y. R., Yang, L. C., Chen, J. K., Mardini, S., Chung, H. Y., Lu, Y. L., Ma, W. C., and Lou, J. (2004). Cranial repair using BMP-2 gene engineered bone marrow stromal cells. *J. Surg. Res.* **119,** 85–91.

Cowan, C. M., Shi, Y. Y., Aalami, O. O., Chou, Y. F., Mari, C., Thomas, R., Quarto, N., Contag, C. H., Wu, B., and Longaker, M. T. (2004). Adipose-derived adult stromal cells heal critical-size mouse calvarial defects. *Nat. Biotechnol.* **22,** 560–567.

Deasy, B. M., Jankowski, R. J., and Huard, J. (2001). Muscle-derived stem cells: Characterization and potential for cell-mediated therapy. *Blood Cells Mol. Dis.* **27,** 924–933.

Erices, A., Conget, P., and Minguell, J. J. (2000). Mesenchymal progenitor cells in human umbilical cord blood. *Br. J. Haematol.* **109,** 235–242.

Friedenstein, A. J., Petrakova, K. V., Kurolesova, A. I., and Frolova, G. P. (1968). Heterotopic transplants of bone marrow. Analysis of precursor cells for osteogenic and hematopoietic tissues. *Transplantation* **6,** 230–247.

Fukuchi, Y., Nakajima, H., Sugiyama, D., Hirose, I., Kitamura, T., and Tsuji, K. (2004). Human placenta-derived cells have mesenchymal stem/progenitor cell potential. *Stem Cells* **22,** 649–658.

Gimble, J. M. (2003). Adipose tissue-derived therapeutics. *Expert. Opin. Biol. Ther.* **3,** 1–9.

Jaiswal, N., Haynesworth, S. E., Caplan, A. I., and Bruder, S. P. (1997). Osteogenic differentiation of purified, culture-expanded human mesenchymal stem cells *in vitro.* *J. Cell Biochem.* **64,** 295–312.

Jorgensen, N. R., Henriksen, Z., Sorensen, O. H., and Civitelli, R. (2004). Dexamethasone, BMP-2, and 1,25-dihydroxyvitamin D enhance a more differentiated osteoblast phenotype: Validation of an *in vitro* model for human bone marrow-derived primary osteoblasts. *Steroids* **69,** 219–226.

Kuznetsov, S. A., Mankani, M. H., Gronthos, S., Satomura, K., Bianco, P., and Robey, P. G. (2001). Circulating skeletal stem cells. *J. Cell Biol.* **153,** 1133–1140.

Mauney, J. R., Jaquiery, C., Volloch, V., Heberer, M., Martin, I., and Kaplan, D. L. (2005). *In vitro* and *in vivo* evaluation of differentially demineralized cancellous bone scaffolds combined with human bone marrow stromal cells for tissue engineering. *Biomaterials* **26,** 3173–3185.

Meinel, L., Fajardo, R., Hofmann, S., Langer, R., Chen, J., Snyder, B., Vunjak-Novakovic, G., and Kaplan, D. (2005). Silk implants for the healing of critical size bone defects. *Bone* **37,** 688–698.

Owen, M. (1988). Marrow stromal stem cells. *J. Cell Sci.* **10**(suppl.), 63–76.

Petite, H., Viateau, V., Bensaid, W., Meunier, A., de Pollak, C., Bourguignon, M., Oudina, K., Sedel, L., and Guillemin, G. (2002). Tissue-engineered bone regeneration. *Nat. Biotechnol.* **18,** 959–963.

Prockop, D. J. (1997). Marrow stromal cells as stem cells for nonhematopoietic tissues. *Science* **276,** 71–74.

Rickard, D. J., Sullivan, T. A., Shenker, B. J., Leboy, P. S., and Kazhdan, I. (1994). Induction of rapid osteoblast differentiation in rat bone marrow stromal cell cultures by dexamethasone and BMP-2. *Dev. Biol.* **161,** 218–228.

Shang, Q., Wang, Z., Liu, W., Shi, Y., Cui, L., and Cao, Y. (2001). Tissue-engineered bone repair of sheep cranial defects with autologous bone marrow stromal cells. *J. Craniofac. Surg.* **12,** 586–593.

Schantz, J. T., Hutmacher, D. W., Lam, C. X., Brinkmann, M., Wong, K. M., Lim, T. C., Chou, N., Guldberg, R. E., and Teoh, S. H. (2003). Repair of calvarial defects with customised tissue-engineered bone grafts II. Evaluation of cellular efficiency and efficacy *in vivo. Tissue Eng.* **9**(Suppl. 1), S127–S139.

Tu, Q., Valverde, P., and Chen, J. (2006). Osterix enhances proliferation and osteogenic potential of bone marrow stromal cells. *Biochem. Biophys. Res. Commun.* **341,** 1257–1265.

Vacanti, C. A., Bonassar, L. J., Vacanti, M. P., and Shufflebarger, J. (2001). Replacement of an avulsed phalanx with tissue-engineered bone. *N. Engl. J. Med.* **344,** 1511–1514.

Vacanti, C. A., Kim, W., Upton, J., Vacanti, M. P., Mooney, D., Schloo, B., and Vacanti, J. P. (1993). Tissue-engineered growth of bone and cartilage. *Transplant Proc.* **25,** 1019–1021.

Vacanti, C. A., and Upton, J. (1994). Tissue-engineered morphogenesis of cartilage and bone by means of cell transplantation using synthetic biodegradable polymer matrices. *Clin. Plast. Surg.* **21,** 445–462.

Warnke, P. H., Springer, I. N., Wiltfang, J., Acil, Y., Eufinger, H., Wehmoller, M., Russo, P. A., Bolte, H., Sherry, E., Behrens, E., and Terheyden, H. (2004). Growth and transplantation of a custom vascularised bone graft in a man. *Lancet* **364,** 766–770.

Weng, Y., Wang, M., Liu, W., Hu, X., Chai, G., Yan, Q., Zhu, L., Cui, L., and Cao, Y. (2006). Repair of experimental alveolar bone defects by tissue-engineered bone. *Tissue Eng.* **12,** 1503–1513.

Yeh, L. C., Tsai, A. D., and Lee, J. C. (2002). Osteogenic protein-1 (OP-1, BMP-7) induces osteoblastic cell differentiation of the pluripotent mesenchymal cell line C2C12. *J. Cell Biochem.* **87,** 292–304.

Zhu, L., Liu, W., Cui, L., and Cao, Y. (2006). Tissue-engineered bone repair of goat-femur defects with osteogenically induced bone marrow stromal cells. *Tissue Eng.* **12,** 423–433.

Zuk, P. A., Zhu, M., Mizuno, H., Huang, J., Futrell, J. W., Katz, A. J., Benhaim, P., Lorenz, H. P., and Hedrick, M. H. (2001). Multilineage cells from human adipose tissue: Implications for cell-based therapies. *Tissue Eng.* **7,** 211–228.

Zuk, P. A., Zhu, M., Ashjian, P., De Ugarte, D. A., Huang, J. I., Mizuno, H., Alfonso, Z. C., Fraser, J. K., Benhaim, P., and Hedrick, M. H. (2002). Human adipose tissue is a source of multipotent stem cells. *Mol. Biol. Cell.* **13,** 4279–4295.

[18] Engineering Three-Dimensional Tissue Structures Using Stem Cells

By JANET ZOLDAN and SHULAMIT LEVENBERG

Abstract

The worldwide status of rapidly increasing demand for organ and tissue transplantation has promoted tissue engineering as a promising alternative, in particular the use of stem cells. Human embryonic stem cells (hESCs) have the advantage of differentiating to all cell types in the body and high proliferation capabilities. Considering their ability to organize into complex multi-cell–type structures during embryonic-like differentiation, hESCs can potentially provide a source of cells for tissue engineering applications and meet the growing demand for viable human tissue structures in therapeutic clinical application. This chapter describes first steps toward realizing this goal gathered from our experience in growing and differentiating hESCs in three dimensions.

Introduction

Tissue engineering combines cell biology with materials science to develop appropriate strategies for repair and regeneration of biological tissues. Biological tissues consist of cells situated within a complex molecular framework known as the *extracellular matrix* (ECM) with an integrated vascular system for oxygen or nutrient supply. Artificial three-dimensional (3D) polymeric scaffolds can mimic the ECM and serve as a physical support, providing tissues with the appropriate 3D architecture for *in vitro* cell culture, as well as *in vivo* tissue regeneration. Many cell types have been successfully cultured on polymer scaffolds, including smooth muscle cells, endothelial cells, hepatocytes and chondrocytes (Langer and Vacanti, 1993; Lanza *et al.*, 2000; Levenberg and Langer, 2004; Niklason and Langer, 1997). Yet, these are usually "single-cell–type" cultures, and attempts to reconstruct tissues with more than one cell type have usually encountered problems. Another critical obstacle in engineering tissue constructs is the limited amount of available human cells. Human embryonic stem cells (hESC) represent a promising source of human cells without a full organ donation that can then be expanded *in vitro* to yield the cells needed for transplantation applications. The advantage of hESC besides their ability to differentiate to broad class of cellular subtypes and their unlimited proliferating capabilities, is their potential to organize

METHODS IN ENZYMOLOGY, VOL. 420
0076-6879/06 $35.00
DOI: 10.1016/S0076-6879(06)20018-1

into complex multi-cell–type structures during their embryonic-like differentiation. *In vitro,* ESCs have been shown to give rise to cells of hematopoietic (Bigas *et al.,* 1995; Kaufman *et al.,* 2001; Palacios *et al.,* 1995), endothelial (Hirashima *et al.,* 1999), cardiac (Fleischmann *et al.,* 1998; Kehat *et al.,* 2001; Rohwedel *et al.,* 1994), neural (Brustle *et al.,* 1999; Reubinoff *et al.,* 2001; Schuldiner *et al.,* 2001; Zhang *et al.,* 2001), osteogenic (Buttery *et al.,* 2001), hepatic (Hamazaki *et al.,* 2001), and pancreatic (Assady *et al.,* 2001; Lumelsky *et al.,* 2001) tissue. Several experiments have demonstrated the therapeutic potential use of ESCs to repair ischemic tissues or treat diseases where damaged cells are not normally repaired or replaced. Creation of dopamine-producing cells in animal models of Parkinson's disease (Bjorklund *et al.,* 2002; Kim *et al.,* 2002); ESCs derived neural precursors incorporated into various regions of the mouse brain differentiated into neurons and astrocytes, as well as migrated within the host brain and differentiated in a region-specific manner (Reubinoff *et al.,* 2001; Zhang *et al.,* 2001); ESC-derived cardiomyocytes could potentially be used for cell therapy in the heart (Kehat *et al.,* 2001, 2002; Klug *et al.,* 1996; Min *et al.,* 2002; Mummery *et al.,* 2003; Yang *et al.,* 2002); Mouse ESCs transfected with an insulin promoter have been shown to give rise to insulin-producing cells that can restore glucose levels in animals (Soria *et al.,* 2000). Another area in which hESC can potentially be beneficial is the engineering of complex tissues where vascularization of the regenerating tissue is essential. Early endothelial progenitor cells isolated from differentiating mouse ESCs were shown to give rise to three blood vessel cell components, hematopoietic, endothelial, and smooth muscle cells (Yamashita *et al.,* 2000). We have recently demonstrated the formation and stabilization of endothelial vessels network *in vitro* in 3D-engineered skeletal muscle tissue (Levenberg *et al.,* 2005).

Porous biodegradable polymer scaffolds are an ideal system for inducing tissue formation, because they can be tailored to modulate cell attachment growth and differentiation. The use of scaffolds provides 3D environments essential for the formation of tissue-like structures. After degradation, the polymers can promote further growth of cells and provide space for remodeling tissue structures (Vacanti and Langer, 1999). These scaffolds are expected to be biocompatible and, with a controlled porous architecture, to allow for rapid and controlled tissue growth and to maximize diffusion parameters allowing nutrient exchange, gas exchange and waste exchange. Desirable features include biocompatibility, biodegradability, ease of fabrication with a range of shapes, and the intrinsic capability to communicate with living cells, thereby facilitating controlled and rapid tissue restoration. α-Polyesters; such as polylactic acid (PLA), polyglycolic acid (PGA), and their copolymers (PLGA), most closely fulfill these criteria. Other polyesters including poly(ε-caprolactones) and polyorthoesters, as well as different polymer families such as polyanhydrides, polycarbonates, and polyfuma-rates, have been studied as intraluminar grafts, stent-like devices, temporary vascular grafts, and temporary conduits for peripheral nerve regeneration (Agrawal and Ray, 2001).

Numerous fabrication techniques have been developed to produce 3D porous scaffolds using solvents (or nonuse of solvents), pressure, heat and porogens (Agrawal and Ray, 2001; Salgado et al., 2004; Wan-Ju Li, 2005). The choice of material and production procedure affects the scaffold's properties (mechanical, crystallinity, and permeability), the degree of po-rosity, and the pore size. It is generally agreed that high open porosity (pores within 100–1000 μm rang) of scaffolds is an important parameter, because it provides space not only for the cells to infiltrate the scaffold and attach but also for the ECM formation. High permeability is also an important feature of scaffolds, allowing inflow of nutrients and the elution of metabolic waste and biodegradation products. Changing the polymer scaffold porosity or permeability (or both) can affect the degradation characteristics (Athanasiou and Agrawal, 1998). The latter can be tailored to meet the proliferation rates of the seeded cells. All these characteristic determine the scaffold's mechanical properties, as well as affect cell growth, differentiation, and organization during tissue formation, leading to the growing evidence on the mechanotransduction between scaffolds and cells on them (Ingber, 2003; Levenberg et al., 2003; Semler et al., 2000).

This chapter will outline our method in differentiating and growing hESCs on 3D scaffolds. We have seeded both undifferentiated and early differentiating hESCs directly onto scaffolds and then differentiated them into various committed embryonic tissues (Levenberg et al., 2005).

Protocols for Differentiating ESCs

Human ES cells have the ability to spontaneously differentiate on 2D culture dishes or within a suspension culture of cell aggregates. These cell aggregates are called *embryoid bodies* (EBs) because they mimic many aspects of embryonic development. Cell–cell interactions are critical to normal embryonic development, so allowing some of these "natural" *in vivo* interactions to occur in the culture dish are a fundamental strategy for inducing hESC differentiation *in vitro*.

In the laboratory, hESCs are maintained and expanded in their undif-ferentiated state by growing on feeder layers (murine or human). This layer secrets chemical signals and molecular cues that sustain the undifferentiat-ed phenotype and at the same time prevents interaction between hESCs. Therefore, the induction of hESCs differentiation involves first the removal of this feeder layer.

EB Formation

EBs can be formed by a number of methods (Levenberg *et al.*, 2006). One of the most versatile methods appropriate for hESCs is suspending the cells within nonadhesive dishes that induce aggregate formation of the cells.

EB Cell Media

> Knockout (KO) serum, 20%
> KO DMEM medium, 80%
> Nonessential amino acid solution, 1%
> 2-mercaptoethanol, 0.3% (55 mM in DPBS)
> L-glutamine, 0.5% (200 mM in 0.85% NaCl)
> Filter the solution using a 0.22-μm filter bottle
> Serum and stock solutions should be stored at $-20°$

Nonadhesive Dishes

1. Add 4 ml of 200 U/ml collagenase solution to 10-cm dishes containing hESCs:
   a. Aspirate the medium from the plates.
   b. Add 4 ml of 200 U/ml collagenase solution to each plate.
   c. Leave the plate in the incubator for 30–45 min.
   d. Add 8 ml of ES medium.
   e. Wash the plate gently to remove the ES colonies without removing MEFs from the bottom of the dishes.
   f. Move the ES colonies to a 15-ml falcon tube.
   g. Wash the plate a second time with 3 ml ES medium to collect any ES colonies that were not taken the first time. Add to the solution in the 15-ml tube.
   h. Spin down at 800 rpm for about 3 min.
2. Resuspend the cells in EB medium and add to nontreated polystyrene dishes.
3. Typically the cells are seeded so that one 10-cm ES plate is split into three 10-cm EB plates (or similar).
4. Put the plates in the incubator.

After several days, the cells typically form clusters that range in size from 50–1000 μm, as can be seen in Fig. 1.

Protocol for Scaffold Seeding

Recently we have demonstrated that hESCs or early differentiating hESCs (EBs) can be differentiated within biodegradable polymer scaffolds (Levenberg *et al.*, 2003).

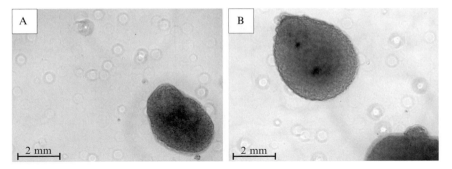

FIG. 1. EBs differentiated from hESC for: (A) 6 days and (B) 8 days.

To facilitate cell attachment to the scaffolds, we mix the cells with matrigel solution and load the cell/matrigel solution onto the scaffolds (Levenberg *et al.*, 2002, 2003). The gel mixture solidifies in 37° and keeps the cells inside the scaffolds.

Scaffold Preparation

The selected biodegradable polymers PLLA and PLGA are most commonly used or studied for medical purposes. Hence, their biocompatibility and degradation is already well known and studied. Blending these polymers combines the high PLLA strength and modulus with the increased hydrolysis rate of the amorphous PLGA, leading to intermediate mechanical properties (Nakafuku and Takehisa, 2004). Furthermore, this blend was found appropriate for hESC attachment and growth (Anderson *et al.*, 2004). To produce porous scaffolds from the synthetic PLGA/PLLA polymer blends, we chose standard technique such as salt leaching. In this procedure, the polymers are dissolved in a solvent, and salt (usually sodium chloride) is added. The solvent is extracted, and then the salt is leached out by immersion in deionized water. Pore size is dictated by the salt particles' size. This technique offers easy fabrication of porous 3D scaffolds at room temperature, achieving more than 90% porosity. Figure 2A depicts a PLLA/PLGA 50/50 scaffold produced by this technique.

1. Dissolve PLLA and PLGA ratio 1/1 in chloroform.
2. Into a conical Teflon mold (20 cm in diameter) add 0.4 g of 212–500 μM diameter salt.
3. Wet the weighed salt with 0.24 μl of 50/50 PLGA/PLLA polymer solution in chloroform and cap to prevent the chloroform from escaping.

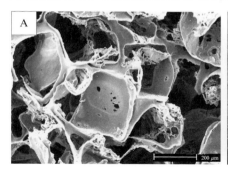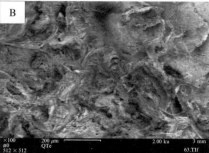

FIG. 2. SEM and HRSEM micrographs of a PLLA/PLGA 50/50 scaffolds: (A) without cells; (B) 2 weeks after seeding the scaffold with 1×10^6 EBs (8 days old).

4. Allow the containers to sit, covered, for 1 h.
5. Take the lids off of the molds and allow the chloroform to evaporate overnight in the hood.
6. Remove the scaffold from the mold.
7. Leach out salt with DDI water (change the water each hour for 6–8 h).
8. Lyophilize overnight to ensure dry scaffolds.

PLLA/PLGA Scaffold Sterilization Before Seeding

1. Cut the scaffolds into squares of 3×3 mm (do not use the outer rims of the scaffold).
2. Place cut scaffolds in a 50-ml flask and add 70% ethanol, so that the scaffolds are fully immersed within the ethanol.
3. Leave overnight. A shorter procedure, yet one with a higher incidence of contamination, involves scaffold immersion for 5 min in 100% ethanol and then for at least 2 h in 95% ethanol.

PLLA/PLGA Scaffold Seeding

The scaffolds can be seeded with hESCs, which will start their differentiation on the scaffold, or seeded with EBs, which will complete their differentiation on the scaffold (Figs. 2B and 3).
For EBs:

1. Transfer EBs, suspended in nonadhesive plates, to 15-ml flasks by *slow* aspiration with 10-ml pipette.
2. Wait for 5 min (the EBs start to sink at the flask bottom) and then aspirate slowly 3 ml of the medium at the flask top and wash the EBs plates to ensure that all EB colonies were removed.

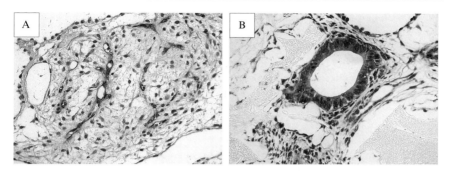

FIG. 3. Human EBs, 8 days old, seeded on PLLA/PLGA 50/50 scaffold after 2 weeks: (A) treated with IGF and stained for CD31; (B) treated with RA and stained for nestin.

3. Wait for 15 min until all EBs sink at the flask bottom.
4. Spin down at 800 rpm for 1 min.
5. Aspirate the medium above the EB pellet slowly with a 10-ml pipette.
6. Add 2 ml trypsin (0.1 M) and resuspend.
7. Place in the incubator for 5 min on a 3D shaker (23 orbits per min).
8. After trypsinization for 5 min, vigorously resuspend the cells with a 1000-μm pipetter tip and add 4 ml TNS (Trypsin neutralizing solution) to neutralize the trypsin.

For hESCs:

1. Aspirate the medium from the plates.
2. Add 4 ml of 200 U/ml collagenase solution to each plate.
3. Leave the plate in the incubator for 20–30 min.
4. Add 5 ml of ESC medium (Levenberg *et al.*, 2006).
5. Wash the plate gently to remove the ES colonies without removing the feeder layer.
6. Move the ESC colonies to a 15-ml falcon tube.
7. Wash the plate a second time with 3 ml ESC medium to collect any ESC colonies that were not taken the first time. Add to the 5 ml medium along with 4 ml collagenase solution in the 15-ml tube.
8. Spin down at 800 rpm for about 3 min.
9. Resuspend the ES cell pellet with fresh 3–4 ml medium and pipette strongly to break the colonies into smaller pieces.

Scaffold seeding:

1. Aspirate the ethanol and add 30 ml sterile PBS (0.05 M) for 30 min (after 15 min, aspirate again the PBS and replace with fresh PBS).

2. Place an ice bucket full of ice within the hood on which is situated an aliquot of matrigel and an Eppendorf tube containing 0.5 ml of EB medium.
3. Count the cells with a hemocytometer. Each scaffold should be seeded with 1×10^6 cells.

> No. of scaffolds to be seeded = No. of cells (according to the hemocytometer) / 1×10^6

4. Spin down at 800 rpm for 3 min.
5. Aspirate the medium above the cell pellet and resuspend with EB medium; the amount of required medium equals the number of scaffolds to be seeded (for each scaffold 1 ml of suspended cells).
6. Divide the suspended cells into Eppendorf tubes, so that each Eppendorf tube for each scaffold contains 1 ml with 1×10^6 cells.
7. Microcentrifuge the Eppendorf tubes at 1000 rpm for 4 min.
8. While the cells are spinning, aspirate the PBS in the scaffold flask and replace with fresh PBS.
9. Place centrifuged Eppendorf tubes on ice.
10. Prepare seeding solution by mixing equal parts of matrigel and ice-cold EB medium (as described in Section 2). Each scaffold should be mounted with 20 μl of seeding solution. *All of this stage should be performed on ice*, keeping all components at ice temperature. Amount of matrigel in seeding solution = Amount of ice-cold EB medium in seeding solution = No. of scaffolds $*$ 20/2 μl.
11. Aspirate the second PBS wash in the scaffold flask and replace with EB medium. Rinse the scaffolds around for a few minutes so that they are soaked in medium.
12. Aspirate the medium from the scaffolds and place each scaffold in a separate well, using non-tissue–culture-treated dishes. Make sure that the scaffolds are dry.
13. Aspirate the medium above the cell pellet in the Eppendorf tubes (make sure that the entire old medium is aspirated) and resuspend with 20 μl seeding solution (containing 10 μl matrigel mixed with 10 μl of EB medium). *All this stage should be performed on ice.*
14. Assuming that 1×10^6 cells will take up 5 μl, take 25 μl of the cells/matrigel/ medium mixture.
15. Place the tip of the pipette on the dry scaffold and slowly release the mixture into the scaffold. Pipette up and down three times, so that the mixture is pushed through the scaffold and evenly distributed. Make sure not to drag the scaffold around the well and avoid air bubbles.
16. Repeat for all scaffolds.

17. Place on the incubator for 30 min (to solidify the matrigel).
18. Put 5 ml EB medium in each well. Do not touch the scaffold directly but instead pour the medium slowly on the side of the well. The matrigel is still fragile, and cells could spray out of the scaffold. If the seeded scaffold is still stuck to the bottom of the well, use a 25-ml pipette and gently push the scaffold until it detaches and floats in the medium.
19. Place seeded scaffolds in the incubator on a 3D shaker.
20. Change medium every 2–3 days. Use 25-ml pipette to replace 4 ml of the medium (leaving the seeded scaffold in 1 ml old medium). Medium withdrawal and addition should be performed at the slowest available velocity.
21. If cells begin to grow at the well bottom, replace the dish.

References

Agrawal, C. M., and Ray, R. B. (2001). Biodegradable polymeric scaffolds for musculoskeletal tissue engineering. *J. Biomed. Mater. Res.* **55,** 141–150.

Anderson, D. G., Levenberg, S., and Langer, R. (2004). Nanoliter-scale synthesis of arrayed biomaterials and application to human embryonic stem cells. *Nat. Biotechnol.* **22,** 863–866.

Assady, S., Maor, G., Amit, M., Itskovitz-Eldor, J., Skorecki, K. L., and Tzukerman, M. (2001). Insulin production by human embryonic stem cells. *Diabetes* **50,** 1691–1697.

Athanasiou, K. A., Schmitz, J. P., and Agrawal, C. M. (1998). The effects of porosity on *in vitro* degradation of polylactic acid polyglycolic acid implants used in repair of articular cartilage. *Tissue Eng.* **4,** 53–63.

Bigas, A., Martin, D. I., and Bernstein, I. D. (1995). Generation of hematopoietic colony-forming cells from embryonic stem cells: Synergy between a soluble factor from NIH-3T3 cells and hematopoietic growth factors. *Blood* **85,** 3127–3133.

Bjorklund, L. M., Sanchez-Pernaute, R., Chung, S., Andersson, T., Chen, I. Y., McNaught, K. S., Brownell, A. L., Jenkins, B. G., Wahlestedt, C., Kim, K. S., and Isacson, O. (2002). Embryonic stem cells develop into functional dopaminergic neurons after transplantation in a Parkinson rat model. *Proc. Natl. Acad. Sci. USA* **99,** 2344–2349.

Brustle, O., Jones, K. N., Learish, R. D., Karram, K., Choudhary, K., Wiestler, O. D., Duncan, I. D., and McKay, R. D. (1999). Embryonic stem cell-derived glial precursors: A source of myelinating transplants. *Science* **285,** 754–756.

Buttery, L. D., Bourne, S., Xynos, J. D., Wood, H., Hughes, F. J., Hughes, S. P., Episkopou, V., and Polak, J. M. (2001). Differentiation of osteoblasts and *in vitro* bone formation from murine embryonic stem cells. *Tissue Eng.* **7,** 89–99.

Fleischmann, M., Bloch, W., Kolossov, E., Andressen, C., Muller, M., Brem, G., Hescheler, J., Addicks, K., and Fleischmann, B. K. (1998). Cardiac specific expression of the green fluorescent protein during early murine embryonic development. *FEBS Lett.* **440,** 370–376.

Hamazaki, T., Iiboshi, Y., Oka, M., Papst, P. J., Meacham, A. M., Zon, L. I., and Terada, N. (2001). Hepatic maturation in differentiating embryonic stem cells *in vitro*. *FEBS Lett.* **497,** 15–19.

Hirashima, M., Kataoka, H., Nishikawa, S., Matsuyoshi, N., and Nishikawa, S. (1999). Maturation of embryonic stem cells into endothelial cells in an *in vitro* model of vasculogenesis. *Blood* **93,** 1253–1263.

Ingber, D. E. (2003). Tensegrity II. How structural networks influence cellular information processing networks. *J. Cell Sci.* **116,** 1397–1408.

Kaufman, D. S., Hanson, E. T., Lewis, R. L., Auerbach, R., and Thomson, J. A. (2001). Hematopoietic colony-forming cells derived from human embryonic stem cells. *Proc. Natl. Acad. Sci. USA* **98,** 10716–10721.

Kehat, I., Gepstein, A., Spira, A., Itskovitz-Eldor, J., and Gepstein, L. (2002). High-resolution electrophysiological assessment of human embryonic stem cell-derived cardiomyocytes: A novel *in vitro* model for the study of conduction. *Circ. Res.* **91,** 659–661.

Kehat, I., Kenyagin-Karsenti, D., Snir, M., Segev, H., Amit, M., Gepstein, A., Livne, E., Binah, O., Itskovitz-Eldor, J., and Gepstein, L. (2001). Human embryonic stem cells can differentiate into myocytes with structural and functional properties of cardiomyocytes. *J. Clin. Invest.* **108,** 407–414.

Kim, J. H., Auerbach, J. M., Rodriguez-Gomez, J. A., Velasco, I., Gavin, D., Lumelsky, N., Lee, S. H., Nguyen, J., Sanchez-Pernaute, R., Bankiewicz, K., and McKay, R. (2002). Dopamine neurons derived from embryonic stem cells function in an animal model of Parkinson's disease. *Nature* **418,** 50–56.

Klug, M. G., Soonpaa, M. H., Koh, G. Y., and Field, L. J. (1996). Genetically selected cardiomyocytes from differentiating embryonic stem cells form stable intracardiac grafts. *J. Clin. Invest.* **98,** 216–224.

Langer, R., and Vacanti, J. P. (1993). Tissue engineering. *Science* **260,** 920–926.

Lanza, R. P., Langer, R., and Vacanti, J. P. (2000). "Principles of Tissue Engineering." Boston: Academic Press. 181–191, 251–279.

Levenberg, S., Golub, J. S., Amit, M., Itskovitz-Eldor, J., and Langer, R. (2002). Endothelial cells derived from human embryonic stem cells. *Proc. Natl. Acad. Sci. USA* **99,** 4391–4396.

Levenberg, S., Huang, N. F., Lavik, E., Rogers, A. B., Itskovitz-Eldor, J., and Langer, R. (2003). Differentiation of human embryonic stem cells on three-dimensional polymer scaffolds. *Proc. Natl. Acad. Sci. USA* **100,** 12741–12746.

Levenberg, S., Khademhosseini, A., Macdonald, M., Fuller, J., and Langer, R. (2006). "Human Embryonic Stem Cell Culture for Tissue Engineering." Wiley & Sons, New Jersey.

Levenberg, S., and Langer, R. (2004). Advances in tissue engineering. *Curr. Top. Dev. Biol.* **61,** 113–134.

Levenberg, S., Rouwkema, J., Macdonald, M., Garfein, E. S., Kohane, D. S., Darland, D. C., Marini, R., van Blitterswijk, C. A., Mulligan, R. C., D'Amore, P. A., and Langer, R. (2005). Engineering vascularized skeletal muscle tissue. *Nat. Biotechnol.* **23,** 879–884.

Lumelsky, N., Blondel, O., Laeng, P., Velasco, I., Ravin, R., and McKay, R. (2001). Differentiation of embryonic stem cells to insulin-secreting structures similar to pancreatic islets. *Science* **292,** 1389–1394.

Min, J. Y., Yang, Y., Converso, K. L., Liu, L., Huang, Q., Morgan, J. P., and Xiao, Y. F. (2002). Transplantation of embryonic stem cells improves cardiac function in postinfarcted rats. *J. Appl. Physiol.* **92,** 288–296.

Mummery, C., Ward-van Oostwaard, D., Doevendans, P., Spijker, R., van den Brink, S., Hassink, R., van der Heyden, M., Opthof, T., Pera, M., de la Riviere, A. B., Passier, R., and Tertoolen, L. (2003). Differentiation of human embryonic stem cells to cardiomyocytes: Role of coculture with visceral endoderm-like cells. *Circulation* **107,** 2733–2740.

Nakafuku, C., and Takehisa, S. Y. (2004). Glass transition and mechanical properties of PLLA and PDLLA-PGA copolymer blends. *J. Appl. Polymer Sci.* **93,** 2164–2173.

Niklason, L. E., and Langer, R. S. (1997). Advances in tissue engineering of blood vessels and other tissues. *Transpl. Immunol.* **5,** 303–306.

Palacios, R., Golunski, E., and Samaridis, J. (1995). *In vitro* generation of hematopoietic stem cells from an embryonic stem cell line. *Proc. Natl. Acad. Sci. USA* **92,** 7530–7534.

Reubinoff, B. E., Itsykson, P., Turetsky, T., Pera, M. F., Reinhartz, E., Itzik, A., and Ben-Hur, T. (2001). Neural progenitors from human embryonic stem cells. *Nat. Biotechnol.* **19,** 1134–1140.

Rohwedel, J., Maltsev, V., Bober, E., Arnold, H. H., Hescheler, J., and Wobus, A. M. (1994). Muscle cell differentiation of embryonic stem cells reflects myogenesis *in vivo*: Developmentally regulated expression of myogenic determination genes and functional expression of ionic currents. *Dev. Biol.* **164,** 87–101.

Salgado, A. J., Coutinho, O. P., and Reis, R. L. (2004). Bone tissue engineering: State of the art and future trends. *Macromol. Biosci.* **4,** 743–765.

Schuldiner, M., Eiges, R., Eden, A., Yanuka, O., Itskovitz-Eldor, J., Goldstein, R. S., and Benvenisty, N. (2001). Induced neuronal differentiation of human embryonic stem cells. *Brain Res.* **913,** 201–205.

Semler, E. J., Ranucci, C. S., and Moghe, P. V. (2000). Mechanochemical manipulation of hepatocyte aggregation can selectively induce or repress liver-specific function. *Biotechnol. Bioeng.* **69,** 359–369.

Soria, B., Roche, E., Berna, G., Leon-Quinto, T., Reig, J. A., and Martin, F. (2000). Insulin-secreting cells derived from embryonic stem cells normalize glycemia in streptozotocin-induced diabetic mice. *Diabetes* **49,** 157–162.

Vacanti, J. P., and Langer, R. (1999). Tissue engineering: The design and fabrication of living replacement devices for surgical reconstruction and transplantation. *Lancet* **354** (Suppl 1), SI32–SI34.

Li, W.J, and Tuan, R. S. (2005). Polymeric scaffolds for cartilage tissue engineering. *Macromol. Symp.* **227,** 65–76.

Yamashita, J., Itoh, H., Hirashima, M., Ogawa, M., Nishikawa, S., Yurugi, T., Naito, M., Nakao, K., and Nishikawa, S. (2000). Flk1-positive cells derived from embryonic stem cells serve as vascular progenitors. *Nature* **408,** 92–96.

Yang, Y., Min, J. Y., Rana, J. S., Ke, Q., Cai, J., Chen, Y., Morgan, J. P., and Xiao, Y. F. (2002). VEGF enhances functional improvement of postinfarcted hearts by transplantation of ESC-differentiated cells. *J. Appl. Physiol.* **93,** 1140–1151.

Zhang, S. C., Wernig, M., Duncan, I. D., Brustle, O., and Thomson, J. A. (2001). *In vitro* differentiation of transplantable neural precursors from human embryonic stem cells. *Nat. Biotechnol.* **19,** 1129–1133.

[19]   Immunogenicity of Embryonic Stem Cells and Their Progeny

By MICHA DRUKKER

Abstract

The ability of pluripotent human embryonic stem cells (hESCs) to differentiate into multiple cell types has led to great excitement about their potential use in the treatment of various degenerative and malignant human diseases. Before such a goal is attainable, however, it must be demonstrated

METHODS IN ENZYMOLOGY, VOL. 420
Copyright 2006, Elsevier Inc. All rights reserved.

0076-6879/06 $35.00
DOI: 10.1016/S0076-6879(06)20019-3

that pure populations of specialized cell types can be isolated and transplanted while simultaneously avoiding possible immune-mediated rejection of these cells. In this chapter, I will discuss the utility of the humanized mouse Trimera model as an *in vivo* experimental system to study the immunological properties of hESCs and their differentiated derivatives.

Introduction

Human embryonic stem cell (hESC) lines are excellent candidates to serve as a valuable source of cells for regenerative medicine because of their capacity to grow indefinitely in culture without losing pluripotency and to generate any cell types of the body on induction of differentiation (Itskovitz-Eldor *et al.*, 2000; Reubinoff *et al.*, 2000; Thomson *et al.*, 1998). For example, detailed differentiation protocols are currently available for the derivation of neurons (Carpenter *et al.*, 2001; Reubinoff *et al.*, 2001; Schuldiner *et al.*, 2001; Schulz *et al.*, 2003; Zhang *et al.*, 2001), cardiomyocytes (He *et al.*, 2003; Kehat *et al.*, 2001, 2002; Mummery *et al.*, 2002, 2003; Xu *et al.*, 2002), endothelial cells (Levenberg *et al.*, 2002), hematopoietic precursors (Chadwick *et al.*, 2003; Kaufman *et al.*, 2001), keratinocytes (Green *et al.*, 2003), osteoblasts (Sottile *et al.*, 2003), hepatocytes (Lavon *et al.*, 2004; Rambhatla *et al.*, 2003), and others. However, there is a major concern that immune responses directed against hESC-derived transplants may severely limit their use in therapeutics.

The initial attempts to determine the antigenicity of hESCs were carried out by examining the expression of MHC molecules before, and after, differentiation (Draper *et al.*, 2002; Drukker *et al.*, 2002). These studies revealed that hESCs express low levels of cell surface MHC class I (MHC-I) molecules, elevated expression in embryoid bodies, and even higher levels of expression in teratomas. MHC class II (MHC-II) molecules, however, were not expressed (Drukker *et al.*, 2002). Importantly, it was found that undifferentiated, as well as the differentiated, hESCs upregulate expression of MHC-I by at least 10-fold in response to interferons (IFNs); however, MHC-II expression was not induced (reviewed in Drukker and Benvenisty [2004]). Although these are important observations, it is important to note that such knowledge does not allow accurate prediction of the immune responses against the cells, because multiple factors apart from MHC expression are involved in such responses. Therefore, it is imperative to develop improved human tissue rejection models to determine whether or not differentiated hESCs will be rejected, and, if so, how these responses are mediated.

Various *in vitro* assays have been developed to evaluate responses of human immune subsets against allogeneic (from another individual) human cells. In the mixed lymphocyte reaction (MLR), lymphocyte subsets from two individuals are mixed together *in vitro* and then cytotoxicity, proliferation, and secretion assays can provide qualitative and quantitative data regarding the avidity of immune recognition. In a similar manner, responses of human lymphocyte subsets against hESCs were tested. By incubating hESCs with a primary human cytotoxic T-cell (CTL) line specifically primed to recognize antigen-loaded cells, the cytotoxic immune response occurred only after MHC-I induction by interferon-γ (IFN-γ) (Drukker *et al.*, 2006). However, a robust response against hESCs did not occur when they were incubated with primary human natural killer (NK) cell line (Drukker *et al.*, 2002). Thus, these studies suggest that hESCs are recognized by T cells only on strong induction of MHC-I and that the NK-cell response is negligible. Although these experiments provide important insights into potential mechanisms of immune recognition, they do not measure other aspects of innate and adaptive immunity *in vivo*.

The use of a humanized mouse model offers the ability to study both the innate and adaptive immune responses against human cells *in vivo*. Early attempts to establish such a model used the severe combined immunodeficient (SCID) mice that were adoptively transferred with human peripheral blood mononuclear cells (PBMCs). By use of this model, it was shown that human B cells efficiently produce antibodies against human viruses (Torbett *et al.*, 1991), but T cells become functionally anergic (Saxon *et al.*, 1991). Preservation of T-cell function was accomplished by use of supralethally irradiated immunocompetent mice radioprotected with SCID bone marrow cells and then adoptively transplanted with human PBMCs, (Trimera model) (Dekel *et al.*, 2003; Lubin *et al.*, 1994). The improvement in the latter model was attributed to the presence of normal lymphoid organs in the recipients.

Given the likelihood of future efforts to develop hESC-derived cellular therapeutics, it is critical to establish models that closely mimic the clinically relevant transplantation settings. I describe here a detailed protocol for the generation of Trimera mice and the transplantation of undifferentiated and differentiated hESCs into these mice. The Trimera model would be useful to study the antigenicity and immunogenicity of purified populations of differentiated hESCs for the development of safe transplantation strategies.

Generation of Trimera Mice

Overview

The generation of Trimera mice involves three steps (Fig. 1): The first is supralethal irradiation of mice from an immunocompetent strain to eliminate

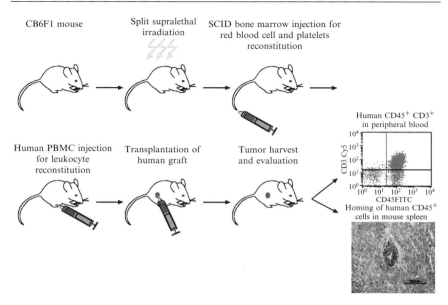

FIG. 1. Construction of human/mouse radiation chimera ("Trimera") model. This model consists of three major components. CB6F1 mice are exposed to a split dose (4 Gy followed 3 days later by 10 Gy) of total body irradiation. Irradiated mice are radioprotected with 3×10^6 bone marrow cells from NOD/SCID mice; 100×10^6 human PBMCs are injected intraperitoneally into recipient mice, and 1–3 days later hESCs or somatic grafts are injected under the kidney capsule. Mice are sacrificed 3–5 weeks later, and the grafts are then evaluated for infiltration by human lymphocytes and tissue damage. Performing FACS analysis to a mouse blood samples validates the state of chimerism. Note the high proportion of human $CD3^+$, $CD45^+$ cells in the mouse peripheral blood. Also, it is possible to see that human $CD45^+$ cells (red staining) populate the spleen in chimera mice (www.StemCells.com [Drukker et al., 2006]).

the mouse lymphocytes that can elicit a xenorejection (between species) response against human cells. The second is radioprotection of the irradiated animals by bone marrow cells that are harvested from SCID mice and serve to produce essential myeloid cells. Because SCID mice carry mutations in genes that are required for lymphocyte development, transplanted bone marrow cells from these mice cannot give rise to lymphocytes, and, therefore, they cannot contribute to immune responses against human cells. Finally, the mice are injected with a high dose of human PBMCs that act as the immune component in this system, and their response against hESCs can then be tested. For best results adhere to the following timetable:

1. Irradiate the mice twice: Use 4 Gy the first time (Day −6); 3 days later, irradiate with a second dose of 10 Gy (Day −3).

2. 24 h later transplant a dose of 3×10^6 SCID bone marrow cells to each mouse (Day -2).

3. 24 h later transplant $80-100 \times 10^6$ human PBMCs to the mice (Day -1). Transplantation of PBMCs within this time range is thought to be ideal, because at this point endogenous lymphocytes are undergoing programmed cell death, but the lymph node architecture is intact.

4. Transplantation of hESCs or their derivatives should be carried out within 1–3 days. It is advisable not to wait more than 5 days because the immune responses are more robust adjacent to the time of PBMC introduction.

Each cell type should be injected into three animals at least. As a control, it is important to inject all cell types into mice that were not reconstituted with human PBMCs. In these mice, all cell types should grow with no signs of rejection. To ensure that the human lymphocytes in the Trimera mice are active, carry out transplantations of fragments of primary human tissue, such as skin fragments, which are available from plastic surgery clinics. These transplants are used to confirm an intact immune response in the Trimera mice. For instance, if you plan to inject two types of cells plus one control tissue, prepare nine PBMC-reconstituted mice and six nonreconstituted mice; you will inject three mice with each cell type (six total) and an additional three with the control tissue. Two nonreconstituted mice will be used as a control for the two cell types and one somatic tissue.

Materials

- Two-month-old immunocompetent mice (e.g., CB6F1). Five animals per cage. Use one gender to avoid mating.
- 70-μm Nylon Cell Strainer (Cat# 352350, BD Falcon).
- PBS wash media: Dulbecco's phosphate-buffered saline without calcium/magnesium (Cat# 14190–144, Invitrogen) supplemented with 2% FBS. Carry out all the washing steps using this solution.
- ACK lysis buffer: 150 mM NH$_4$Cl, 10 mM KHCO$_3$, 0.1 mM EDTA.
- Histopaque-1119 (Cat# 1119, Sigma). Store at $4°$.
- 1.077 g/ml Ficoll-Paque PLUS (Cat# 17-1440-02, GE Healthcare). Store at $4°$ in the dark.
- 300 ml of human peripheral blood anticoagulated with heparin.

Step 1: Irradiation of Mice and Bone Marrow Transplantation

As noted previously, conditioning mice to carry human PBMCs involves supralethal total body irradiation to eliminate all endogenous leukocytes. Different mouse strains may vary in their response to this shock, and thus irradiation conditions should be adjusted according to the strain. To avoid excessive loss of mice because of irradiation, it is recommended that F1 mice (e.g. from BALB/c × C57BL cross) be used, because they are usually more resilient to irradiation. After the first dose of irradiation, maintain the animals on antibiotic-containing water (10×10^6U/l polymyxin B sulfate and 1.1 g/l neomycin sulfate) for 6 weeks.

One day after the second irradiation dose (i.e., Day -2), prepare bone marrow cells from SCID mice. In selecting a donor mice strain, it is important to pick an immunodeficient strain that will not be able to contribute to the immune response towards transplanted human cells. The NOD/SCID/γc^{null} (common gamma chain of the IL2 receptor complex) mouse represents one potential donor strain because it has multiple immunological impairments and no detectable NK cell function (Ito et al., 2002). SCID and NOD (non-obese diabetic)/SCID mice are suboptimal, because both strains have residual NK cell activity that can mediate rejection of human cells. Alternately, the RAG2/γc^{null} double knockout strain may be used because of their T, B, and NK cell deficiencies (Goldman et al., 1998). To harvest bone marrow cells for rescue of irradiated animals, perform the following steps:

1. Humanely euthanize the mice by terminal CO_2 inhalation.

2. Cut out the femur and tibia bones and remove the muscles. Place the bones into PBS to prevent tissue drying.

3. Cut off the ends of the bones (it is recommended to cut as far toward the end as possible; in case of distal femur and proximal tibia, dislocation of the joint surface is sufficient). Flush the shafts into a 50-ml conical tube with PBS using a short (5/8 inch) 25-gauge needle and a 10-ml syringe. Pass the isolated bone marrow cells through an 18-gauge needle to disaggregate the larger bone marrow pieces.

4. Centrifuge the suspension at 400g for 5 min at room temperature (RT) and resuspend in 300 ml of ACK solution. After lysing for 1–3 min, restore osmolarity by filling the tube with PBS. Filter the suspension into another 50-ml conical tube through a 70-μm cell strainer to remove clots and bone fragments. Spin the suspension at 400g for 5 min (RT).

5. Pour 5 ml Histopaque (Ficoll density 1.119) into a 15-ml conical tube. Before layering the cell suspension on the Ficoll, make sure the Ficoll is at RT. Resuspend the cell pellet in 5 ml PBS and carefully layer it over the Ficoll. Centrifuge for 5 min at 800g (RT) without braking. Using a 5-ml pipette, carefully collect the mononuclear cell band at the Ficoll/PBS interface, avoiding the Ficoll as much as possible. Then transfer the cells to a new 15-ml tube. Add one volume of PBS and centrifuge at 400g for 5 min (RT).

6. Discard the supernatant, resuspend the cell pellet in 15 ml PBS, and spin again for 5 min in 400g (RT). Repeat this washing step twice.

7. Discard the supernatant, resuspend the cell pellet in 1 ml PBS, and count the cells using a hemocytometer. There should be a total of 30–60 $\times 10^6$ BM mononuclear cells from one mouse.

8. Adjust the cell suspension to a concentration of 30×10^6 cells/ml with PBS and intravenously inject 100 μl into the tail vein of each recipient using a 27-gauge needle. To facilitate visualization and injection of the tail vein, use a heat lamp to warm the mice.

Step 2. Preparation and Transplantation of Human Peripheral Blood Mononuclear Cells (PBMCs)

Human PBMCs are prepared to serve as the human functional immune-component cells in Trimera mice. Typically, 500–1500 $\times$ 10^6 PBMCs are isolated from 300 ml of peripheral blood, and thus could be used for a group of six animals or more. Do not pool PBMCs from different individuals, because it will lead to a severe allogeneic response.

1. PBMCs are prepared by density gradient centrifugation. Place 15 ml Ficoll-Paque PLUS (density 1.077) in a 50-ml conical tube, tilt the tube, and gently overlay up to 30 ml of human blood diluted 1:1 with PBS. Do not disrupt the interface between the lower Ficoll and upper cell suspension phase.

2. Centrifuge at 800g for 30 min (RT) with the brake off. Using a 10-ml pipette, carefully collect the mononuclear cell band at the Ficoll-Paque/serum interface and transfer the cells into a fresh 50-ml tube. Make sure that you take as little of the Ficoll as possible. Add one volume of PBS and centrifuge at 400g for 5 min (RT).

3. Discard the supernatant, resuspend the cell pellet in 50 ml PBS, and spin under the same conditions. Repeat this step twice.

4. Discard the supernatant and resuspend all the PBMCs from one donation in 1 ml PBS and count the cells using a hemocytometer. The yield should be a total of 500–1500 $\times$ 10^6 PBMCs from 300 ml of starting material.

5. Adjust the cell suspension to a concentration of 500×10^6 cells/ml with PBS and inject 500 μl of into the peritoneum of each mouse using a 27-gauge needle.

Once the mice have been prepared, they can be used as recipients for human grafts for up to 5 days. Injection at later time points increases the chance of inducing T-cell anergy.

Transplantation of hESCs and Derivatives into Trimera Mice

Overview

The Trimera mouse model may be used to assay the immunological properties of undifferentiated hESCs, as well as differentiated cells. I will describe here the generation and transplantation of undifferentiated cells, teratoma fragments, and skin fragments into recipient mice. In these experiments, teratomas serve as representatives of mature, disorganized differentiation, while skin fragments serve as immunogenic controls.

The protocol begins with culturing hESCs to produce teratomas by injecting them into the kidney capsule of SCID mice (described later). After sufficient time elapses to allow for teratoma formation, recipient mice and human PBMCs are prepared to generate Trimera mice and controls. Preparation of recipient mice and initiation of undifferentiated hESC culture should be appropriately timed to coincide with the development of teratomas.

It is important to note that this system may be used to examine the immune response against any type of human cell. With the advancement of differentiation protocols for hESCs, it will be critical to assay immune responses against purified hESC–derived populations as part of their evaluation for therapeutic use.

Materials

• hESC maintenance media: 400 ml Dulbecco's modified Eagle medium: Nutrient Mix F-12 (D-MEM/F-12) (1×), liquid, 1:1, with L-glutamine and HEPES buffer (Cat# 11330–032) supplemented with 100 ml Knockout Serum Replacement (Cat# 10828–028), 5 ml MEM nonessential amino acids 100× solution (Cat# 11140–050), 5 ml GlutaMAXI Supplement (Cat# 35050–061), 5 ml penicillin-streptomycin (Cat# 15140–122), 0.5 ml 2-mercaptoethanl (Cat# 21985–023) (all from Invitrogen), and one vial of 200 μl FGF-basic (see later). Filter the medium using a 0.22-μm filter unit and store refrigerated in the dark.

• Recombinant human FGF-basic (Peprotech Inc) is dissolved in 5 mM Tris, pH 7.6, to a concentration of 25 μg/ml and stored as 200 μl aliquots in –80°. Add one aliquot per 500 ml hESC media to reach a final concentration of 10 ng/ml. Avoid repeated freezing and thawing.

• Mouse embryonic fibroblasts (MEF) media: 500 ml Dulbecco's modified Eagle medium high glucose (Cat# 11965–092, Invitrogen) supplemented with 50 ml characterized fetal bovine serum (FBS, Cat# SH30071, HyClone) and 5 ml penicillin-streptomycin (Cat# 15140-122, Invitrogen). Filter the medium using 0.22-μm filter unit and store refrigerated.

• Solution of trypsin (0.25%) and 1 mM ethylenediaminetetraacetic acid (EDTA) (Cat# 25200-056, Invitrogen).

• Gelatin solution: Prepare 1% autoclaved gelatin type A solution (Cat# 0 G-1890, Sigma) in distilled water.

• Dulbecco's phosphate-buffered saline without calcium/magnesium (Cat# 14190-144, Invitrogen).

• Sterile 1 mg/ml collagenase type IV (Cat# 17104-019, Invitrogen) solution in D-MEM/F-12.

- Basement membrane matrix (matrigel), phenol red-free, 10 ml (Cat#356237, BD). Thaw vial overnight on ice in a cold room (4°). In the hood, while the vial remains on ice, transfer 1-ml aliquots into chilled 1.5-ml microtubes. Store in –20°.
- Basement membrane matrix, working solution. Thaw 1-ml aliquot overnight on ice in a cold room (4°). In the hood on ice, transfer aliquot to a 50-ml conical tube containing 19 ml D-MEM/F-12 medium. Mix briefly and keep on ice. Store in –20°.
- Dimethylsulfoxide (DMSO) (Cat# D2650, Sigma, St Louis, MO).
- Avertin stock solution: In 20 ml glass vial, dissolve 25 g of 2,2,2-tribromoethanol (Cat# T48402, Sigma) with 15.5 ml of tert-amyl alcohol (Cat# 152463, Sigma). Store at room temperature wrapped with aluminum foil in a glass jar for up to 6 months.
- Avertin working solution: Add 1 ml of stock solution to 49 ml of PBS. Maintain constant stirring of PBS that is warmed to 37° while adding Avertin to avoid formation of crystals in the final solution. Aliquot and store protected from light at 4°.
- 70% ethanol, surgical scissors, sharp dissecting scissors, surgical forceps, and wound closing clips and forceps.
- Scalpel no. 11 (Cat# 373911, BD).
- Hamilton removable needle syringe capacity 25 μl (Cat# 80230) fitted with a 30-gauge removable needle (Cat# 7762-03).

Step 1. hESC Culture and Differentiation*

This protocol assumes that the hESC culture starts from one plate of approximately 1×10^6 cells.

1. Transfer approximately 1×10^6 mouse embryonic fibroblasts (irradiated at 4000 rad) in 10 ml MEF media into a 10-cm tissue culture dish precoated for 10 min with 6 ml 1% gelatin solution. Incubate overnight.

2. Aspirate MEF media. Transfer approximately 1×10^6 hESCs to the MEF-coated plate in 10 ml hESC culture medium. Incubate overnight.

3. Change culture medium every day for 2–5 days. The cells should form medium size colonies (of approximately 100–200 cells, or 150 μm in diameter).

4. 3 h before splitting the cells, coat one 10-cm plate by adding 2 ml diluted matrigel. Swirl the plate until it is uniformly covered with matrigel. Leave the plate in the hood for 3 h.

---

*Detailed protocols for hESC propagation can be found at http://www.wicell.org/forresearchers/index.jsp?catid=12&subcatid=20.

5. Aspirate the medium from the hESC plate, wash with 6 ml PBS, and aspirate again. Add 3 ml collagenase type IV solution to the cells. Incubate in 37° for 15 min.

6. Aspirate the solution and add 2 ml of fresh collagenase solution. Incubate for additional 10 min.

7. The edges of the colonies should become loose. Gently add 5 ml of hESC media to the colonies, and pipette up and down until they become loose. Transfer the suspended cells into a 15-ml conical tube and spin 5 min at 400g (RT). Discard the medium and resuspend in 1 ml of hESC media. Count the cells using a hemocytometer. There should be approximately $2–5 \times 10^6$ cells.

8. Aspirate the remaining matrigel solution, add 10 ml hESC maintenance media and transfer the hESC cell suspension to the new plate.

9. Change culture medium every day for 2–3 days until medium-large colonies form.

10. To transplant the cells, they should be trypsinized. Aspirate the medium from the plate, wash with 6 ml PBS, aspirate PBS, and add 1 ml 0.25% trypsin/EDTA to each plate. Incubate at RT for 5 min, and wash the cells using 4 ml hESC media to quench the trypsin. Transfer the cells into a new 15-ml tube.

11. Spin 5 min at 400g (RT). Resuspend in 1 ml PBS and count the cells using hemocytometer. There should be a total of $5–10 \times 10^6$ cells. Spin again under the same conditions. Aspirate the PBS carefully and adjust the concentration of the cells to 1×10^6 cells/20 μl by adding PBS to the cells while gently tapping on the tube. Transfer the cell suspension to a 0.6-ml microcentrifuge tube. Incubate the cells on ice until ready for transplantation into recipients.

Step 2. Transplantation of Human Grafts into the Kidney Capsule

1. Mouse anesthesia: Inject 15 μl Avertin (working solution) per 1 g of mouse body weight into the peritoneum. After about 2 min, the mouse will be immobilized and will remain so for about half an hour.

2. Preparation of tissues and cells for transplantation:
   a. hESCs: Wash the Hamilton syringe using 70% ethanol, then with sterile PBS, before loading with cells. Resuspend the cells briefly and pull the plunger to load 20 μl of cells. Avoid the formation of bubbles by pulling slowly. Place the syringes on ice.
   b. Teratoma fragments: Humanely sacrifice the SCID mice by terminal CO_2 inhalation. Remove the tumor together with the kidney. Separate the tumor from the kidney using forceps. Using a scalpel, dice the tumor into small fragments ($\sim$1 mm^3). Keep the fragments in PBS on ice until used.

c. Skin fragments: using a sharp scalpel cut small pieces of approximately 1 mm^3 and keep on ice in PBS.

3. Pinch the mouse hind limb to verify that the mouse is fully anesthetized. If the mouse is still conscious, it will reflexively withdraw its leg from your grasp. Do not commence surgery until there is no reflex reaction.

4. To ensure sterility, wipe the left side of the back with 70% ethanol and part the hair to allow clean incision of the skin. Make a small (1 cm) transverse cut in the skin in the midline region between the ribs and pelvis (Fig. 2A).

5. Make a small transverse incision in the muscle perpendicular to spine approximately 0.5 cm below the last rib (Fig. 2B). Place a pair of closed scissors under the muscle and open them to enlarge the opening up to 1.5 cm (Fig. 2C). Locate the kidney and using delicate forceps gently pull the kidney through the abdominal wall defect and hold it above the skin (Fig. 2D).

6. Moisten the kidney capsule with a few drops of PBS to prevent it from drying. Slowly inject 20 μl of cells into the space between the capsule and the surface of the kidney (Fig. 2E). To transplant the teratoma and skin fragments, using a 19-gauge needle make a small hole in the capsule and then gently inset the fragment through the hole using delicate forceps. Some hemorrhage may result from the procedure. Ideally, if bleeding is limited, the capsule should remain translucent and the injected cells can easily be seen (Fig. 2F).

7. Gently reposition the kidney into the abdominal cavity and suture the muscle (not essential). Close the skin with two wound clips. If the muscle suture is not performed, the muscle should be clamped simultaneously with the skin using the wound clips.

8. To prevent infections that might occur because of surgery, it is recommended to provide prophylaxis with antibiotics. Subcutaneously inject the penicillin–streptomycin stock solution (5 μl per 1 g body weight) while the mouse is still anesthetized.

9. Wrap the mouse in a tissue to help keep it warm. Use a heating pad postoperatively until the animal regains consciousness. Return the animal to the cage.

Assessing the Immune Response against Engrafted hESCs

Overview

Once hESCs or their differentiated progeny have been transplanted into recipient mice, several assays are used to assess whether or not a functional immune response was mounted against the graft. The first assay measures the extent of hESC-derived tumor growth, comparing tumor size in the Trimera mice with control group (-PBMC) mice. If transplants in the

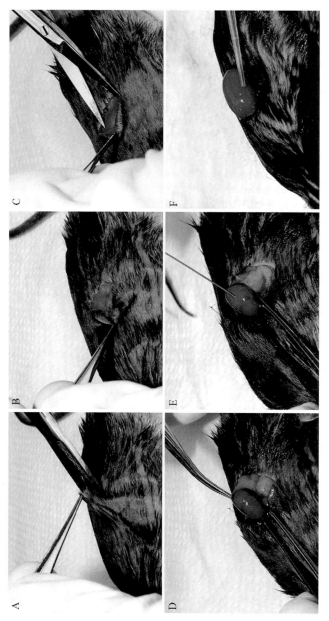

FIG. 2. Cell injection into the mouse kidney capsule. Wipe the left side of the back with 70% ethanol. (A) Make a small (1 cm) transverse cut in the skin in the midline region between the ribs and pelvis. (B) Make a small transverse incision in the muscle perpendicular to the spine, approximately 0.5 cm below the last rib. (C) Place a pair of closed scissors under the muscle and open them to enlarge the opening up to 1.5 cm. (D) Expose the kidney using delicate forceps that were placed under it. Moisten the kidney capsule with few drops of PBS to prevent it from drying. (E) Inject 20 μl of cells into the space between the capsule and the surface of the kidney. (F) If bleeding is limited, the capsule should remain translucent, and the injected cells can be seen easily.

control animals are larger than the Trimera transplants, it suggests that the cells were robustly rejected. Qualitative aspects of the immune response may be evaluated using histological sections. Such sections may reveal clues about the nature of the immune response (e.g., signs of cytotoxic responses as indicated by graft necrosis). In addition, the composition of the immune cell infiltrate may be evaluated with immunohistochemical stains using markers specific to different immune cell lineages or functional subsets. For instance, if a large number of $CD8^+$ T cells are found, it is very likely that alloreactive cytotoxic T lymphocytes mediate the immune response. This section describes some of the assays that may be used to assess immune responses against the transplants and discusses the mechanisms that might be involved in rejection of hESCs and their derivatives.

Materials

- Scalpel no. 11 (Cat# 373911, BD).
- Mouse restraining chamber (Cat# 01-288-31A, Fisher).
- Heat lamp.
- Solution 2% dextran T-500 (Cat# 31392, Sigma) in PBS.
- ACK lysis buffer: 150 mM NH$_4$Cl, 10 mM KHCO$_3$, 0.1 mM EDTA.
- FACS media: Dulbecco's phosphate-buffered saline without calcium/ magnesium (Cat# 14190-144, Invitrogen) supplemented with 2% FBS.
- PBS/EDTA: 10 mM EDTA in Dulbecco's phosphate-buffered saline without calcium/magnesium.
- Human serum (Cat# 14-490E, Cambrex)

Step 1. Estimating PBMC Engraftment

Two weeks after transplantation, leukocyte engraftment is tested by bleeding the transplanted animals and analyzing the percentage of human PBMCs in the peripheral blood using FACS analysis.

1. Place mice (in their cage with the top off) under a heating lamp for approximately 2–3 min. Transfer each mouse in the restraining chamber with the tail toward you.

2. Using the sharp scalpel, make a small incision in one of the two lateral tail veins about an inch away from the base of the tail. Collect 3–5 drops of blood in 1.5-ml microcentrifuge tubes containing 500 μl PBS/ EDTA and immediately invert to mix. If the tail continues to bleed, apply a small amount of pressure to the area before returning the mouse to its cage (not under the heat lamp).

3. Add 500 μl dextran solution and mix by inverting. Incubate for 25 min at 37°. Transfer 800–900 μl of supernatant to a new Microfuge tube,

discarding the red cell pellet. Centrifuge at 400g for 5 min (RT). Aspirate the supernatant and add 200 μl ACK lysis solution to the cell pellet. Incubate for 4 min at RT for lysis of the remaining red blood cells.

4. Add 500 μl FACS staining media and centrifuge again at 400g for 5 min (RT). At this point, there should be a small white pellet with few to no red blood cells in the pellet.

5. Resuspend the pellet in 50 μl staining media containing 10% human serum (to block the Fc receptor) and incubate on ice for 15 min. Fill the tube with staining media and spin down at 400g for 5 min (4°). Discard the supernatant, incubate with a fluorophore conjugated anti-human CD45 antibody in a total volume of 50 μl, and incubate on ice for 30 min.

6. Fill the tube with FACS staining media and spin down at 400g for 5 min (4°). Discard the supernatant, add 200 μl staining media and analyze by fluorescent-activated cell sorter (FACS).

7. Mouse peripheral blood should contain approximately 5% human PBMCs. If the level is lower than 1% 2 weeks after transplantation of human PBMCs, engraftment is considered poor, and this specimen should be excluded from the experiment.

Step 2. Examining Lymphocyte Infiltration

Three weeks after transplanting hESCs and their derivatives to the Trimera mice, harvest the tumors and analyze the human lymphocytic infiltrate.

1. Humanely sacrifice the mice by terminal CO_2 inhalation.

2. Remove the tumor together with the kidney. Small tumors are easily separated from the kidney, but larger ones may penetrate the parenchyma, making it difficult to separate the kidney tissue completely.

3. Measure the tumor and take a photograph as a record.

4. To examine infiltration of human cells in the tumors, fix the tissues and prepare paraffin-embedded sections or frozen sections according to standard histological procedures. It is recommended that mouse anti human CD3, CD4, CD8, and CD45 antibodies be used for detection of human T cells.

Results and Discussion

Transplantation of hESCs and transplanted teratoma fragments into immunodeficient mice results in rapid cell growth and differentiation. Tissue structures that resemble epithelia, neural tube, cartilage, bone, and other mature tissue types are expected. Tumors derived from teratomas may contain a greater proportion of confluent sheets of monotonous cell types, particularly immature neuroepithelium, relative to cystic areas, indicating malignant transformation of the cells. By transplanting hESCs and teratoma fragments into the Trimera model, one may assess the allogeneic immune response of PBMCs against undifferentiated cells (hESCs) and compare it with differentiated cells (teratomas). When undifferentiated cells are transplanted into Trimera mice, the allogeneic lymphocytes do not mount a significant immune response against the cells, evident by tumor size, which is not affected and infiltration of human leukocytes into the graft is limited (Fig. 3A). As expected, when transplanted in this model, skin grafts show clear signs of rejection such as heavy leukocyte infiltration and deformed structures (Fig. 3C). Interestingly, transplanting hESC-derived tumors into Trimera mice do not result in overt graft rejection, even though in this case T cells encounter differentiated cell types when they infiltrate the graft (Fig. 3B).

Two explanations may account for the reduced capacity of the immune system to reject hESCs and transplanted teratomas in contrast to somatic tissues. One possibility is that hESCs express active immune suppressive signals that inhibit the immune response against them. The normal function of such signals may be to protect embryonic cells from the risk of rejection by maternal lymphocytes. For example, it was suggested that rat embryonic stem cell–like cells (rESCs) prevent immune responses against them by presenting the proapoptotic signal Fas Ligand (FasL) to allogeneic lymphocytes (Fandrich et al., 2002). Another inhibitory signal that was shown to protect the embryo from maternal NK cells is the HLA-G molecule that is expressed exclusively at the fetomaternal interface of the placenta (Jurisicova et al., 1996). However, it is unlikely that inhibition of lymphocytes by FasL and/or HLA-G can account for the reduced immune response, because hESCs and their in vitro differentiated derivatives do not express these molecules (Drukker et al., 2002, 2006).

Another possibility is that hESCs and undifferentiated derivatives are ignored by lymphocytes because of their inability to provide strong stimulatory signals that are required for the initiation and progression of the immune response. There are several lines of evidence to support this hypothesis: (1) hESCs express low levels of MHC-I molecules, and they are not recognized in vitro by CTLs unless MHC-I expression is strongly stimulated by IFNs; (2) hESC-derived cells do not express detectable levels of MHC-II proteins, even after differentiation; (3) they are not recognized by NK cells in vitro; and, (4) they are not rejected in Trimera mice in vivo. Furthermore, it was recently shown that hESCs and their derivatives do not express multiple immune stimulating genes, including the costimulatory molecules CD80 and CD86 (Drukker et al., 2006). Hence, it is likely that

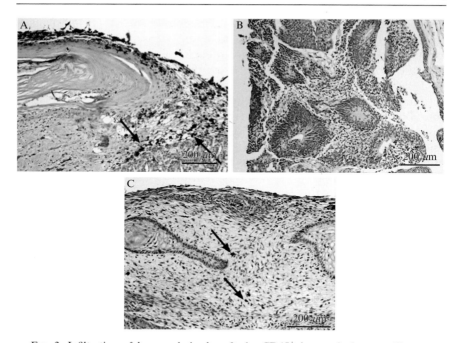

Fig. 3. Infiltration of human derived grafts by CD45$^+$ human leukocytes. Shown are histological sections of 3-week-old kidney subcapsular grafts stained by human specific anti-CD45 antibody (original magnification ×10, counter staining by H&E). (A) After transplantation into Trimera mice, human skin grafts show clear signs of rejection; the epithelium is degenerated and infiltrated with human leukocytes (arrows). (B) Transplantation of undifferentiated hESCs resulted in teratoma formation in Trimera mice with no signs of growth interruption and infiltration by human leukocytes. (C) Differentiated tissue fragments cut from a hESC-induced teratoma continued to develop on transfer to new hosts. No tissue damage was evident in the presence of human leukocytes, and only scattered leukocytes could be detected (arrows) (www.StemCells.com [Drukker *et al.*, 2006]).

the undifferentiated cells and transplanted teratomas are not recognized by allogeneic lymphocytes because they do not effectively deliver stimulatory signals to them.

With the development of increasing numbers of differentiation protocols for hESCs, it is likely that hESC-derived, mature cell types will eventually be tested in clinical setting. Examining their immunological properties would be an essential part of their preclinical evaluation. Because such allogeneic responses cannot be tested in human subjects, the Trimera model provides a unique, and important, opportunity to test immunological responses that cannot be analyzed *in vitro*. In contrast to *in vitro* assays that typically evaluate one immune cell subset, the Trimera mouse allows human immune cell subsets to interact with human grafts in a dynamic, physiological setting. Furthermore, this system may be modified to investigate specific components of the immune response that may mediate rejection. For example, injection of fusion proteins that block costimulation of T cells has demonstrated T-cell involvement in rejection of human kidney transplants (Dekel *et al.*, 2003). Other improvements to the model may include transplantation of cord blood hematopoietic stem cells, because they have the capacity to self-renew for the life of the mouse, thereby creating a more stable immunological environment suitable for studying long-term immune responses (Traggiai *et al.*, 2004).

Although such improvements will expand the power of the Trimera system, it is important to note that the current Trimera model primarily evaluates direct interactions between transplanted cells and human immune cells (i.e., interactions between donor-derived antigen presenting cells [APCs] and allogeneic leukocytes [reviewed in (Rogers and Lechler, 2001]). Indirect pathways of allorecognition (i.e., donor-derived antigens processed and presented by human APCs to human leukocytes) are inefficient in the Trimera model, and, therefore, such interactions cannot be evaluated. Nevertheless, the Trimera mouse model represents an important advancement in the study of human allogeneic responses, because it allows investigators to use a robust, *in vivo*, functional immune assay to understand the immune processes that may limit the effectiveness of hESC–derived cell therapeutics. Ultimately, systems such as the Trimera mouse model will accelerate the use of hESCs in clinical setting, bringing hope to patients who once had no expectation of cures for their ailments.

Acknowledgments

I wish to thank my collaborators Dr. Helena Katchman and Prof. Yair Reisner from the Weizmann Institute of Science for their kind help and encouragement and to Drs. Christopher Park, Yoav Soen, and Yoav Mayshar and for their critical review of the manuscript. Micha Drukker is a Human Frontier Science Program fellow.

References

Carpenter, M. K., Inokuma, M. S., Denham, J., Mujtaba, T., Chiu, C. P., and Rao, M. S. (2001). Enrichment of neurons and neural precursors from human embryonic stem cells. *Exp. Neurol.* **172,** 383–397.

Chadwick, K., Wang, L., Li, L., Menendez, P., Murdoch, B., Rouleau, A., and Bhatia, M. (2003). Cytokines and BMP-4 promote hematopoietic differentiation of human embryonic stem cells. *Blood* **102,** 906–915.

Dekel, B., Burakova, T., Arditti, F. D., Reich-Zeliger, S., Milstein, O., Aviel-Ronen, S., Rechavi, G., Friedman, N., Kaminski, N., Passwell, J. H., and Reisner, Y. (2003). Human and porcine early kidney precursors as a new source for transplantation. *Nat. Med.* **9,** 53–60.

Draper, J. S., Pigott, C., Thomson, J. A., and Andrews, P. W. (2002). Surface antigens of human embryonic stem cells: Changes upon differentiation in culture. *J. Anat.* **200**, 249–258.

Drukker, M., and Benvenisty, N. (2004). The immunogenicity of human embryonic stem-derived cells. *Trends. Biotechnol.* **22**, 136–141.

Drukker, M., Katchman, H., Katz, G., Even-Tov Friedman, G., Shezen, E., Hornstein, E., Mandelboim, O., Reisner, Y., and Benvenisty, N. (2006). Human embryonic stem cells and their differentiated derivatives are less susceptible to immune rejection than adult cells. *Stem Cells* **24**, 221–229.

Drukker, M., Katz, G., Urbach, A., Schuldiner, M., Markel, G., Itskovitz-Eldor, J., Reubinoff, B., Mandelboim, O., and Benvenisty, N. (2002). Characterization of the expression of MHC proteins in human embryonic stem cells. *Proc. Natl. Acad. Sci. USA* **99**, 9864–9869.

Fandrich, F., Lin, X., Chai, G. X., Schulze, M., Ganten, D., Bader, M., Holle, J., Huang, D. S., Parwaresch, R., Zavazava, N., and Binas, B. (2002). Preimplantation-stage stem cells induce long-term allogeneic graft acceptance without supplementary host conditioning. *Nat. Med.* **8**, 171–178.

Goldman, J. P., Blundell, M. P., Lopes, L., Kinnon, C., Di Santo, J. P., and Thrasher, A. J. (1998). Enhanced human cell engraftment in mice deficient in RAG2 and the common cytokine receptor gamma chain. *Br. J. Haematol.* **103**, 335–342.

Green, H., Easley, K., and Iuchi, S. (2003). Marker succession during the development of keratinocytes from cultured human embryonic stem cells. *Proc. Natl. Acad. Sci. USA* **100**, 15625–15630.

He, J. Q., Ma, Y., Lee, Y., Thomson, J. A., and Kamp, T. J. (2003). Human embryonic stem cells develop into multiple types of cardiac myocytes: Action potential characterization. *Circ. Res.* **93**, 32–39.

Ito, M., Hiramatsu, H., Kobayashi, K., Suzue, K., Kawahata, M., Hioki, K., Ueyama, Y., Koyanagi, Y., Sugamura, K., Tsuji, K., Heike, T., and Nakahata, T. (2002). NOD/SCID/gamma(c)(null) mouse: An excellent recipient mouse model for engraftment of human cells. *Blood* **100**, 3175–3182.

Itskovitz-Eldor, J., Schuldiner, M., Karsenti, D., Eden, A., Yanuka, O., Amit, M., Soreq, H., and Benvenisty, N. (2000). Differentiation of human embryonic stem cells into embryoid bodies comprising the three embryonic germ layers. *Mol. Med.* **6**, 88–95.

Jurisicova, A., Casper, R. F., MacLusky, N. J., Mills, G. B., and Librach, C. L. (1996). HLA-G expression during preimplantation human embryo development. *Proc. Natl. Acad. Sci. USA* **93**, 161–165.

Kaufman, D. S., Hanson, E. T., Lewis, R. L., Auerbach, R., and Thomson, J. A. (2001). Hematopoietic colony-forming cells derived from human embryonic stem cells. *Proc. Natl. Acad. Sci. USA* **98**, 10716–10721.

Kehat, I., Gepstein, A., Spira, A., Itskovitz-Eldor, J., and Gepstein, L. (2002). High-resolution electrophysiological assessment of human embryonic stem cell-derived cardiomyocytes: A novel *in vitro* model for the study of conduction. *Circ. Res.* **91**, 659–661.

Kehat, I., Kenyagin-Karsenti, D., Snir, M., Segev, H., Amit, M., Gepstein, A., Livne, E., Binah, O., Itskovitz-Eldor, J., and Gepstein, L. (2001). Human embryonic stem cells can differentiate into myocytes with structural and functional properties of cardiomyocytes. *J. Clin. Invest.* **108**, 407–414.

Lavon, N., Yanuka, O., and Benvenisty, N. (2004). Differentiation and isolation of hepatic-like cells from human embryonic stem cells. *Differentiation* **72**, 230–238.

Levenberg, S., Golub, J. S., Amit, M., Itskovitz-Eldor, J., and Langer, R. (2002). Endothelial cells derived from human embryonic stem cells. *Proc. Natl. Acad. Sci. USA* **99**, 4391–4396.

Lubin, I., Segall, H., Marcus, H., David, M., Kulova, L., Steinitz, M., Erlich, P., Gan, J., and Reisner, Y. (1994). Engraftment of human peripheral blood lymphocytes in normal strains of mice. *Blood* **83,** 2368–2381.

Mummery, C., Ward, D., van den Brink, C. E., Bird, S. D., Doevendans, P. A., Opthof, T., Brutel de la Riviere, A., Tertoolen, L., van der Heyden, M., and Pera, M. (2002). Cardiomyocyte differentiation of mouse and human embryonic stem cells. *J. Anat.* **200,** 233–242.

Mummery, C., Ward-van Oostwaard, D., Doevendans, P., Spijker, R., van den Brink, S., Hassink, R., van der Heyden, M., Opthof, T., Pera, M., de la Riviere, A. B., Passier, R., and Tertoolen, L. (2003). Differentiation of human embryonic stem cells to cardiomyocytes: Role of coculture with visceral endoderm-like cells. *Circulation* **107,** 2733–2740.

Rambhatla, L., Chiu, C. P., Kundu, P., Peng, Y., and Carpenter, M. K. (2003). Generation of hepatocyte-like cells from human embryonic stem cells. *Cell Transplant.* **12,** 1–11.

Reubinoff, B. E., Itsykson, P., Turetsky, T., Pera, M. F., Reinhartz, E., Itzik, A., and Ben-Hur, T. (2001). Neural progenitors from human embryonic stem cells. *Nat. Biotechnol.* **19,** 1134–1140.

Reubinoff, B. E., Pera, M. F., Fong, C. Y., Trounson, A., and Bongso, A. (2000). Embryonic stem cell lines from human blastocysts: Somatic differentiation *in vitro. Nat. Biotechnol.* **18,** 399–404.

Rogers, N. J., and Lechler, R. I. (2001). Allorecognition. *Am. J. Transplant.* **1,** 97–102.

Saxon, A., Macy, E., Denis, K., Tary-Lehmann, M., Witte, O., and Braun, J. (1991). Limited B cell repertoire in severe combined immunodeficient mice engrafted with peripheral blood mononuclear cells derived from immunodeficient or normal humans. *J. Clin. Invest.* **87,** 658–665.

Schuldiner, M., Eiges, R., Eden, A., Yanuka, O., Itskovitz-Eldor, J., Goldstein, R. S., and Benvenisty, N. (2001). Induced neuronal differentiation of human embryonic stem cells. *Brain Res.* **913,** 201–205.

Schulz, T. C., Palmarini, G. M., Noggle, S. A., Weiler, D. A., Mitalipova, M. M., and Condie, B. G. (2003). Directed neuronal differentiation of human embryonic stem cells. *BMC. Neurosci.* **4,** 27.

Sottile, V., Thomson, A., and McWhir, J. (2003). *In vitro* osteogenic differentiation of human ES cells. *Cloning Stem Cells* **5,** 149–155.

Thomson, J. A., Itskovitz-Eldor, J., Shapiro, S. S., Waknitz, M. A., Swiergiel, J. J., Marshall, V. S., and Jones, J. M. (1998). Embryonic stem cell lines derived from human blastocysts. *Science* **282,** 1145–1147.

Torbett, B. E., Picchio, G., and Mosier, D. E. (1991). hu-PBL-SCID mice: A model for human immune function, AIDS, and lymphomagenesis. *Immunol. Rev.* **124,** 139–164.

Traggiai, E., Chicha, L., Mazzucchelli, L., Bronz, L., Piffaretti, J. C., Lanzavecchia, A., and Manz, M. G. (2004). Development of a human adaptive immune system in cord blood cell-transplanted mice. *Science* **304,** 104–107.

Xu, C., Police, S., Rao, N., and Carpenter, M. K. (2002). Characterization and enrichment of cardiomyocytes derived from human embryonic stem cells. *Circ. Res.* **91,** 501–508.

Zhang, S. C., Wernig, M., Duncan, I. D., Brustle, O., and Thomson, J. A. (2001). *In vitro* differentiation of transplantable neural precursors from human embryonic stem cells. *Nat. Biotechnol.* **19,** 1129–1133.

[20] Manufacturing Considerations for Clinical Uses of Therapies Derived from Stem Cells

By DARIN J. WEBER

Abstract

Manufacturing a therapeutic cell-based product from a stem cell source is far from simple. Regulatory authorities expect that the donor source of the stem cells is appropriately screened and tested for human pathogens. All of the synthetic or animal-derived ancillary materials must be appropriately qualified and tested before use in clinical manufacturing. The manufacturing process used to generate the therapeutic cells from the stem cells must be aseptic, consistent, and scalable. Finally, a robust quality program is necessary to ensure that appropriate quality procedures for the manufacturing process are in place and a quality assurance function that verifies the intended therapeutic cellular product has been prepared in a manner that is compliant with all regulatory expectations for clinical use in patients. This chapter discusses regulatory issues for manufacturing of therapeutic cells derived from stem cells and provides approaches for successfully addressing them.

Introduction

Worldwide there is tremendous research activity on the basic biology of stem cells from a variety of sources, including embryonic, fetal, and "adult" sources such as those isolated from bone marrow and other tissue and organs. Those contemplating translating these research findings into potential human clinical therapies must understand that regulatory authorities have high standards for establishing biosafety (Weber, 2004) and demonstrating proof of concept before human clinical studies can be initiated. In the United States, regulatory authorities have been proactive in developing the regulatory framework for therapies containing living cells and tissues that are directly relevant to developers of therapies derived from stem cells. In addition, the U.S. Food and Drug Administration, which regulates clinical uses of these therapies, has issued guidelines (US FDA, 1998, 2003) and held meetings of its advisors to discuss issues for specific clinical therapies involving living cells that are likely therapeutic targets for stem cell–derived therapies (US FDA, 2000, 2003, 2004, 2005).

The purpose of this chapter is to provide an overview of the regulatory approval process in the United States for developers of therapeutic cells

METHODS IN ENZYMOLOGY, VOL. 420
0076-6879/06 $35.00
DOI: 10.1016/S0076-6879(06)20020-X

derived from stem cells, discuss areas of concern with the manufacturing of stem cells therapies that must be addressed either before or concurrent with human clinical studies, and provide general recommendations as to how to address many of these issues.

U.S. Regulatory Framework for Therapies Derived from Stem Cells

Living cellular and tissue products derived from stem cells fall within the definition of human cells, tissues, or cellular or tissue-based products (HCT/P) under section 361 of the Public Health Service Act (Weber, 2004) under the statutory authority of the Food and Drug Administration (FDA) and are subject to donor eligibility determination and good tissue practice (GTP) requirements. In most cases, the manufacturing process used to create a therapeutic product derived from stem cells exceeds the FDA's definition of minimal manipulation and, therefore, also falls within the definition of somatic cell therapy (Kessler et al., 1993; US FDA, 1993) and requires premarket approval as a biological product under the Public Health Service Act (PHS Act). Therapies derived from stem cells also meet the definition of a drug under the Federal Food, Drug and Cosmetic Act and are subject to applicable provisions of that law (FD&C Act). Therefore, clinical studies are needed to gather safety and effectiveness data in accordance with FDA investigational new drug regulations (IND). As a somatic cell therapy requiring premarket approval, a biologics license would be issued on demonstration that a cell-based therapy derived from stem cells "meets standards designed to assure that the biological product continues to be safe, pure, and potent..." (PHS Act). It is conceivable that some therapies derived from stem cells will consist of cells combined with a variety of biomaterials, such as natural or synthetic matrices. Although the scientific community frequently refers to these constructs as tissue engineering or regenerative medicine, in U.S. regulatory parlance, they are designated as biologic-device combination products (Combination Product Regulations) and are frequently regulated under both the biologic and medical device authorities (Medical Device Regulations). If the stem cells or the therapeutic cells derived from the stem cells are genetically modified, transiently or permanently, they will be regulated under additional guidelines established for gene therapy products.

If the stem cells must be cocultured with cells of animal origin, such as is commonly the case for human embryonic stem cells, the FDA has determined that therapeutic products derived from such cells may be used clinically (US FDA, 2001). Such cells will be considered xenotransplantation products (US FDA, 2003) and have additional testing requirements, as well as clinical monitoring requirements. It is of interest to note that the

FDA has already granted marketing approval to a xenotransplantation product (Genzyme Biosurgery, 2002), suggesting that it is, indeed, possible to develop therapies in which human cells have been cocultured with animal cells. It should be recognized that in the European Union and elsewhere, regulations might differ on the acceptability of using animal feeder cells for embryonic stem cells.

Development of a therapy derived from stem cells necessarily requires expertise in preparing the therapeutic cells (manufacturing), establishment of preclinical proof of concept and safety (pharmacology and toxicology), and an understanding of clinical trial expectations. Only issues related to manufacturing of stem cell–based therapies are discussed in this chapter.

The Need for a Science-Based Approach for the Product and the Process

The term *manufacturing* encompasses all the steps from where and how the cells are isolated, the steps involved in culture expansion and/or differentiation into the final therapeutic product, transport of the final product from the manufacturing facility to the clinical site, and preparation steps before patient administration. Unlike small molecules or synthetic medical devices, developers of cellular therapies, such as those derived from stem cells, face unique manufacturing challenges. Some of these challenges relate to the nature of the source cells or tissue in that they are generally complex mixtures obtained from living sources. If the source cells/tissue is obtained from donors (allogeneic), it can be difficult to control the availability, quantity, and quality necessary to maximize the yield of the stem cell population. This can be particularly problematic for cells or tissue sourced from fetal tissue or "surplus" embryos. There is also an absolute need to prevent the transmission or introduction of infectious agents while preserving the desired therapeutic attributes, primarily because it is not possible to effectively sterilize the final cell-based product without degrading or destroying its potential therapeutic benefits. In many cases, changes in the manufacturing process can impact product safety, identity, purity, potency, consistency, and stability in unforeseen ways.

To successfully address these various challenges, it is essential to establish a science-based product development process that emphasizes product safety, product characterization, and the importance of good manufacturing practices (GMPs) for these complex mixtures to obtain a final product with the desired properties and to prevent the introduction of adventitious agents (US FDA, 1998). A recommended approach for achieving this is to qualify each of the components that are used in the manufacturing process; to anticipate the need to establish a process for "manufacturing" of the therapeutic cells that is both consistent and scaleable; and to perform all of these activities under the umbrella of a quality program that is appropriate for the state of product development. Each of these areas is discussed further.

Qualify the Source of Cells and Ancillary Materials Used to Create the Therapeutic Product

In general, the starting materials for creating a therapeutic product derived from stem cells consists of the both the source cells or tissue and the various ancillary materials (culture media, cytokines, and growth factors, etc.) needed to manufacture the desired product.

Source of Cells and Tissue

For stem cells, sources typically include embryonic, fetal, or adult tissues, such as hematopoietic stem cells. Because these cells or their derivatives will be administered to patients, careful attention must be given to fully document the methods by which the source cells are collected, including verifying the "eligibility" of the donor. In addition, creating a bank of cryopreserved cells that can be further tested and characterized is advised.

Donor Eligibility Determination

A necessary starting point for qualification of human cells and tissues is to perform *donor eligibility determination* (Donor Eligibility Regulation, 2004). This FDA term means that a screen of the donor's medical history must be performed and a blood sample must be tested for specific human pathogens, such as human immunodeficiency viruses, human T-cell lymphotropic viruses, herpes viruses, hepatitis viruses, cytomegalovirus, and parvovirus, among others (US FDA, 2004). Autologous donors are not required to undergo donor eligibility determination. For some sources of stem cells, such as fetal tissue or donated embryos, it may be difficult to comply with the FDA requirements, because of limited availability of donor information. The FDA expects that every effort will be made to obtain donor screening and testing information; however, in situations in which this proves to be impossible, it may be possible to provide alternative assurances of donor eligibility, such performing screening and testing on the cells once they have been established in culture. The feasibility of pursuing such an alternative approach should be discussed with the FDA and may require a specific exemption or waiver as permitted under the regulations (Exemptions and Alternatives Regulation).

Cell Bank System

When possible, it is advisable to establish a cell bank of the stem cells soon after they are isolated from the source cells or tissue. A typical cell bank system consists of a master cell bank (MCB) and working cell bank (WCB). The advantages of a cell bank system from a manufacturing perspective is to provide for a means to reproducibly generate the therapeutic cellular product from the same stem cell source, thus avoiding the need to repeatedly procure a new population of stem cells from a new donor source, as a culture of stem cells is depleted or exhibits chromosomal abnormalities. From a biosafety standpoint, a cell bank provides the opportunity to extensively characterize the stem cells and test them for a variety of endogenous and adventitious agents (ICH Q5A and Q5D, 1997). Table I contains a list of types of pathogen testing generally expected for a master cell bank (MCB). Not all tests may be necessary, depending on the specific characteristics of the cells. Regulatory authorities in other regions of the world may require additional tests for human pathogens. A subset of the tests in Table I is usually also performed on the working cell bank (WCB), if created. There is an ever-growing list of contract testing organizations (CTO) that can perform cell bank testing. Surprisingly, there is wide variability in the tests recommended by these organizations and

TABLE I
EXAMPLES OF PATHOGEN TESTING FOR A MASTER
CELL BANK (MCB)

Sterility with bacteriostasis/fungistasis
Mycoplasma
In vitro assay for adventitious viruses
In vivo assay for viral contaminants
Electron microscopy for viruslike particles
Mouse antibody production (MAP) assay
PCR-based reverse transcriptase assay (PBRT)
Xenotropic retrovirus by S+L- assay
Murine retrovirus by XC plaque assay
HIV-1/-2
HTLV-I/II
Herpes 6, 7, & 8
Hepatitis B & C
Parvovirus (B-19)
Cytomegalovirus
Epstein Barr virus
Detection of bovine viruses
Detection of porcine viruses

corresponding costs. Therefore, developers of therapies derived from stem cells are advised to obtain cost estimates from several CTOs. AppTec, Charles River Laboratories, and Invitrogen (BioReliance) are examples of CTOs with varying degrees of experience in this area.

It is conceivable that in some cases, several cell banks could be established. For example with human embryonic stem cells (hESCs) a hypothetical scenario for cell banking may include a MCB/WCB for the hESCs and separate cell banks for therapeutic cells that are subsequently differentiated from the stem cells. This might include cell banks of lineage-specific cell lines, as well as banks of the fully differentiated therapeutic cells that are intended to be administered to patients. It should be understood that the number and types of cell banks that could be established are largely at the discretion of the developer of the intended clinical therapy. Because performing the virus testing that is expected as part of establishing the biosafety of the stem cells and/or therapeutic cells is not inexpensive, careful consideration should be given for the timing of such testing. After the stem cells or its derivatives have shown efficacy in a relevant animal model of disease would be a reasonable time to perform at least limited virus testing, assuming the original cell or tissue source of the stem cells was appropriately screened and tested for donor eligibility as previously discussed. If adequate donor eligibility information is not available, serious consideration should be given to reisolating the stem cells from an appropriate donor source. The ideal situation would be to perform full cell bank testing on the stem cells and little or no additional virus testing on subsequently derived therapeutic cells. However, this scenario is only feasible if from that point on the cells are only exposed to components that have also been appropriately tested and qualified, including any feeder cells (see discussion of ancillary materials following). If that strategy is chosen, careful documentation would be necessary and readily available to demonstrate to regulatory authorities that this, in fact, is the case. Along those same lines, consideration could be given performing the level of virus testing for a master cell bank (MCB) on the undifferentiated stem cells and at some point later, on the subsequently derived therapeutic cells, virus testing equivalent to that expected for a working cell bank (WCB) could be performed. Again, this scenario presumes that any ancillary materials that the cells from the tested MCB are exposed have also been appropriately tested and qualified.

In some cases, such as therapies derived from autologous stem cells, or where yields of stem cells from the donor source tissue are limiting, it may not be desirable or feasible to establish a formal cell bank system. In these situations, increased emphasis on characterization is usually necessary, because when isolating stem cells from multiple donors, one often has little control of the "quality" of these starting materials and thus must assess the impact of various parameters, such as gender, gestational age (if applicable), genetic background, storage, and handling of the tissue before receipt on the ability to generate a therapeutic product with the desired functional characteristics.

If human or animal feeder cells are used for maintaining the human stem cells, the same attention to details with respect to qualification the source of the tissue, cell bank testing, and characterization are expected as for the human stem cells. If animal feeder cells are obtained from primary tissue, rather than established cell lines, additional information on animal husbandry should be obtained (US FDA, 2003).

Ancillary Materials

It is frequently the case that the manufacturing process used to create a therapeutically useful product from stem cells encompass steps in which enzymes, cell selection, or depletion with antibodies, and *ex vivo* culture in media supplemented with a cocktail of cytokines and growth factors, are routinely used. These components are examples of ancillary materials, because they are only transient in the manufacturing process and are not intended to part of the final product. Additional examples of ancillary materials are listed in Table II. A well-established qualification program for the use of these ancillary materials is required because they come in contact with cells that will be subsequently administered to patients. The extent of qualification necessary to satisfy regulatory authorities depends largely on its origin (synthetic vs. animal derived or human derived) and the manufacturing standards used by the supplier of the ancillary material. In many cases, FDA approved or so-called GMP grade ancillary

TABLE II

EXAMPLES OF ANCILLARY MATERIALS USED IN
MANUFACTURING OF CELL-BASED THERAPIES

Monoclonal antibodies used in cell selection/depletion
Cytokines, growth factors, and other supplements used to
 regulate/activate/differentiate cells in culture
Feeder cells, human or animal
Antibiotics
Serum
Culture media
Enzymes used to passage cells
Plastic ware and attachment substrates (e.g., matrigel)

materials do not exist, requiring the use of "research only": materials that were never intended by the supplier to be used to produce cells for use in clinical studies. In such cases, review of a certificate of analysis (COA) is unlikely to provide sufficient information on how the material was manufactured and whether or not the purification process for the ancillary material involved the use of untested animal components. For example, some recombinant ancillary materials are purified using affinity chromatography. In some cases, murine antibodies, which have not been previously tested for murine viruses, are used. The FDA would likely consider the recombinant protein to be contaminated with murine viruses and ask for test results verifying the absence of adventitious agents. Alternately, testing or viral clearance studies on the murine antibodies could be provided. Regardless of the regulatory status of an ancillary material, ultimately the manufacturer of the therapeutic product is responsible for developing procedures to qualify the ancillary material as acceptable for use in the manufacturing process used to create the cell-based product. Depending on the criticality of the particular ancillary material to the success of the manufacturing process, consideration should be given to establishing custom manufacturing agreements with suppliers to ensure the ancillary material meets the necessary quality standards. For ancillary materials of animal or human origin, documentation must be provided that the material was appropriately tested and found to be free of human or animal pathogens. Table III provides a basic outline of a qualification program for ancillary materials.

The United States Pharmacopoeia (USP) has recently issued an information chapter (USP <1043>, 2006) specifically addressing the use of

TABLE III
BASIC OUTLINE OF QUALIFICATION PROGRAM FOR ANCILLARY MATERIALS

Verify from vendor certificates of analysis (COA) that material meets acceptance criteria

Perform audits of suppliers and other partners, especially if material is custom manufactured/tested

Verify that purification process of material does not use untested components, such as affinity chromatography using untested murine monoclonal antibodies

Verify or perform adventitious agent testing of materials containing human or animal derived components

Obtain documentation that confirms all ruminant derived materials are from BSE-free countries

Perform analyses verifying identity, purity, and performance of key materials in manufacturing system ancillary materials for cell-based products; this is a recommended resource for better understanding the concerns of regulatory authorities and potential approaches for addressing them.

Residual Ancillary Materials in Final Product

The presence of low levels of ancillary materials in the final cell-based product is a frequent area of concern for regulatory authorities given that certain materials, such as cytokines and growth factors, can be bioactive or toxic in patients independent of the cellular product. There are also concerns because of potential hypersensitivity reactions. One widely recognized example is the use of beta-lactam antibiotics because some patients have allergic reactions. There is also the potential for hypersensitivity reactions in subjects previously exposed to monoclonal antibody therapy who are subsequently administered a cellular therapy in which residual levels of monoclonal antibody are adherent to the cell surface. In some cases, when there is likely to be significant levels of a ancillary material in the final product, the FDA may require that the manufacturing standards meet those equivalent for direct therapeutic use in humans, even though they are intended only to be used as ancillary materials. In several instances, this has been required for cell-based products using cell selection just upstream of final formulation, because detectable levels of antibody remains bound to the cells. As a result of these concerns, regulatory authorities frequently request that calculations and measurements for residual levels in the final product be determined. In some cases, they may request that limits on the amounts of residual ancillary materials be established. In other cases, clinical monitoring for adverse reactions to a residual ancillary material may be requested. One example in which clinical monitoring may be requested is if a monoclonal antibody is used to purify the cellular product late in the manufacturing process, upstream of final formulations. If a murine antibody is used in the cell selection, the FDA may request that the patient be serologically monitored for human anti-mouse antibody (HAMA) reactions.

Genetic Modification

Genetic modification of stem cells or subsequently derived therapeutic cells is acceptable, if warranted, but will result in the final product being regulated as *ex vivo* gene therapy (US FDA, 1993). Consequently, additional information will need to be provided regarding the vector used and how it was manufactured (US FDA, 2004). In addition, the FDA will likely request additional testing for cells transduced with retroviral vectors, as well as additional clinical monitoring (US FDA, 2000, 2005).

Combination Products

If the therapeutic cells derived from the stem cells are seeded onto a natural or synthetic matrix or are encapsulated, it is likely they will be regulated as a biologic-device combination product (Combination Product Regulation). Most natural or synthetic biomaterials are regulated as medical devices and, consequently, are expected to meet medical device standards. Examples include bovine collagen, alginate, and biodegradable polymers such as polyglycolic acid (PGA). In situations in which novel biomaterials are used, biocompatibility testing is expected (ISO 10993-1, 1997) along with other typical medical device testing, such as assessments of mechanical strength, *in vitro* and *in vivo* performance, and possibly tumorigenicity. The specific combinations of cells and biomaterial should also be assessed according to the intended use of the biomaterial. For an encapsulated cell product this might include determination of effectiveness as an immunoisolation barrier or barrier to transmission of adventitious agents. More generally, information should be provided on the interactions between the cells and biomaterials; for example, genotypic or phenotypic changes that occur in the cells after seeding onto the biomaterial or changes in the rate of degradation of the biomaterial because of metabolic activity of the cells. In recent years, the FDA has made significant strides in harmonizing its expectations for these types of combination products to ensure consistency between those that will be approved as biologics versus those that may be approved as medical devices. In general, both sets of regulatory statutes are applicable to combination products.

Developing a Manufacturing Process That Is Consistent and Scalable

Clearly, there is much to be considered in qualifying the cells or tissue and the various ancillary materials used to create therapeutic cells from stem cell sources. However, ultimately, the stem cells and critical ancillary materials must be brought together in a process that leads to the generation of the desired therapeutic cell type(s). For clinical uses, regulatory authorities expect the development of a well-defined, aseptic manufacturing process that provides for a pure and potent population of therapeutic cells. Additional considerations must be given to develop a manufacturing process that is also scalable to provide sufficient quantities of cells to meet increasing demand for animal studies, clinical trials, and possibly commercialization. This is easier said than done in large part because of the variability that is inherent in the starting materials, as well as the fact that often the procedures for deriving and/or differentiating therapeutic cells from stem cells are more art than science. In general, regulatory authorities recognize that for early-phase clinical studies, the process for manufacturing therapeutic cells will continue to evolve, albeit in a well-controlled fashion. However, demonstrating that the initial manufacturing process does not introduce external contaminants, such as adventitious viral agents, and reproducibly yields the cell population of therapeutic interest is of paramount importance before the use of the cells in human subjects. In addition, regulatory authorities expect that significant effort will be devoted to characterization of the cells to understand the biological and physiochemical changes the cells undergo as they differentiate or otherwise mature from stem cells to the desired therapeutic cells. Such characterization data will be need to establish specifications for key parameters of the therapeutic product, as well as demonstrating sufficient control over the manufacturing process as it is further optimized.

Aseptic Processing

Because it is not possible to effectively sterilize the final cell-based product without degrading or destroying its potential therapeutic benefits, an aseptic manufacturing process must be used (US FDA, 2004). This requires that the components, such as the stem cells and all ancillary materials, that are brought together in the manufacturing process be previously tested for freedom from microbiological agents, such as bacteria, fungi, mycoplasma, pyrogens, and viruses, as appropriate. Such testing is typically done as part of the materials qualification program, as discussed previously. In addition, during the manufacturing process, appropriate controls must be in place to prevent the introduction of contaminants into the final therapeutic cellular product. Presuming the cells and ancillary materials have been previously tested for freedom from microbiological contamination, the most frequent source of subsequent contaminants is the surrounding environment, including personnel, in which the manufacturing process occurs. To minimize the potential for contamination of the final product, regulatory agencies encourage the development of closed systems and expect that "open" processes, such as feeding and passaging of cells, will only occur in a appropriately prepared biological safety cabinet (BSC) that maintains a class 100 (ISO 5) environment. Furthermore, for manufacturing of a clinical product, the environment surrounding the BSC should also be a controlled class 10,000 (ISO 7) clean room environment. Both the BSC and the surrounding clean room should be routinely monitored to verify the quality. In addition to the quality of the air to which the cells are exposed, the personnel must also be appropriately gowned and trained in aseptic processing to "protect" the product from the personnel. Additional considerations regarding aseptic processing are discussed in the FDA

Aseptic Processing Guidance (US FDA, 2004). Demonstrating acceptable aseptic processing practices is expected before initiating clinical studies in humans.

Characterization

Regulatory authorities expect that data will be routinely collected on the biological and physiochemical changes the cells undergo as they differentiate or otherwise mature from stem cells to the desired therapeutic cells. One of the main purposes of these data is to demonstrate control of the purity and impurity profiles of the final product. Because the final therapeutic cell product may be a mixed cell population of more than one cell type, these data would be used to demonstrate that each time therapeutic cells are derived from stem cells, one consistently and reproducibly obtains the expected cell types in the same proportion. As developmental data and manufacturing experience is accumulated, the collected data should be assessed and specification established to ensure product integrity and stability. These characterization data play an essential role as the manufacturing process is optimized, the technology is transferred, or changes are made to facilitate process scaling, because one must demonstrate that changes made to the process do not adversely impact the safety or functional characteristics of the therapeutic cells. These assessments are typically done as part of a comparability protocol, which requires knowledge of the characteristics of the cells before and after the manufacturing change (US FDA, 2003).

Examples of expected routine characterization to be done periodically throughout the manufacturing process, as well as more specialized assessments to encompass key parameters of the therapeutic cells or precursors, are listed in Table IV.

In addition to performing these characterization activities to collect data on the dynamic processes evoked in the cells as they develop into the therapeutic cells of interest, a secondary goal is to monitor for signs of aberrant growth, inappropriate phenotypes, or other reasons to preclude the cells from clinical use.

In-Process and Release Testing

Many of the characterization activities just described overlap with regulatory authorities' expectations for in-process and final product release testing. The overarching purpose of in-process and release testing is to verify that the manufacturing process for the cells remains aseptic and that the cells are exhibiting the specific properties expected at the point in the

TABLE IV

TYPICAL EXAMPLES OF EXPECTED CELL CHARACTERIZATION

Growth kinetics/population doubling time
Morphological assessment
Percent confluence at passage
Cell counts
Viability
Sterility
Endotoxin
Mycoplasma testing
Phenotypic expression of desired and undesired cell types
Monitoring of unique biochemical markers
Assessments of functional activity
Gene and protein expression analysis
Expression of immune antigens (HLA/MHC)

process at which they are being monitored. Because the final cellular product cannot be terminally sterilized and culture times can extend to several weeks, it is recommended that periodic monitoring for sterility and mycoplasma be performed at regular intervals such as at the time of media exchange or cell passaging. Other in-process testing should include assessment of morphology and viable cell count at time of passage. Monitoring of the loss of stem cell–specific markers, as well as the appearance of expected markers representative of the final therapeutic cells and potential cellular contaminants, is also recommended at defined intervals during the manufacturing. These assessments typically coincide with cell passaging. More intensive interrogation of the cells as they are manufactured into the final therapeutic cellular product is expected at earlier phases of preclinical and clinical studies. These extensive characterization and in-process testing data are intended to be evaluated and the data trended toward develop meaningful specifications for a subset of the broader set of parameters initially monitored. This subset of characterization data will continue to be monitored for later stages of clinical development. A typical approach for establishing specifications for in-process tests is to set fairly broad specifications for the initial human clinical study on the basis of the experience gained during preclinical animal studies. As mentioned previously, the adequacy of these initial specifications would be assessed at the conclusion of the initial human clinical study and, if warranted, the specifications may be tightened or broadened on the basis of the collected data. It is acceptable to eliminate some of the initial characterization assessments if collected data indicate the test is redundant or provides no meaningful information.

In the United States, therapeutic cells are regulated as biological products and, therefore, are required to undergo lot release testing on the final product (General Biological Product Standards). These tests include sterility, mycoplasma, purity, identity, and potency. An additional set of testing specific for the desired therapeutic cells is usually also performed, along with testing for other cell types that may be present in the final therapeutic product. General examples of lot release tests are identified in Table V. It should be understood that other than mandatory tests for microbiological safety and identity, purity, and potency, there is some flexibility regarding the extent of testing for other product parameters because it is highly dependent on the characteristics of the final therapeutic cellular product. It is frequently the situation that a potency assay is not in place for early-phase clinical studies; however, some assessment of product functionality is strongly encouraged to provide a correlation to any subsequent potency assay that is developed at a later time. The FDA recently held an advisory committee meeting to discuss its current thinking on potency (US FDA, 2006). If the product is cryopreserved, release testing should be performed on a thawed vial of the final product, whenever possible, because post-thaw viability and expression of phenotypic markers may be altered. Before the initiation of a Phase III clinical trial in the United States, the FDA will require that specifications for all tests, including potency, be established on the basis of available data.

Although it is beyond the scope of this chapter, it is generally recognized by regulatory agencies that obtaining timely results to some release tests are problematic. For example, the sterility assay requires 14 days, and the mycoplasma assay requires 28 days. These lengthy time frames often exceed the shelf life of final product if they are to be administered fresh. In such cases, the FDA encourages the development of more rapid alternative test methods, such as PCR testing for mycoplasma and automated sterility testing. In lieu of these tests, the FDA will request that preliminary test results be read before release of the final product. In the specific case of sterility, the FDA often requests that a Gram stain be performed to detect any gross contamination before release. The value of such a test is the subject of much debate within industry and academia, but at the present time no other rapid screening test is currently available.

By the time a pivotal clinical study is initiated, regulatory authorities expect that a well-defined manufacturing process is in place and supported by the monitoring of a set of essential parameters with meaningful specifications as part of in-process and final release tests.

TABLE V
EXAMPLES OF FINAL PRODUCT RELEASE TESTS

Test	Typical test method	Typical specification
Sterility	USP <71> or 21 CFR 610.12	Negative
Mycoplasma	Culture method[a]	Negative
Purity (pyrogenicity)	(LAL) endotoxin	<5 EU/Kg (nonintrathecal) <0.2 EU/kg (intrathecal)
Identity	Not specified	Product specific[b]
Potency (functional assay)	Not specified	Product specific[b]
Viability	Not specified; propidium iodide or trypan blue	Product specific,[b] minimally >70%; lower with justification
Cell dose	Not specified; manual or automated cell counter	Product specific[b]; specific number depends on dosing indicated in clinical protocol
Desired Therapeutic Cells		
Specific marker A	Not specified; flow cytometry, immunohistochemistry, PCR	Product specific[b]; often a minimum % of detectable expression
Specific marker B	Not specified; flow cytometry, immunohistochemistry, PCR	Product specific[b]; often a minimum % of detectable expression
Specific marker C	Not specified; flow cytometry, immunohistochemistry, PCR	Product specific[b]; often a minimum % of detectable expression
Other Cellular Constituents		
Specific marker D	Not specified; flow cytometry, immunohistochemistry, PCR	Product specific[b]; often a maximum % of detectable expression
Specific marker E	Not specified; flow cytometry, immunohistochemistry, PCR	Product specific[b]; often a maximum % of detectable expression
Specific marker E	Not specified; flow cytometry, immunohistochemistry, PCR	Product specific[b]; often a maximum % of detectable expression
Potency	Not specified; secretion of a biologically relevant factor or marker	Product specific[b]; for early phase clinical studies a specification of "or information only" is acceptable

[a] Recommend testing at cell harvest.
[b] To be developed by product manufacturer.

Shipment

Once the final therapeutic cellular product has been manufactured and release testing indicates it is suitable for clinical use, the product must be distributed from the manufacturing facility to the clinical site under a well-planned chain of custody to ensure that when the cells are administered to the patient, they are still sterile, viable, and potent (functional). The final cellular product is likely to be shipped "fresh" or in a cryopreserved state. In either instance, the shipping container should be validated to maintain the necessary temperature well beyond the expected shipping duration. Typically, manufacturers of shipping containers will have already performed such studies and can provide the results. Verifying these data is recommended, and in some cases the conditions under which the validation of the container occurred should be further challenged. A basic example would entail placing a temperature-monitoring device inside an appropriately configured shipping container and exposing it to a variety of simulated environmental conditions, such as in a cold room or incubator. These data should form a baseline for how long the final product can be held within the shipping container at the clinical site under specified conditions. For cryopreserved products, accommodations at the clinical site may be necessary for longer term storage if there is a delay in administration of the cells to the patient that exceeds the established hold time within the shipping container. For final products that are shipped fresh, subsequent studies should be performed with developmental lots of the putative final product to establish how long the cellular product is stable, that is, how long it remains sterile, viable, and potent. On the basis of these data, an expiration-dating period should be established, after which time the quality of the final product is considered questionable and, consequently, not suitable for clinical use. Similar types of studies should also be done on the source of the stem cells if repeated procurement is necessary to support the manufacturing process and the procurement site is remote from the manufacturing facility. This would form the basis for establishing acceptance criteria that the incoming cells or tissue should meet to be used in the manufacturing process.

Handling of Cellular Product at Clinical Site

In many cases, on receipt at the clinical site, the final product will undergo additional preparation before administration to the patient. For example, a cryopreserved product would be thawed and is often washed to remove the cryoprotectants and then formulated in a suitable infusion media. In other instances, the thawed cells may need to be cultured for several additional days to obtain the required number of viable cells. Performing additional manipulations on the final product at the clinical site is an area of concern for the FDA. Because manipulations at the clinical site typically occur outside of a clean room environment, although usually at least within a class 100 BSC, there is the potential it could become contaminated either from the environment or from the media used to wash the cells. Thus, the FDA will likely request that one retest the formulated cells for parameters such as sterility, endotoxin, viable cells, and possibly potency. To minimize the amount of testing, it is recommended to supply the clinical site a pretested "kit" of components needed to wash the cells, along with data showing the wash steps can be done aseptically.

If, on thawing, the cryopreserved cells do need to be cultured more than a few hours, it is likely that all the release testing listed in Table V would need to be repeated.

The Need for a Quality Program

Anyone contemplating developing a therapy derived from stem cells should be aware of the need to develop a supporting quality control and quality assurance function. This is clearly described in the good tissue practice (GTP) regulations, which encompasses donor eligibility determination of the starting cells or tissue, as well as the good manufacturing practices (GMP) (Good Manufacturing Practices Regulation) that cover cell-based therapies regulated as biological products. Most of the information described in this chapter, such as the necessary qualification program for source cells/tissue and ancillary materials, as well as the procedures and processes used to prepare and test the therapeutic cells, need to be done under the auspices of a quality program.

Because much of the innovation and development of stem cell–based therapies is occurring in academic laboratories or small biotech startups, often a formal quality program is more a concept than a reality. However, it is essential that basic concepts of quality be established even from the earliest stages. The most fundamental quality concept can be loosely referred to as "good documentation practices" (GDP). From a regulatory perspective, this can summarized as, *if it wasn't written down, it did not happen...* even if it did. If one cannot produce the underlying primary data to support a statement made to regulatory authorities regarding the safety or efficacy of your therapeutic cells, then it must be repeated. In general, regulatory authorities do not expect one to submit raw data; however, if they decide to perform an audit of one's program, they may very well ask to see the raw data supporting a table, figure, or statement. Therefore, a practical approach for building a quality program, where one does not yet exist, is to ensure commonly accepted practices, such as documentation of experiments and results in a bound laboratory notebook using indelible ink are happening concurrent with the experiment. Associated graphs or outputs from equipment should be permanently attached to the laboratory notebook or clear reference made to its location. Each page should be signed and dated by the scientist who did the work. Results should be checked, signed, and dated or witnessed by another scientist or supervisor. It should be understood that these data have multiple purposes, ranging from intellectual property claims, due diligence assessments by outside partners, and regulatory compliance. Clearly, there are very good reasons to consider good documentation practices at the earliest stages, beyond the need for regulatory compliance.

As a research discovery is developed into a potential therapeutic product, experimental protocols should be written down in the form of draft standard operating procedures (SOPs). The findings of each experiment, or series of experiments, should be summarized in a research report, which describes the purpose of the experiment(s), methods of assessments, results, and conclusions. Such a document provides for traceability to primary data and may prevent the need to repeat experiments to support regulatory filings. It also could facilitate the writing of one or more scientific articles for publication. As protocols are refined, SOPs should be updated to reflect current practices. Document control procedures should be implemented to ensure everyone is using the current procedures, as well as to prevent the loss of intellectual property. As proof of concept data is developed, additional emphasis should be given to a qualification program of all materials being used to generate the data to ensure that uncontrolled changes in one or more materials do not lead to inconsistent results. Any work performed in animals to assess the safety of the cellular product requires following good laboratory practices (GLP), which are beyond the scope of this chapter.

In the United States, the FDA recognizes that the manufacturing process is likely to continue to be optimized as experience is gained during clinical studies. Consequently, full validation of the process and analytical methods is not expected until the end of pivotal clinical studies. However, developmental data verifying that the manufacturing process can consistently yield the therapeutic cellular product with the desired characteristics is expected. The analytical methods used to characterize and test the product at various points in the manufacturing process should be qualified and appropriate controls used to verify the validity of the results. Other important aspects of the quality program extend to the facility; installation, qualification, and maintenance of equipment; validation of equipment including heating, ventilation, and air conditioning (HVAC); cleaning; changeover procedures; environmental monitoring; and manufacturing records. All equipment used should undergo installation, operational and process qualification (IQ, OQ, PQ) and have associated preventative maintenance programs and equipment use and cleaning logs. All of these activities must be performed under written SOPs with associated documentation that verifies these activities were performed.

To attempt to implement all of these quality program activities in a short time frame would be overwhelming and would likely divert significant resources from the development of the therapeutic cells. Consequently, it is important to methodically plan out the implementation of these various activities with involvement of someone with a background in quality assurance at an early stage. In some cases, the use of the services of a contract manufacturing organization (CMO) that has already implemented a quality program for its manufacturing facility can relieve the pressure on resources that building a quality program from scratch may cause.

Summary

Because of the frequent heterogeneity of the starting cells or tissue used to isolate stem cells, the need to use "research-only" ancillary materials, and the fact that manufacturing of a cell-based therapy is often more art than science, regulatory authorities have high expectations that you will make a significant investment in ensuring the quality of the therapeutic product being developed. This requires a qualification program for the components used in the manufacturing process and includes verification of biosafety and fitness for use of the stem cells and ancillary materials to be used in the manufacturing process. It requires the development of a scalable and aseptic manufacturing process that consistently yields the desired therapeutic cells from the stem cell source. One must demonstrate to regulatory authorities that the manufacturing process is controlled by establishing analytical methods that allow one to characterize the cells as they develop into the final product. Finally, one must provide evidence that the product maintains its essential therapeutic characteristics from the time it is released from manufacture to the time of treatment of the patient. The information necessary to address regulatory concerns regarding the use of therapeutic cells derived from a stem cell source is necessarily extensive. The information conveyed in this chapter covers the core issues frequently raised by the FDA for clinical studies involving cell-based therapies. The applicability of this information to a specific stem cell–based therapy depends, of course, on the specific attributes of the planned therapy, including the source and intended recipient. However, if a developer of a stem cell–based therapy is able to successfully address most of these issues, the likelihood that regulatory authorities will find the proposed manufacturing process to be acceptable is high.

References

Combination Products Regulation. Title 21 US Code of Federal Regulations, Part 3.2(e).

Donor Eligibility Regulation. Title 21 US Code of Federal Regulations, Part 1271.45.

Exemptions and Alternatives Regulation. Title 21 US Code of Federal Regulations, Part 1271.155.

Federal Food, Drug and Cosmetic Act, Title 21, USC §321(g), §201(g).

General Biological Product Standards Regulation. Title 21 US Code of Federal Regulations, Part 610.

Genzyme Biosurgery (2002). Epicel Package Insert. http://www.genzymebiosurgery.com/pdfs/epicel_package_insert.pdf

Good Manufacturing Practices Regulation. Title 21 US Code of Federal Regulations, Parts 210 and 211.

International Conference on Harmonization. (1997). Q5A: Viral Safety Evaluation of Biotechnology Products Derived from Cell Lines of Human or Animal Origin.

International Conference on Harmonization. (1997). Q5D: Derivation and Characterization of Cell Substrates Used for Production of Biotechnological/Biological Products.

International Organization for Standardization. (1997). "Biological Evaluation of Medical Devices—Part 1: Evaluation and Testing," 2nd ed. ISO 10993–1. ISO, Geneva.

Investigational New Drug Applications. Title 21, US Code of Federal Regulations, Part 312.

Kessler, D. A., Siegel, J. P., Noguchi, P. D., et al. (1993). Regulation of somatic cell therapy and gene therapy by the Food and Drug Administration. N. Engl. J. Med. **329**, 1169–1173.

Medical Devices Regulation. Title 21 US code of Federal Regulations, Part 814.

Public Health Service Act. Title 42, USC §262, §351.

US Food and Drug Administration. (1993). Application of current statutory authorities to human somatic cell therapy products and gene therapy products: Notice. Federal Register 58FR, 53248.

US Food and Drug Administration. (1998). Guidance for industry: Guidance for Human Somatic Cell Therapy and Gene Therapy.

US Food and Drug Administration. (2000). Guidance for Industry Supplemental Guidance on Testing for Replication Competent Retrovirus in Retroviral Vector Based Gene Therapy Products and During Follow-up of Patients in Clinical Trials Using Retroviral Vectors.

US Food and Drug Administration. (2000). Biologics Response Modifiers Advisory Committee. Human Stem Cells as Cellular Replacement Therapies for Neurological Disorders. FDA briefing document. 2000 July 13–14. Available at: http://www.fda.gov/ohrms/dockets/ac/00/backgrd/3629b1.htm

US Food and Drug Administration. (2001). Letter from B. Schwetz, Office of the Commissioner, to Senator Edward Kennedy, 8 September 2001. Available at: http://www.fda.gov/oc/stemcells/kennedyltr.html

US Food and Drug Administration. (2003). Biologics Response Modifiers Advisory Committee. Allogeneic pancreatic islets for the treatment of type 1 diabetes, FDA briefing document. 2003 Oct. 09–10. Available at: www.fda.gov/ohrms/dockets/ac/03/briefing/3986b1.htm

US Food and Drug Administration. (2003). Guidance For Industry: Comparability Protocols—Chemistry, Manufacturing, and Controls Documentation.

US Food and Drug Administration. (2003). Guidance for Industry Source Animal, Product, Preclinical, and Clinical Issues Concerning the Use of Xenotransplantation Products in Humans.

US Food and Drug Administration. (2003). Draft Guidance for Reviewers: Instructions and Template for Chemistry, Manufacturing, and Control (CMC) Reviewers of Human Somatic Cell Therapy Investigational New Drug Applications (INDs).

US Food and Drug Administration. (2004). Draft Guidance for Industry Eligibility Determination for Donors of Human Cells, Tissues, and Cellular and Tissue-Based Products (HCT/Ps).

US Food and Drug Administration. (2004). Biologics Response Modifiers Advisory Committee. Cellular products for the treatment of cardiac disease, FDA briefing document. 2004 Mar 18. Available at: www.fda.gov/ohrms/dockets/ac/04/briefing/4018b1.htm

US Food and Drug Administration. (2004). Guidance for Industry Sterile Drug Products Produced by Aseptic Processing—Current Good Manufacturing Practice.

US Food and Drug Administration. (2005). Draft Guidance for Industry: Gene Therapy Clinical Trials—Observing Participants for Delayed Adverse Events.

US Food and Drug Administration. (2006). Cellular, Tissue and Gene Therapies Advisory Committee. Potency Measurements for Cellular and Gene Therapy Products. FDA briefing document. 2006 Feb. 09–10. Available at: http://www.fda.gov/ohrms/dockets/ac/06/briefing/2006-4205B1-index.htm

US Food and Drug Administration. (2005). Cellular, Tissue and Gene Therapies Advisory Committee. Cellular Products for Joint Surface Repair. FDA briefing document. 2005 Mar 03. Available at: http://www.fda.gov/ohrms/dockets/ac/05/briefing/2005-4093b2.htm

United States Pharmacopoeia. (2006). <1043> Ancillary Materials for Cell, Gene, and Tissue-engineered Therapy Products. USP 29–NF 24.

Weber, D. J. (2004). Biosafety considerations for cell-based therapies. *BioPharm. Int.* **17,** 48–55.

Weber, D. J. (2004). Navigating FDA regulations for human cells and tissues. *BioProcessing Int.* **2**(8), 22–26.

Author Index

A

H

Subject Index

A

ACCESS, DNA microarray analysis, 180
Adipocyte, mesenchymal stem cell
    differentiation
    adipogenic stimulants, 351–352
    culture, 352
    markers, 352–353
Adipose-derived stem cell, bone
    engineering, 364
AffylmGUI, DNA microarray analysis, 170,
    177–178, 200–201
AffyPLM, DNA microarray analysis, 169
Alkaline phosphatase, human embryonic
    stem cell detection, 27
Amniotic fluid stem cell, tissue
    engineering, 298
Ascorbic acid 2-phosphate, osteogenic
    stimulation from mesenchymal stem
    cells, 349

B

Blastocyst, morphological classification, 4–5
BMPs, *see* Bone morphogenetic proteins
BMSC, *see* Bone marrow stromal cell
Bone
    autologous transplantation, 362–363
    engineering
        adipose-derived stem cells, 364
        adult stem cells, 294–295
        bone marrow stromal cells
            clinical trials, 371–373
            dog cranial model, 366, 368–369, 371,
                373–375
            goat femur model, 369, 371,
                375–376, 378
            mouse model, 364
            osteogenic differentiation, 364
            rabbit model, 365
        cell sources, 363–364
Bone marrow stromal cell, *see* Bone;
    Mesenchymal stem cell

Bone morphogenetic proteins, osteogenic
    stimulation from mesenchymal stem
    cells, 349
BrdU, *see* Bromodeoxyuridine
Bromodeoxyuridine, human embryonic stem
    cell labeling, 29

C

Cardiac tissue engineering
    adult stem cells as donors, 296–297
    liquid collagen-based engineering
        cell sheets
            cardiomyocyte sheet manipulation
                into layered constructs, 334, 337
            culture dish preparation, 331–332, 334
            cell–collagen mix preparation, 321
            lattice system, 321, 324
            optimization, 337
            principles, 317–318, 321
            ring system, 324, 327–329, 331
        scaffold seeding, 317
        therapeutic applications and prospects,
            316–317
Cartilage tissue, engineering from adult stem
    cells, 295–296
CD117, *see* c-Kit
CD133, human embryonic stem cell marker,
    24
CD9, human embryonic stem cell marker, 24
Cell bank, stem cell product manufacturing
    considerations, 414–416
Cell reprogramming
    cell extract induction
        extract preparation, 278–280
        overview, 269–270
        reaction assembly, 274–275
        resealing and recovery of permeabilized
            cells, 275–276
        streptolysin O-mediated cell
            permeabilization
            permeabilization reaction, 275
            principles, 270–271

469

55 Tissues

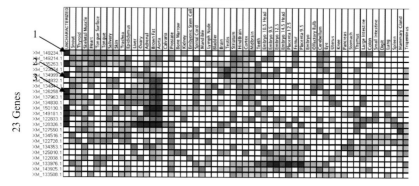

1. Zinc finger protein 106 (Zfp106)

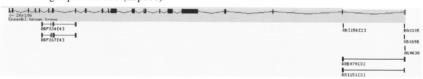

2. Expressed sequence AV340375

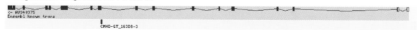

3. Acety-coenzyme A carboxylase alpha (Acaca)

STANFORD *ET AL.*, CHAPTER 8, FIG. 4. Expression patterns of 23 genes known or predicted to be involved in insulin receptor signaling (GO:0008286). Predictions were made at a precision of 25% or greater as described (Zhang, 2004). Of the nine predicted genes (indicated by colored boxes in the left column), three have been trapped by members of the IGTC (arrows). The genomic structure of these three genes, together with the position of gene trap sequence tags are illustrated in the bottom panel.

A   Wnt signaling pathway

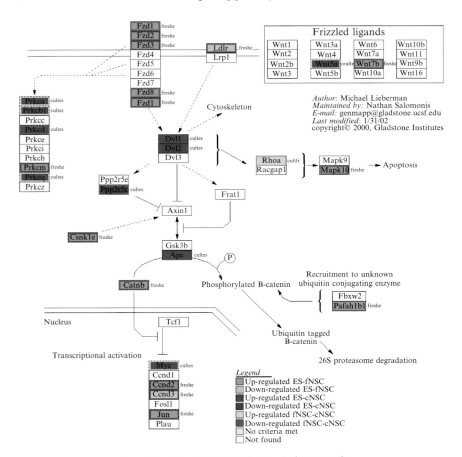

HIPP AND ATALA, CHAPTER 9, FIG. 6. (*continued*)

B

Translation factors

Initiation

Eif2b1
Eif2b2
Eif2b3
Eif2b4
Eif2b5

Eif3s1 freshe
Eif3s2
Eif3s3
Eif3s4 cultes
Eif3s5
Eif3s6 cultes
Eif3s7 freshe
Eif3s8
Eif3s9 freshe
Eif3s10 cultes

Eif1a freshe

IF2

40S Subunit

43S pre-initiation complex

Guanine nucleotide exchange

Eif2ak1
Prkr
Eif2ak3

Eif2s1 cultes
Eif2s2 freshe
Eif2s3x
Eif2s3y freshe

Recruitment of 43S
pre-initiation complex

m7G

Eif4e

Eif4g1
Eif4g2
Eif4g3 freshe

Cap binding complex

Eif4ebp1 freshe
Eif4ebp2
Eif4ebp3

(AAAAAAAAAAAA)

Pabpc1 freshe
Pabpc2
Paip1

Su1-rs1

Scanning

AUG

Eif4a1 cultes
Eif4a2 freshe
Eif4b freshe
Wbscr1

mRNA

Itgb4bp

Recruitment of 60S subunit
and first peptide bond

Eif5
Eif5a

60S Subunit

Translocation

Binds aminoacyl-tRNA

Elongation

Eef1a1
Eef1a2 freshe
Eef1b2
Eef1g
Eef1d

Eef2k cultes

Eef2

Termination

Eef1 freshe
cRF3

Author: Kam Dahlquist, Meredith Braymer
E-mail: genmapp@gladstone.ucsf.edu
Last modified: 12/4/2003
Copyright © 2001, gladstone institutes

Legend
Up-regulated ES-fNSC
Down-regulated ES-fNSC
Up-regulated ES-cNSC
Down-regulated ES-cNSC
Up-regulated fNSC-cNSC
Down-regulated fNSC-cNSC
No criteria met
Not found

HIPP AND ATALA, CHAPTER 9, FIG. 6. (*continued*)

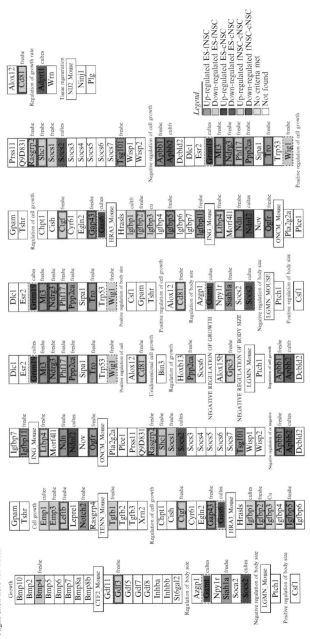

Hipp and Atala, Chapter 9, Fig. 6. Genes that were identified as being up-regulated and down-regulated on *in vivo* mouse ESC differentiation into NSCf and those that were further cultured for 5 days NSCc. (A) GenMapp Wnt pathway. (B) GenMapp translation factors pathway. (C) GenMapp growth pathway.

A

Chromatin

Author: Adapted from Gene Ontology
Maintained by: GenMAPP.org
E-mail: genmapp@gladstone.ucsf.edu
Last modified: 7/15/2005
Right click here for notes.

Legend
Up-regulated in HESC Sato et al.
Down-regulated in HESC Sato et al.
Up-regulated in PGESC
Down-regulated in PGESC
Up-regulated in HESC Sperger et al.
Down-regulated in HESC Sperger et al.
Up-regulated in HESC Brandenberger et al.
Down-regulated in HESC Brandenberger et al.
Binds to SOX2-NANOG-OCT4
Binds to SOX2 or NANOG or OCT4
No criteria met
Not found

HIPP AND ATALA, CHAPTER 9, FIG. 8. (*continued*)

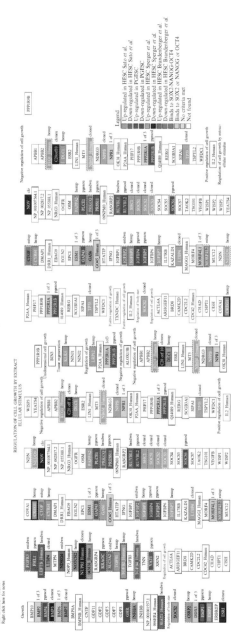

Extracellular matrix (sensu Metazoa)

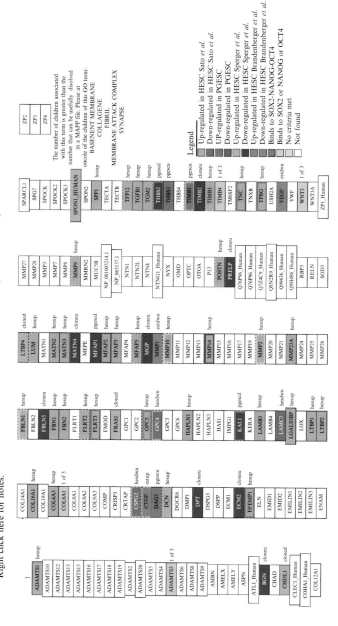

HIPP AND ATALA, CHAPTER 9, FIG. 8. Genes that were up-regulated and down-regulated in the Sperger *et al.*, Sato *et al.*, PGESC *et al.*, Brandenberger *et al.* data sets, and in the Boyet *et al.* (SOX2-NANOG-OCT4), and Boyet *et al.* (SOX2 or NANOG or OCT4) data sets. (A) GenMAPP chromatin pathway. (B) Genmapp growth pathway. (C) GenMapp extracellular matrix pathway.

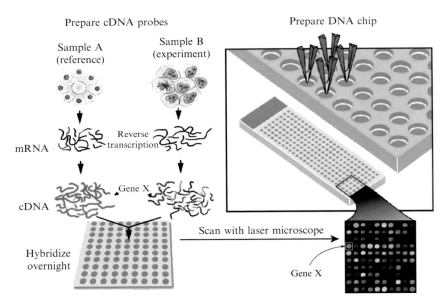

Prepare cDNA probes

Sample A
(reference)

Sample B
(experiment)

mRNA

Reverse
transcription

cDNA

Gene X

Hybridize
overnight

Prepare DNA chip

Scan with laser microscope

Gene X

CHANG *ET AL.*, CHAPTER 10, FIG. 1. Principle of cDNA microarrays. PCR products are printed onto glass slides to produce high-density cDNA microarrays. RNA is extracted from experimental samples and reference samples and differentially labeled with Cy5 and Cy3, respectively, by reverse transcriptase. The subsequent cDNA probes are mixed and hybridized to cDNA microarray overnight. The slides are washed and scanned with fluorescence laser scanner. The relative red/green ratio of gene X indicates the relative abundance of gene X in experimental samples versus reference.

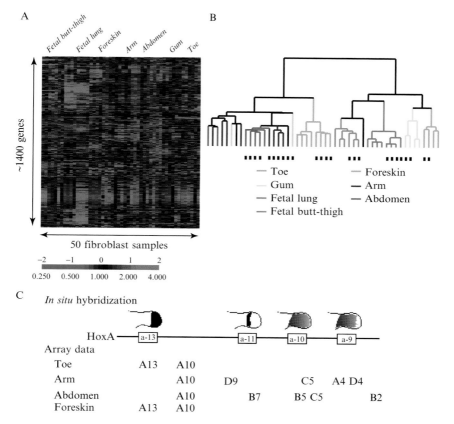

CHANG *ET AL.*, CHAPTER 10, FIG. 3. Topographic differentiation of fibroblasts identified by microarray analysis. (A) Heat map of fibroblast gene expression patterns. Fibroblasts from several anatomical sites were cultured, and their mRNAs were analyzed by cDNA microarray hybridization (Chang *et al.*, 2002). Approximately 1400 genes varied by at least threefold in two samples. The fibroblast samples were predominantly grouped together on the basis of site of origin. (B) Supervised hierarchical clustering revealed the relationship of fibroblast cultures to one another. Site of origin is indicated by the color code, and high or low serum culture condition is indicated by the absence (high) or presence (low) of the black square below each branch. Because fibroblasts from the same site were grouped together irrespective of donor, passage number, or serum condition, topographic differentiation seemed to be the predominant source of gene expression variation among these cells. (C) *HOX* expression in adult fibroblasts recapitulates the embryonic Hox code. In a comparison of *HOX* expression pattern in secondary axes, schematic of expression domains of 5′ *HoxA* genes in the mouse limb bud at approximately 11.5 days after coitus is shown on top. The *HOX* genes up-regulated in fibroblasts from the indicated sites are shown below. *HoxC5* is expressed in embryonic chick forelimbs, and *HoxD9* functions in proximal forelimb morphogenesis. (Discussed in detail in Chang *et al.* [2002]).

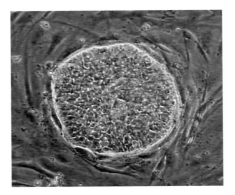

COHEN *ET AL.*, CHAPTER 14, FIG. 1. The appearance of a high-quality human embryonic stem cell (hESC) colony. Note round-shaped, well-defined edges, and high nucleus/cytoplasm ratio of cells within the colony.

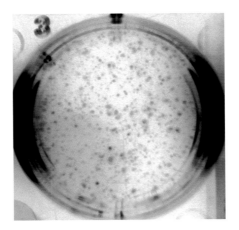

COHEN *ET AL.*, CHAPTER 14, FIG. 2. The optimal density of human embryonic stem cell (hESC) colonies.

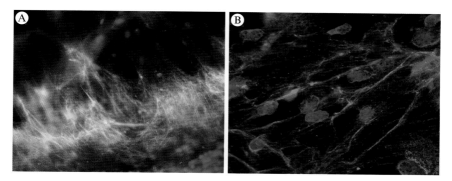

COHEN *ET AL.*, CHAPTER 14, FIG. 3. CTPs stained with antibody against type I collagen (A) and type II collagen (B). DAPI was used for nuclear visualization. Note cells embedded in self-produced extracellular matrix.

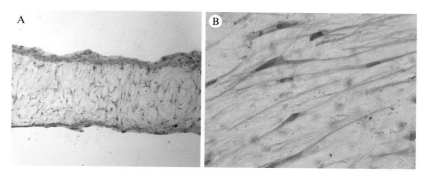

COHEN *ET AL.*, CHAPTER 14, FIG. 5. Hematoxylin-eosin–stained histological images of cross-sectioned CTPs seeded on nanofiber scaffolds at low (A) and high (B) power magnifications.

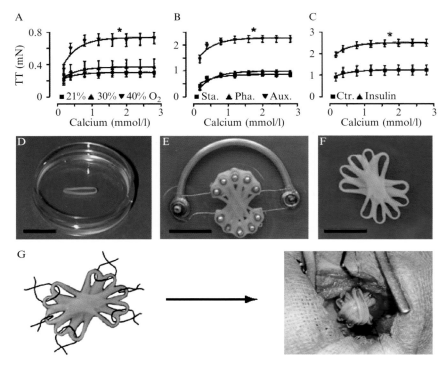

GUO *ET AL.*, CHAPTER 15, FIG. 1. Construction of optimized EHTs. Effects of oxygen, load, and insulin were analyzed by isometric contraction experiments in EHT rings. TT, twitch tension. Direct comparison of calcium response curves showed that EHTs benefited from oxygen supplementation (O_2, $n = 11$ at 21%; $n = 5$ at 30%; $n = 10$ at 40%; (A) auxotonic (Aux.; $n = 8$) in contrast to static (Sta.; $n = 8$) or phasic (Pha.; $n = 8$) load (B), and addition of insulin (10 μg/ml; $n = 4$) compared with untreated controls ($n = 3$); (C). Stacking five single EHTs (D) on a custom-made device facilitated EHT fusion and allowed contractions under auxotonic load (E), resulting in synchronously contracting multiloop EHTs (F) ready for *in vivo* engraftment. (G) Six single-knot sutures served to fix multiloop EHTs on the recipients' hearts. *$p < 0.05$ vs. 21% O_2, static load, and culture in the absence of insulin (Ctr.), respectively, by repeated ANOVA. Scale bars, 10 mm (Zimmermann *et al.*, 2006).

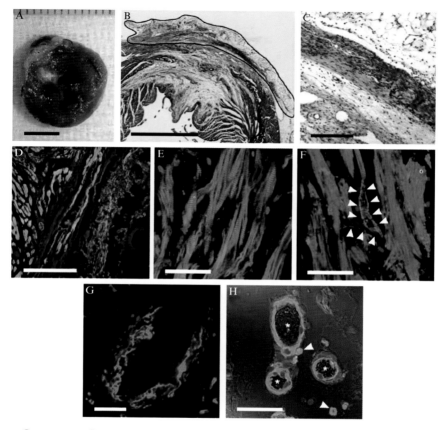

Guo *et al.*, Chapter 15, Fig. 2. EHT morphology 4 weeks after engraftment. (A) Midventricular cross-section 28 days after implantation showed that engrafted EHTs remained pale but firmly attached to the infarct scar. (B and C) H&E staining of paraffin sections through the infarcted left ventricular free wall 4 weeks after EHT engraftment showed the formation of thick cardiac muscle on top of the infarct scar (B; EHT circled). High-power magnification of the infarct area showed that engrafted EHTs formed compact and oriented heart muscle (C) spanning the transmural infarct. (D) Engrafted EHTs could be identified by DAPI-labeled nuclei (blue; actin, green; background, red). (E) Laser scanning microscopy showed the highly differentiated sarcomeric organization of engrafted cardio-myocytes (actin, green; nuclei, blue). (F–H) EHT grafts were vascularized *in vivo* (F; actin, green; nuclei, blue; arrows indicate a putative vessel in a reconstituted confocal image). Newly formed vessels contained DAPI$^+$ endothelial (G; lectin, red; nuclei, blue) or smooth muscle cells (H; actin, green; nuclei, blue). Macrophages (ED2, red; highlighted by arrows in H) with blue nuclei were found in close proximity to newly formed vessels. Asterisks indicate erythrocytes visualized by differential interference contrast imaging (H). Scale bar in A,B, 5 mm; in C,D, 500 μm; in E–H, 50 μm (Zimmermann *et al.*, 2006).

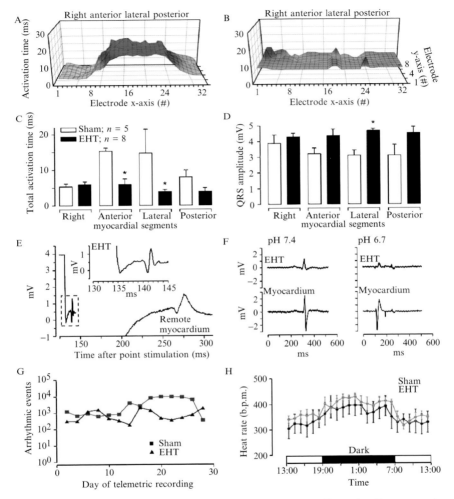

GUO ET AL., CHAPTER 15, FIG. 3. Electrical integration of EHTs *in vivo*. Representative plots of epicardial activation times in sham-operated (A) and EHT-engrafted (B) hearts. Total activation time (C) and QRS-complex voltage (D) in right, anterior, lateral, and posterior segments of the investigated hearts. (E) Point stimulation of an implanted EHT with simultaneous recording of the propagated potential in the EHT and in remote myocardium showed retrograde coupling. EHT could be uncoupled after acidification of the hearts (F). Telemetric ECG recordings showed a similar frequency of arrhythmias in sham-operated and EHT-grafted groups ($n = 5$ per group; G). (H) Circadian rhythm in sham-operated and EHT groups. *$p < 0.05$ vs. sham-operated rats by ANOVA with Mann–Whitney U test (Zimmermann *et al.*, 2006).

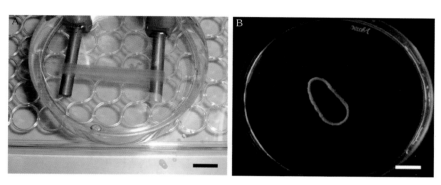

Guo *et al.*, Chapter 15, Fig. 6. Macroscopy of ECT. (A) Mechanical stretching of ECTs. The ECTs were fixed between the two rods of the stretching machine and given a unidirectional and cyclic stretch (10%, 2 Hz) in culture medium for 7 days. The medium was changed every day. Scale bar 11 mm. (B) Microscopic view of spontaneously contracting ECT constructed by seeding cardiomyocytes derived from mouse ES cells into liquid type I collagen. Note the vigorous contraction of the ECT in organ bath solution, with a frequency of more than 1 Hz (Guo *et al.*, 2006).

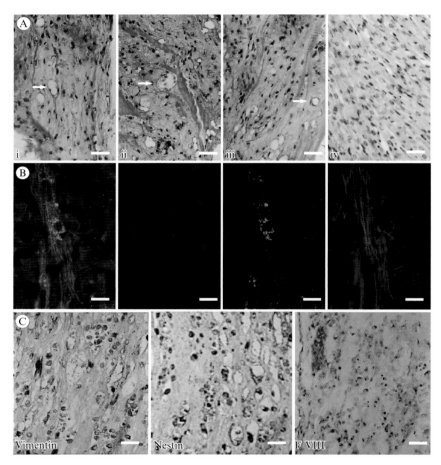

G U O *ET AL.*, C H A P T E R 15, F I G. 8. Histology of and distinct cell types in ECT. Photo-micrographs of H&E–stained paraffin sections from ECTs showed formation of complexes of multicellular aggregates and longitudinally oriented cell bundles (A, i–iii). Vascular vessels were notable in the ECTs (arrow). The histological morphology of the ECTs resembles that of immature neonatal cardiac tissue (A, iv). Immunolabeling indicates formation of cardiac cell bundles with significant striations of sarcomeres in the ECT. (Actin appears red; α-sarcomeric actin, green; and nuclear, blue.) (B) Distribution of fibroblasts (vimentin), vascular endothelial cells (F VIII), and neural cell–like cells (nestin) were also observed as indicated by immunolabeling (green) (C) Scale bars, 30 μm (A), 15 μm (B), or 30 μm (C) (Guo *et al.*, 2006).

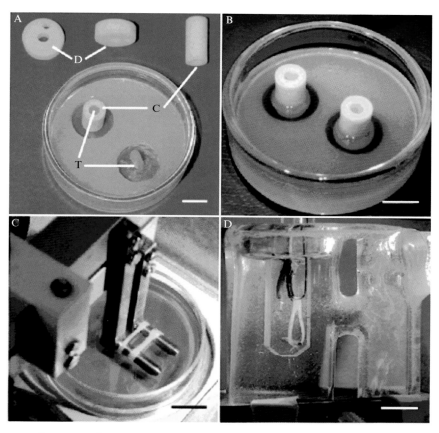

GUO *ET AL.*, CHAPTER 15, FIG. 11. The ring system (Zimmermann *et al.*, 2002).

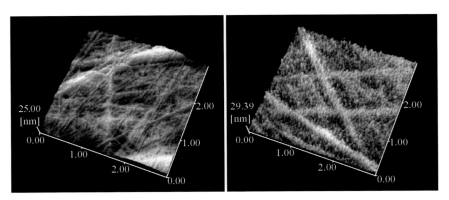

GUO *ET AL.*, CHAPTER 15, FIG. 12. Atomic force microscope images of temperature-responsive culture dish surfaces. Nongrafted, polystyrene culture dish surfaces (left) and poly (N-isopropylacrylamide)-grafted culture dish surfaces (right) were examined in air. Defects and scratches were observed on both surfaces. Small prickles can be seen on the grafted surface. Image size is 3 μm × 3 μm. Height is 25 nm (left) and 30 nm (right) (Yamato and Okano, 2004).

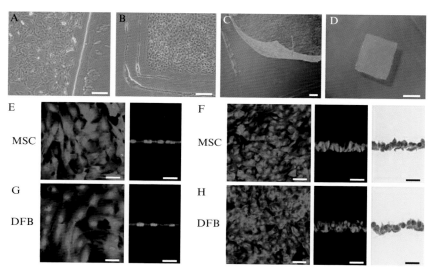

Guo *et al.*, Chapter 15, Fig. 14. Preparation of monolayered MSCs. (A) MSCs 2 days after seeding on a temperature-responsive dish. (B) Cultured MSCs expanded to confluence within the square area of the dish by day 3. (C) The monolayered MSCs detached easily from the culture dish at 20°. (D) The completely detached monolayered MSCs were identified as a 12 × 12 mm square sheet. (E–H) Cross-sectional analysis of GFP-expressing monolayered MSCs and DFBs before detachment (E and G, confocal images) and after detachment (F and H, left and center, confocal images; right, Masson trichrome). The thickness of both monolayers was 3.5-fold greater than the thickness before detachment, and constituent cells were compacted. Scale bars in A–C, 100 μm; in D, 5 mm; in E–H, 20 μm (Miyahara *et al.*, 2006).

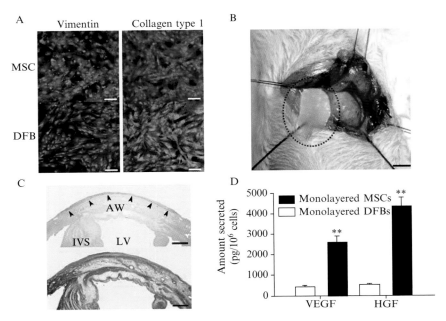

GUO *ET AL.*, CHAPTER 15, FIG. 15. Characteristics of monolayered MSCs. (A) Properties of constituent cells in the monolayered grafts. Compared with DFBs (green), MSCs (green) are positive for vimentin (red) and slightly positive for collagen type 1 (red). (B) Monolayered MSCs (in the dotted circle) transferred to the infarcted heart. (C) Extent of monolayered MSCs 48 h after transplantation (arrows). AW, anterior wall; LV, left ventricle; RV right ventricle; IVS, interventricular septum. (D) Comparison of secretion of growth factors between monolayered MSCs and DFBs. $**p < 0.01$ vs. DFBs. Scale bar in A, 20 μm; in B, 5 mm; in C, 100 μm (Miyahara *et al.*, 2006).

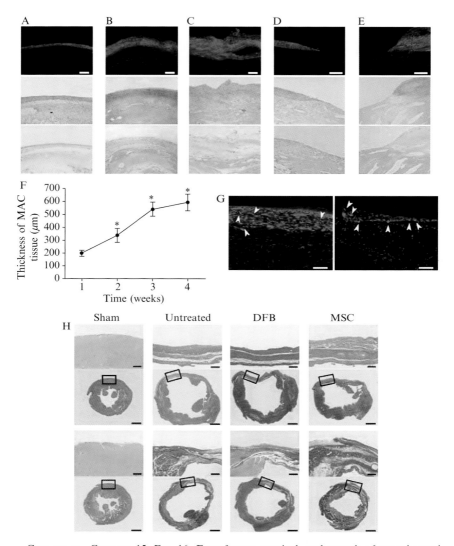

Guo *et al.*, Chapter 15, Fig. 16. Engraftment, survival, and growth of monolayered MSCs. To identify the transplanted cells within myocardial sections, we used GFP-expressing cells derived from GFP-transgenic Sprague-Dawley rats. (A–C) MSC tissue above the anterior scar at day 2 (A), day 14 (B), and day 28 (C). GFP-expressing monolayered MSCs were grafted to the native myocardium and grew gradually *in situ*, resulting in increased wall thickness. (D and E) MSC tissue above the surrounding area of the scar at day 2 (D) and day 28 (E). In A–E, upper row shows immunofluorescent staining of MSC tissue (green); nuclei are stained with DAPI (blue). Middle row shows identical sections stained with antibody to GFP and DAB by bright-field microscopy. Lower row shows hematoxylin and eosin–stained sections. (F) Time course of growth of MSCs expressing GFP. *$p < 0.05$ vs. thickness of GFP[+] MSC tissue at 1 week. (G) TUNEL staining of transplanted MSCs (green, left) and DFBs (green, right) 48 h after transplantation. Nuclei are stained with DAPI (blue). Arrows indicate TUNEL-positive nuclei (red). (H) Photomicrographs show two cases of representative myocardial sections stained with Masson trichrome in the individual groups. Left ventricle enlargement was attenuated by the transplantation of monolayered MSC. Scale bars in A–E and upper panels of H, 100 μm; in g, 20 μm; in lower panels of H, 1 mm (Miyahara *et al.*, 2006).

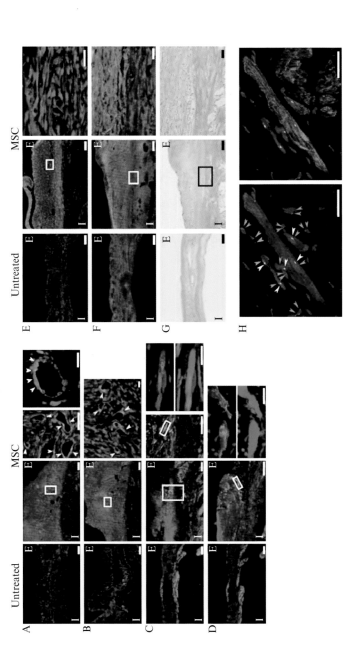

Guo ET AL., CHAPTER 15, FIG. 17. Differentiation of MSCs within the MSC tissue after growth *in situ*. (A and B) GFP-expressing MSCs (green) were identified as a thick stratum at the epicardial side of the myocardium. The MSC tissue contained a number of vascular structures positive for vWF (red, A) and αSMA (red, B). MSCs that did not participate in blood vessel formation were only rarely positive for αSMA, a marker for myofibroblasts. Arrows indicate transplanted MSCs positive for vWF or αSMA. (C and D) Some MSCs within the MSC tissue were positive for cardiac markers cardiac troponin T (red, C) and desmin (red, D). (E) Most of the MSC tissue was positive for vimentin (red). (F) The MSC tissue modestly stained for collagen type 1 (red). (G) Collagen deposition was also detected by picrosirius red staining. (H) FISH analysis. Newly formed cardiomyocytes (desmin, red) that were positive for GFP (green) had only one set of X (purple) and Y chromosomes (white), whereas two X chromosomes were detected exclusively in GFP⁻ host–derived cells. Nuclei are stained with DAPI (blue, A–F and H). Scale bars in left three panels of A and C in two left panels of B and D–G, 100 μm; in H and far right panels of A–G, 20 μm. E, epicardial side; I, intimal side (Miyahara *et al.*, 2006).